INTERNATIONAL SERIES IN EXPERIMENTAL PSYCHOLOGY

GENERAL EDITOR : H. J. EYSENCK

VOLUME 23

SLEEP AND DREAMING: ORIGINS, NATURE AND FUNCTIONS

NOTICE TO READERS

Dear Reader

If your library is not already a standing order customer or subscriber to this series, may we recommend that you place a standing or subscription order to receive immediately upon publication all new issues and volumes published in this valuable series. Should you find that these volumes no longer serve your needs your order can be cancelled at any time without notice.

The Editors and the Publisher will be glad to receive suggestions or outlines of suitable titles, reviews or symposia for consideration for rapid publication in this series.

ROBERT MAXWELL
Publisher at Pergamon Press

SLEEP AND DREAMING: ORIGINS, NATURE AND FUNCTIONS

by

DAVID B. COHEN

*Department of Psychology,
University of Texas at Austin*

PERGAMON PRESS

OXFORD · NEW YORK · TORONTO · SYDNEY · PARIS · FRANKFURT

U.K.	Pergamon Press Ltd., Headington Hill Hall, Oxford OX3 0BW, England
U.S.A.	Pergamon Press Inc., Maxwell House, Fairview Park, Elmsford, New York 10523, U.S.A.
CANADA	Pergamon of Canada, Suite 104, 150 Consumers Road, Willowdale, Ontario M2J 1P9, Canada
AUSTRALIA	Pergamon Press (Aust.) Pty. Ltd., P.O. Box 544, Potts Point, N.S.W. 2011, Australia
FRANCE	Pergamon Press SARL, 24 rue des Ecoles, 75240 Paris, Cedex 05, France
FEDERAL REPUBLIC OF GERMANY	Pergamon Press GmbH, 6242 Kronberg-Taunus, Hammerweg 6, Federal Republic of Germany

First edition 1979
Reprinted 1980

British Library Cataloguing in Publication Data
Cohen, David B
Sleep and dreaming.
1. Sleep — Physiological aspects
I. Title
612'.821   QP425   78-40567
ISBN 0-08-021467-3 hardcover
ISBN 0-08-027400-5 flexicover

Printed in the United States of America

For LESLIE KAREN
and
JASON AARON

CONTENTS

CONTENTS

ACKNOWLEDGEMENTS

Acknowledgement seems paltry recompense for valuable commentary and support. Nevertheless, I do wish to express my appreciation to a number of people. First, I am deeply grateful that I had the privilege to know and to be influenced by the late Arthur Shapiro. My interest in sleep and dream research was kindled largely by the force of his personality, intellect, and research.

To Marty Seligman and Augustine de la Peña I owe a special debt. Each read earlier versions of the book, and provided me with valuable feedback as well as encouragement. Al Rechtschaffen must be credited, not only for his commentary on drafts of some of the chapters, but also with providing a model of achievement toward which I have aspired. I am grateful to many others who read and commented on various parts of the book: Bill Fishbein, Ray Greenberg, Ernest Hartmann, Al Hobson, Milt Kramer, Dan Kripke, Bob McCarley, Howard Roffwarg, Joe Salamy, N. Sitaram, and Del Thiessen. I have benefited from the singular opportunity to work in an intellectually stimulating environment. I am especially indebted to the following of my colleagues: Joe Horn, Lee Willerman, Del Thiessen, Arnold Buss, Jan Bruell, Phil Gough, John Belknap, Dave Hakes, Mike Gabriel, John Loehlin, and Peter MacNeilage. I take full responsibility for straying from the collective wisdom of all the individuals acknowledged here.

Much of the work discussed in this book would not have been possible without the dedicated efforts of many students, both experimenters and subjects, who worked and slept under extraordinary research conditions. In this respect, Gary Wolfe, Randy McCaslin, Merrill Hiscock, Charlie Cox, Mike McGrath, Mike Hanlon, and Naomi Simon have made significant and invaluable contributions. A special acknowledgement is due Les Bell whose technical and organizational skills are matched only by an extraordinary degree of enthusiasm and expertise. His contribution to our overall research program is inestimable. Finally, I would like to thank Tami Booher and Michelle Kean who labored heroically to transcribe into polished form the preliminary drafts of the manuscript.

I would like to acknowledge the contribution made by The National Institute of Mental Health and The University of Texas Research Institute in the form of research grants whose funds supported much of the research described in the book.

I want to thank and acknowledge the following publishers and authors for the use of quotations, data, and graphic and tabular material for which they retain copyright:

Academic Press, *Journal of Research in Personality* 7, 179–188 (1973), Fig. 1.

Aldine-Atherton, Inc., Quotations from S.L. Garfield, *Clinical Psychology: The Study of Personality and Behavior*, 1974.

Aldus Books Ltd., C.G. Jung's *Man and His Symbols*, 1964. Quote from Jung's essay "Approaching the Unconscious".

American Association for the Advancement of Science, and R.W. McCarley and J.A. Hobson, *Science* 189, 58–60 (1975), Fig. 2A; also T. Pivik and D. Foulkes, *Science* 153, 1282–1284 (1966). Graphic display of data.

American Psychological Association, *Journal of Personality and Social Psychology* 32, 1090–1093 (1975), Fig. 1; also *ibid.* 36, 741–751 (1978), Table 1; *Journal of Clinical and Consulting Psychology* 41, 349–355 (1973), Table 1; also *ibid.* 42, 699–703 (1974), Table 2; *Journal of Abnormal Psychology* 82, 246–252 (1973), Tables 1, 2, 3, and 4; also *ibid.* 82, 368–371 (1973), Table 1; also *ibid.* 83, 45–51 (1974), Table 1; also *ibid.* 83, 151–156 (1974), Table 1 and Fig. 1; also *ibid.* 84, 91–108 (1975), Tables 3 and 5 and Fig. 2.

Cambridge University Press, *British Journal of Social and Clinical Psychology* 16, 153–163 (1977), Figs. 3, 4, and 5. Also quotation from K.J.W. Craik, *The Nature of Explanation*, 1952.

Elsevier North-Holland, Quotation from R. Greenberg *et al.*, *Psychosomatic Medicine* 34, 257–262 (1972).

W.H. Freeman and Company, and R.T. Bakker, "Dinosaur Renaissance", *Scientific American*, April, 1975, Figure on p. 77; and H.J. Jerison, "Paleoneurology and the Evolution of Mind", *Scientific American*, January, 1976, Material from figure on p. 94. All rights reserved by *Scientific American*.

Holt, Rinehart & Winston, Quotation from A. Paivio, *Imagery and Verbal Processes*, 1971.

S. Karger A.G., Basel, and Zepelin and Rechtschaffen, *Brain, Behavior and Evolution* 10, 425–470 (1974), Table III.

N. Kleitmen, Quotation from *Sleep and Wakefullness*, 1963.

Perceptual and Motor Skills, *Perceptual and Motor Skills* 44, 1267–1277 (1977), Tables 1, 2, 3, 4, and 5.

Pergamon Press, Inc. and Fishbein, *Physiology and Behavior* 14, 409–412 (1975), Fig. 1.

Plenum Publishing Corporation, *Consciousness and Self-Regulation: Advances in Research*, Vol. 1, Ch. 8, Figs. 2 and 4.

Schenkman Publishing Company, Quotation of Rechtschaffen in W.A. Hunt, *Human Behavior and Its Control*, 1971.

Scott, Foresman Company, and Webb, Quotation of Brooks in W.B. Webb, *Sleep: An Active Process*, 1973.

Spectrum Publications and Anders, Quotation of Anders in E. Weitzman, *Advance in Sleep Research*, Vol. 2, 1975.

Universitá degu Studi di Pisa, and Allison, *Archives Italiennes de Biologie* 110, 145–184 (1922), Fig. 16.

The Williams and Wilkins Company, Baltimore, Quotation of F.J. Evans *et al.* in *Journal of Nervous and Mental Disease* 150, 171–187 (1970). Also graphic material from Nakazawa *et al.*, *Journal of Nervous and Mental Disease* 161, 18–25 (1975).

INTRODUCTION

(Square) Again, was I not taught that as in a Line there are *two* bounding Points, and in a square there are *four* bounding Lines, so in a Cube there must be *six* bounding Squares? Behold once more the confirming Series 2, 4, 6: is not this an Arithmetic Progression? And consequently, does it not necessarily follow that the more divine offspring of the divine Cube in the Land of Four Dimensions, must have 8 bounding Cubes . . .?

(Sphere) But men are divided in opinion as to the facts . . . no one has adopted or suggested a theory of a Fourth Dimension.

(Square) Those who have thus appeared — no one knows whence — and have returned — no one knows whither have they also contracted their sections and vanished somehow into that more Spacious Space, whither I now entreat you to conduct me?

(Sphere) They have vanished, certainly — if they ever appeared. But most people say that these visions arose from the thought — you will not understand me — from the brain; from the perturbed angularity of the Seer.

(Square) Say they so? Oh believe them not. Or if it indeed be so, that this other Space is really Thoughtland, then take me to that blessed Region where I in Thought shall see the insides of all solid things.

E. A. Abbott

Sleep and wakefulness are manifestations in higher organisms of a fundamental "circadian rhythm" of inactivity-activity. Sleeping is as common as wakefulness (virtually all of us do it virtually every night) and yet it is a most curious phenomenon. Consider that a person who lives 70 years will spend about 27 of them asleep, and at least 5-6 of these will include vivid dreaming experiences. Can it be that nature has played some kind of malicious trick by periodically requiring organisms to forego those activities which appear to maximize pleasure and survival: feeding, fleeing, fighting, and sex? Why is it not sufficient for us periodically to remain in a state of quiet wakefulness without having to lose touch with our environments? During the past 30 years research has provided a great deal of new information about the phenomena and phenomenology of sleep and the relationship between sleep and wakefulness. No longer can the textbooks of psychology ignore the dark third of existence with its full complement of behavioral, cognitive, and experiential characteristics. My goal is to describe, organize, and interpret some of this new knowledge in order to stimulate a greater appreciation of the role of sleep and dreaming in human adaptation.

Learning through assimilation refers to selection, retention, and modification of information that readily fits a pre-existing knowledge. It is the latter which largely explains the speed, complexity, range, and novelty of information processing. However, by concentrating on opportunity and training, we have underestimated or ignored biological factors which determine, in a general sense, what the individual knows before he shows evidence of learning. Thus, we have erroneously placed the locus of explanation for learning in the more readily observable and comprehensible external environment. However, evidence combines

1

with common sense to suggest that the parameters of learning are largely determined by endogenous capacities that differ among individuals and across species. Language learning, despite minimal exposure to information and little systematic training, is remarkably easy for the average child (compared to his application of language). The process accelerates about the time that the rate of brain maturation approaches asymptotic levels (about two years). This is not the place to discuss it, but the evidence clearly indicates that understanding precedes the accurate use of language, and no amount of training can induce the child to communicate something that he does not already intuitively know. Likewise, there is evidence that no amount of experience with, or training on, a mirror can induce a monkey to learn that the mirror-image represents himself. In contrast, the chimp readily learns to appreciate the image for what it is. As Gallup says, "a mirror simply represents a means of mapping what the chimpanzee already knows" though, of course, "it provides him with a new and more explicit dimension of knowing about himself . . ." (1977, p. 335).

I am explicitly subscribing to the idea that much of what is learned is based on prior "knowledge" which characterizes the nervous system. Thus, we learn through experience to speak a language, to produce creative ideas, to be skilled in movement, to be sensitive about things or people, because we are endowed differently with the ability to assimilate experience into prior structures that are in large part biologically (not necessarily in the narrow sense of genetically) determined. These structures or capacities are not static. They mature, just as our bodies do, and are affected by experience. This approach to learning, which, in contrast to much contemporary psychological theory, tends to give more weight to assimilation of, than to accommodation to, the environment, is made explicit in order to provide the reader with a fair indication of two major themes of this work: the biological basis of experience, and the importance of individual differences to the understanding of psychological phenomena.

The study of sleep and dreaming provides a very special perspective on human functioning. In many ways it stands in direct contrast to more traditional paradigms utilized in psychology that place the locus of explanation of human behavior in the external environment. What I would call the militant environmentalism of American psychology reflects two characteristics of American cultural tradition: *pragmatism*, emphasizing the conventional, concrete situational, immediately observable, ostensibly controllable, eminently practical; and *egalitarianism*, elevating to an ideal the notion that "all men are created equal". Pragmatism has led psychology toward defining itself as the study of behavior rather than the study of mind and brain function (the two fundamental constituents of the "black box"). Egalitarianism has encouraged suspicion of the very idea of individual differences ("error variance") especially when these turn out to reflect organismic differences. The result is somewhat embarrassing: naive and unnatural theories about normal and abnormal psychological phenomena: naive because they are "mindless", unnatural because they are "gutless". Contemporary psychology is moving closer to the view that, for organisms with even a modest claim to phylogenetic sophistication, what is learned is less movement than acts, that learning is rule more than stimulus governed, that information more than tension (drive) reduction is motivating, that individual differences in basic processes (e.g. ability to detect, identify, remember, innovate, and the ability to regulate affect, experience and behavior) reflect individual differences in constitution as much as or more than individual differences in opportunity or training. I suspect that the psychology of learning is most hampered when "the influence of the environment is nonsensically overrated . . . the essential factor in the process of life is precisely the tremendous inner power to shape and to create forms which merely *uses, exploits* 'environment'" (F. Nietzsche).

No wonder that, until recently, American psychology has contributed so little to the problem of sleep. To the casual observer, sleep has three characteristics that are either uninteresting or positively offensive to behaviorists: an *absence* of behavior (e.g., it is noninstrumental), an absence of responsiveness to external stimuli (i.e., it is resistant to control), and the presence of mental phenomena (i.e., nonobjectifiable, private events). If anything, sleep would appear to be a problem for the physiologists (who, until recent times, have borne the major burden of describing it). But, as I hope this book will demonstrate, sleep *is* a psychological problem whose investigation may tell us much about wakefulness. Despite its limitations, research on sleep and dreaming serves to remind us of the importance of cognition and the organismic basis of experience and individual differences. This point is sufficiently important, both to an appreciation of sleep and dream research as well as to the broader field of psychology, to justify further elaboration.

Learning is generally conceptualized as a process of accommodation to the environment. The individual is stimulated and guided by cues, held by reinforcements (inducements), and gradually "shaped" according to the demands and requirements of the external environment. In this accommodation of psychological structure to environmental structure, the individual is conceived to be a "dependent variable".

An alternative view, which should be thought of as supplemental rather than competitive, holds that learning is a cognitive process by which information is extracted, transformed, and assimilated according to the given and acquired properties of the organism. This latter view is commensurate with the idea that learning is an organismic process which reflects the cumulative influence (degrees of freedom as well as constraints) of telencephalic evolution as much as the controlling and informational properties of the environment (Jerison, 1973). And further, it would seem that while the accommodation view of learning might be more appropriate to explain the behavior of phylogenetically primitive organisms, explaining the behavior of more advanced organisms requires that we pay more attention to learning as invention. Explanations of human behavior in particular, which traditionally have relied so heavily on concepts like classical conditioning, operant learning, modeling (concepts which give little or reluctant consideration to cognitive processes) have surely missed the mark.[1]

The study of sleep and dreaming as organismic processes provides a perspective from which both kinds of learning can be evaluated. In the case of dreaming, while it clearly reflects some degree of accommodation, more than any other cognitive process it represents the epitome of assimilation. It is mind as reconstruction as much as representation. But more, it provides a "window" through which an appreciation, if not an understanding, of cognitive mediation may be achieved. It demonstrates the organism to be continuously active, flexible, inventive. And it suggests, as Klinger (1971) has ably argued, that such a process is part of and influences the learning of the waking state. In addition, as Marty Seligman has impressed upon me, it provides additional experience to which the organism accommodates. If we concede that cognition is what is most special about the human organism (that which permits psychological freedom from direct external control), if the

---

[1] After writing this, I came across Brewer's literature review (1974) which supports his thesis that "there is no convincing evidence for operant or classical conditioning in adult humans". Resonating to this review, Halwes remarked that "we find that the behaviorists have told us nothing of significance" but warns "that the 'cognitive explanations' are just common sense" (in Weimer and Palermo, 1974, p. 57).

highest form of cognition is creative and productive ideation, and if we believe that such ideation mediates behaviors that are fundamental to cultural achievement, then the study of sleep and dreaming takes on a special relevance. If we are to pay more than lip service to the concept of incubation when we try to explain creativity, then we need to pay more scientific attention to *the* fundamental form of incubation. For me, the highest and best property of human functioning, what we so very appropriately call giftedness, is not a property of the social environment (though it does, of course, develop within the social context). Rather it is a property of what I would call "organismic inventiveness", the ability to *extract* information from the "raw material" provided by the environment, recognize its possibilities, and invent new forms. And this is accomplished with a facility, celerity, and dexterity that can not be explained in terms of the language of accommodation. So, whatever else it says about the nature of the organism, sleep and dream research is to some extent commensurate with a romantic view of human nature. It provides evidence of the active, spontaneous, self-determining, self-confronting, and self-revising qualities of human functioning. This view is not antiscientific. Rather it challenges the scientific method to accommodate to its physiological and phenomenological properties. The present book represents, in part, an attempt to assess the degree to which the scientific method has been successful.

Research on sleep and dreaming suggests another characteristic of human functioning, a tendency to return periodically to one's roots. I mean this in both the physiological as well as the psychological sense. Data and speculation scattered throughout the vast literature suggest that dreaming (perhaps more specifically, REM sleep) constitutes a reactivation of ontogenetically early forms of information processing. According to Freud, Piaget, and Werner, the initial stage of intelligence is characterized by information processing that is largely sensorimotor and affective in nature (i.e., primary, preoperational, syncretistic, physiognomic). What we are learning about the nature of dreaming, and the neurophysiological activity which underlies REM dreaming, is in the broadest sense consistent with the view that, whatever else it does, dreaming is a kind of "return to the basics". More specifically it is a more direct expression of phylogenetically older, ontogenetically earlier mental functioning which is normally concurrent with, but latent and only indirectly expressed in, the mental functioning of normal wakefulness.

I have suggested that dreaming is a return to roots. I would like to pursue this notion one step further by looking at the relationship between the phylogeny and the phenomenology of dreaming from the perspective of dream meaning. My brief discussion rests heavily on a paper by Franks (1974) that begins with the question: "Why are psychologists, linguists, philosophers, etc. so dumb when it comes to the problem of meaning?" (p. 231). For Franks, the answer has much to do with our inability to extricate ourselves from "surface structures" (e.g., words, images, behaviors) when attempting to develop hypotheses about the nature of the deep structure which generates those surface structures. "If images are seductive, then words are insidious. The ever-present play of words in awareness, on paper, and in speech seems to make it well-nigh impossible for us to resist inserting them as units of our meaning knowledge structures" (p. 256). The heart of Franks' argument is that images, like other kinds of surface (observable, manifest) structures, are derivations from tacit meanings which, themselves, are derived from a more general background called tacit knowledge. Further, the organization of these levels of deep structure is *not* obviously revealed by the content and organization of the surface structures. Alas, we can at best only infer the nature of deep structure from our understanding of the nature of observables (to which Franks says we have paid too much attention). Formulations about tacit knowledge and situation-specific derivations or tacit meanings on the basis of observable surface structures is at best a theoretical convenience, at worst, misleading and erroneous.

So how do we gain access to deep structure? Franks suggests that we pay more attention to intuition. Along with other forms of surface structure, intuition is defined, in part, as a characteristic of consciousness which most closely embodies the qualities of tacit meaning. "Images, language expressions, and responses are clues to properties of particular derived meanings. In contrast, intuitions seem to be clues to more general relations in tacit knowledge. Intuitions of similarity and difference, of novelty, familiarity, anomaly, etc., are impressions of general, more global, structural relationships among events." Franks goes on to suggest that intuitions may be "a golden road to tacit knowledge" (p. 259).

Let us take some liberties with this idea. Perhaps intuition is a manifestation of know-ledge that does not require, but most certainly is enriched and educated by, the ability to imagine and to verbalize. That is, intuition is a representation of the phylogenetically more primitive intelligence from which animal behavior is derived. It is related to the sensorimotor intelligence of the preverbal infant and to the preoperational intelligence of the child. (It is what paleocortical structures "know".) During dreaming, it is perhaps the deep structures of intuition more than the more recently acquired deep structures of syntax which generate the hallucinated experience. In this sense, both Freud and Jung appear to be profoundly correct in emphasizing a regression to ontogenetically and phylogenetically earlier meanings.

However, I would add that the tacit meanings which generate dream experiences are not merely primitive cognitive expressions of paleocortical activity. Both tacit knowledge in general, and tacit meanings in particular, are modified by maturation and development such that their products in human adulthood are different from those of infancy and childhood. These products are then the joint function of preoperational and operational processes. The obvious point is that intuition should not be maligned as merely "subjective". Intuition may sometimes represent the best fit for reality as exemplified by "solutions" arrived at nonlogically (e.g., common sense decisions, creative insights, clinical judgments, dreams) and subsequently demonstrated to be both valid and useful. If it is true that dream-ing is an intensely intuitive process, and if Franks is correct to emphasize the importance of intuition as the best clue to the ultimate problem of tacit knowledge, then the study of the surface structures of dream content ought to have a special status within cognitive psychology. That it does not is as much the fault of academic psychology, which is only now moving back toward a productive appreciation of cognitive processes after its long bout with behaviorism, as it is the fault of sleep research, with its burden of establishing an objective and scientifically respectable framework for the study of dreaming.

In 1969 the late Arthur Shapiro thought that there was a sufficient data base for a general theory of sleep and dreaming. Neither the data nor hypotheses which continue to be published at a geometrically increasing rate appear to confirm such optimism. And I would add that this is especially true in the area of dream research which is still burdened by an unfavorable ratio of theory vs. data. Consider the following two statements (whose order of presentation I have taken the liberty to reverse): "the richer the theoretical network, the richer the network of theoretical relationships it will generate", and "the greater the richness of a network of experimental relationships, the narrower the range of available theories that will predict this network of experimental relationships *without recourse to highly implausible* auxiliary assumptions" (Dulany, 1974, p. 55). Such an ideal state of affairs does

S.D.— B

not currently exist, especially in the area of dream research. In the present book, I have tried to advance an effective mix of data, theory and speculation. If I have erred in permitting myself the luxury of indulging too much in the latter, it is out of a conscious subscription to Charles Darwin's comment that "false views, if supported by some evidence, do little harm, for everyone takes a salutary pleasure in proving their falseness: and when this is done, one path towards error is closed and the road to truth is often at the same time opened".

A word about the organization of the book. I have decided to develop my discussion about the dreaming process from a biological perspective wherever possible. This bias is derived from my interest in sleep *per se*, the obvious fact that dreaming is part of the fabric of sleep, and the fact that there is precious little discussion of the biological foundations of dreaming in the literature. I do not for one instant minimize the importance of dream symbolism. Rather, I wish to provide a forum for a countervailing contrast to what appears to be an unfortunate imbalance in the dream literature. My bias accounts for two aspects of the organization of this book, one that is immediately obvious from a superficial perusal of the table of contents, the other more subtle. First, I discuss data and theory on rapid eye movement (REM) sleep: electrophysiological characteristics, cyclic rhythmicity, neurophysiology, ontogeny, and phylogeny. I also deal with questions regarding the cognitive capacity of the organism during REM sleep as well as the effects of REM deprivation on both sleep and waking behaviors. I do this in order to provide a broader perspective regarding the biological roots of a process that is usually thought of as purely "psychological". Modern sleep research has yielded far more information about REM than NREM dreaming. Therefore, in the interest of developing an effective rather than a necessarily comprehensive discussion, I have chosen to emphasize dreaming largely as a REM process despite compelling evidence that NREM (in particular, sleep onset) dreaming is phenomenologically similar to REM dreaming (Foulkes and Vogel, 1965). I have allowed myself to be guided by a biological bias regarding the electrophysiologically unique state of REM (Johnson, 1973a). Much of what I have to say, however, will undoubtedly turn out to be more or less true for NREM dreaming as well.

Second, within each of the chapters in the first ("biological") part of the book, I try to draw out where possible implications for the dreaming process. In short, the organization of the book is such that wherever possible, dreaming is approached as a psychobiological process which is manifested at cellular, physiological, psychological and phenomenological levels.

A third objective of this book is to draw attention to the potentially useful implications of individual differences in the phenomena. These crop up in both the animal and human data at all levels of investigation. We will not be in a position to say much that is conclusive because so little attention has been paid to this aspect of the problem. The material in Chapter 4 provides a fair example of the limitations in the current state of knowledge regarding individual differences in REM phenomena. Nevertheless, I am convinced that we will be able to strengthen significantly sleep and dreaming theory by exploiting analyses of correlational and interaction effects derived from the data of individual differences. I hope that one contribution of this book will be to demonstrate how on the one hand, individual difference theory can reveal more about sleep processes while, on the other, sleep phenomena can reveal something about the organismic basis of individual differences. After all, in the last analysis, what is important is explaining how the organism works, not merely how it sleeps or what it does during wakefulness. So in a sense, this book is about more than just sleep and dreaming. It is about adaptation in the broadest sense: survival of species through individual accommodation to and influence on the environment, and reflected in psychobiological functions such as reception storage, organization, transformation, and expression, through consciousness and behavior, of relevant information. Throughout the book I will be suggesting that dream consciousness reflects such processes, that it is a kind of "window" through which an appreciation of psychobiological function can be gained. But further, I will suggest the merits of the hypothesis that dreaming can be an adaptive form of information processing that contributes to the affective and intellectual development in the individual. This adaptive hypothesis represents perhaps the single most formidable empirical challenge to dream research.

Since this book is a monograph, there is greater emphasis on the work of the author than would be appropriate for a textbook. Nevertheless, I hope that the effect is to make useful points about sleep and dreaming rather than merely to make points. The result is only one of many alternative perspectives on the problems and challenges which confront the investigator.

Part A

Psychobiological Characteristics
of REM Sleep and Dreaming

Let us remain in nature when we wish to account for the phenomena of nature. . . . let us be persuaded that, by going beyond nature, we shall never solve the problems which nature presents.

Baron d'Holbach

The cautious and laborious classification of facts must have proceeded much farther than at present before the time will be ripe for drawing conclusions.

Karl Pearson

CHAPTER 1

PHYSIOLOGICAL NATURE OF REM SLEEP

1. ELECTROPHYSIOLOGICAL ASPECTS OF REM AND NREM SLEEP

Defining sleep

Sleep is typically defined operationally with respect to electroencephalogram (EEG), electro-oculogram (EOG), and electromyogram (EMG); that is, "brain waves", eye movement, and muscle tonus, respectively. Recordings are made by a polygraph which receives and amplifies changes in microvolts detected by electrodes attached to the scalp (EEG), on the skin to the right of the right eye and to the left of the left eye (horizontal EOG), and just under the chin (EMG). After amplification, the information of each "channel" is fed to the galvos of the polygraph which then activate ink writing pens. The deflection of the pens is determined by the amplitude of the voltage changes (e.g., 1 mm per 7 μv). A continuous record is produced by these pens on paper that moves at a slow and constant rate (e.g., 15 mm per second) beneath them.[1]

When this is done, a rhythmic pattern of changing sleep stages is revealed. Convention has determined that these stages be divided into two general categories: Non rapid eye movement (NREM) and REM. There are four NREM stages (1, 2, 3 and 4; the latter two are often combined and called "delta" sleep). Examples of these stages are given in Figure 1-1. Each panel represents a 20 second epoch of sleep which is defined in terms of EMG (top channel), EEG (second and fifth from top), and EOG (third and fourth from top) in each example.

The first panel shows a transition from wakefulness to stage 1 (NREM) sleep. Notice that the EMG voltage is relatively high and that there is a subtle diminution as stage 1 ensues. Also, the alpha (8-12 cps) pattern (bracketed) in the EEG of relaxed wakefulness becomes the "low voltage-fast", theta (4-7 cps)-dominated pattern of stage 1 sleep. Finally, notice the wavy pattern in the EOG channels which denotes the slow rolling eye movements characteristic of the beginning of stage 1. Some investigators interpret stage 1 as a transitional stage rather than as true sleep. Unfortunately, in many studies, estimates of total sleep time or latency to REM sleep are ambiguous because the inclusion or exclusion of stage 1 as "sleep" is not made explicit.

The second panel shows an epoch of stage 2 (NREM). Notice that the EMG has flattened out. The background pattern is stage 1 in character but there are two kinds of phasic events

[1] A typical subject run in our laboratory on a single night will require roughly 1462 feet (over a quarter of a mile) of polygraph paper during an eight hour night. Thus, a typical experiment, including as it does about 150 subject-nights, will generate about 200,000 feet (42 miles) of polygraph record.

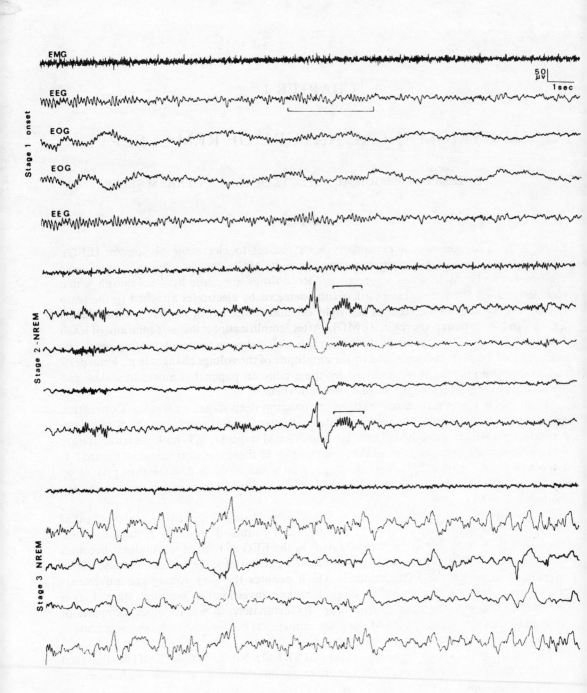

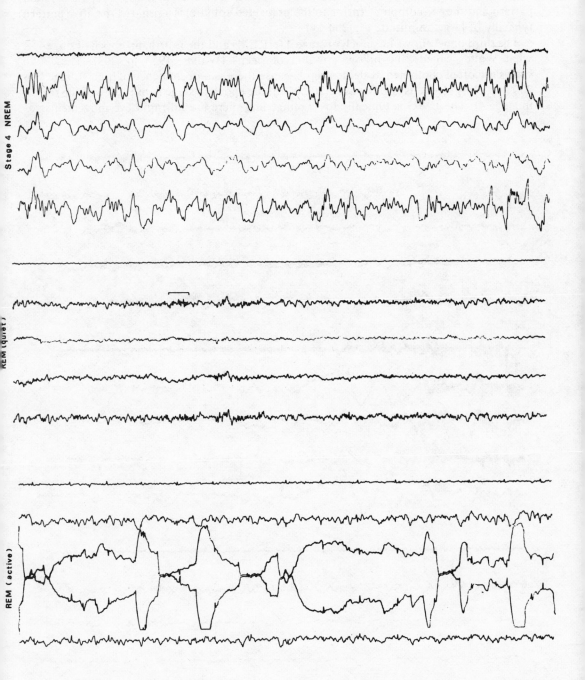

Figure 1-1   Examples of sleep stages. These are here defined in terms of EEG (second and fifth channels) per example, EOG (third and fourth channels) and EMG (first channel). Calibration is 50 microvolts, 1 second.

which indicate that this is a stage 2 EEG: the "spindle" (bracketed) is a 12-14 cps sinusoidal pattern and the "K-complex" (prior to the bracketed spindle) is a negative-positive pattern typically of large amplitude (75-200 μv).

The third panel shows an epoch of stage 3 (NREM) and the fourth, an epoch of stage 4 — what Walter called "the billowy rhythm of sleep" (Walter, 1953, p. 203). These two stages are often combined as delta sleep because there is a prominence of high voltage (75-200 μv) "slow" (1-3 cps) EEG waves (20-50% of the epoch in stage 3, over 50% of the record in stage 4). The EMG is typically low voltage and there are no rapid eye movements.

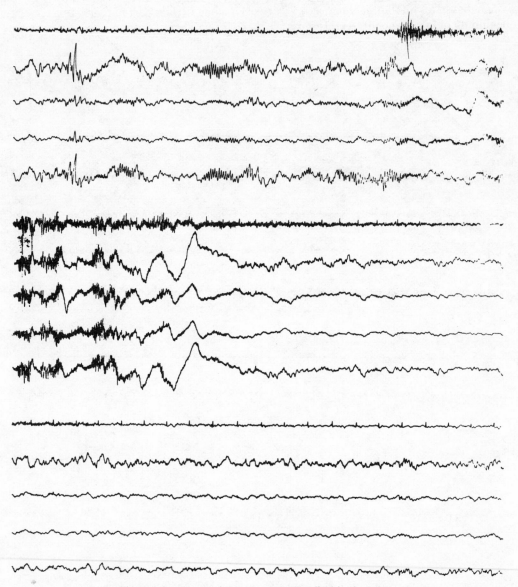

Figure 1-2   Changes in sleep stages (described in the text).

The fifth and sixth panels show epochs of REM sleep. There is a paradoxical flattening of the EMG (the lowest it will get during the night). The background EEG is typically of a stage 1 variety though there are brief phasic events such as the beta burst bracketed in the upper EEG channel of the fifth example. The difference between these two examples of REM sleep is in the activity of the EOG. In the fifth example, there are no rapid eye movements. Rapid eye movement is not required to define an epoch as REM sleep (the flat EMG and typical REM EEG are sufficient). The sixth example shows vigorous rapid eye movement.[2]

Figure 1-2 shows three consecutive 20 second epochs during which there was a transition from stage 2 (at the left of the first epoch) to a moment of transitory wakefulness or tension which dissipates into approximately 15 seconds of stage 1 (right part of the middle epoch to beginning of lower epoch). At this point, note the rather abrupt drop in EMG which signals the onset of REM sleep.

While I have chosen clean examples of sleep stages, one should be alerted to the fact that scoring sleep is not always easy. Under certain naturally occurring (e.g., transition from stage 3 to stage 4) or artificially imposed conditions, ambiguities in the record may be manifest. For example, consider the epoch shown in Figure 1-3. Here is a rather inelegant combination of stage 2 EEG (spindles and K-complex-like wave forms) and stage REM (rather low EMG and rapid eye movement). What is it? Convention dictates that we call it stage 2, since the preceding and subsequent epochs clearly indicate stage 2 characteristics. It is interesting to note that this epoch occurred 55 minutes after stage-2 sleep onset at about the time one would expect the appearance of a REM period. It is as though, organismically speaking, the individual cannot make up his mind. Under conditions of experimentally imposed REM deprivation, a subject may, immediately upon lights out, show a drop-out of the EMG (to levels characteristic of REM) despite the fact that the EEG is filled with the alpha waves of wakefulness. It is as though part of the organism is in REM while part is in

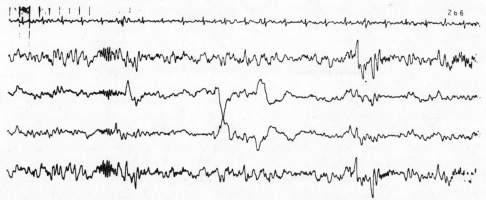

Figure 1-3   Example of an ambiguous stage of sleep marked by REM and stage 2 characteristics.

---

[2] Notice that the two EOG polygraphic tracings of REM sleep shown in Figure 1-1 appear to be mirror images of one another. This is the mark of *conjugate* eye movements. The reason that the tracings are equal and "opposite" is that the electrodes which pick up signals from the two eyes are subject to electrically opposite signals. The electrode for each eye is attached to the skin just to the right or left of the right and left eye respectively. Each electrode detects voltage changes caused by the 1 mV "corneo(+)-retinal(−) potential". When the front of one eye (+) moves toward its electrode, the back of the other eye (−) moves closer to its electrode. Therefore, in the recording shown in Figure 1-1, a right eye movement yields a "negative" EOG for the left eye and a "positive wave" for the right eye.

wakefulness. (The subject's EEG will soon become that of REM which will cause the experimenter to enter the sleeping cubicle to induce yet another awakening.) Investigators have commented on the dissociability of the components of sleep stages, and I will discuss this phenomenon later. However, it should be noted that events such as those shown in Figure 1-3 are not extremely rare. When appropriate recording procedures are utilized, a surprising amount of eye movement (sometimes even rapid eye movement) occurs during NREM sleep (Jacobs, Feldman, and Bender, 1971).

Let us consider further the data of the Jacobs *et al.* (1971) paper. By using D.C. recording procedures, they found a great deal of eye movement during both REM and NREM sleep. Except for REM sleep, while the eyes are closed, they drift upward and remain above the normal line of gaze most of the time. In addition, the two eyes drift divergently, the right eye tending to gaze in a rightward direction, the left in a leftward direction (wall-eyed). Slow eye movements are not only a characteristic of descending stage 1 (at sleep onset), but are also observable during stage 2 and immediately after most REM periods. In addition, *rapid* eye movements occasionally occur during all NREM stages, and, in the subjects of this study, these were vertical rather than horizontal.

During REM sleep, the eyes shift immediately to, or below, the level of forward gaze where they tend to remain during rolling and rapid movement. Actually, most of the eye movement of REM sleep is *slow and rolling*, with the more familiar rapid eye movement superimposed on this activity. About 10% of the rapid eye movement observed in the subjects of this study was horizontal, about 30% vertical, and about 60% oblique (the latter tending more toward the vertical than the horizontal). However, during the first REM period, there is relatively less oblique and relatively more vertical movement (the percentage of horizontal movement tending to remain constant across REM periods).

There is now good evidence that sleep characteristics such as amount of REM (expressed as a number of minutes or percent of total sleep time) are quite reliable within subjects across nights. Eye movement activity (REM density) is particularly reliable. (See Feinberg, 1974, for an excellent discussion of data and methodological problems in assessing reliability of sleep characteristics.)

Characteristics associated with stages of sleep

Before discussing the changes that occur throughout the night in the electrophysiological characteristics of sleep stages, a few points need to be made about some stage-related phenomena. During sleep onset stage 1 (NREM) sleep, individuals are rather easily awakened and often report dreamlike, hallucinatory fantasy which is sometimes indistinguishable from REM dreaming (Foulkes and Vogel, 1965). (For an excellent review of research on the hypnogogic period of sleep onset, which includes stage 1, see Schacter, 1976.) Waking thresholds are somewhat higher during stage 2, mental content has a more thoughtlike and fragmentary form, and recall of this is rather sparse and less reliable. However, there are important individual differences. For example, Zimmerman (1970) reported that while deep sleepers and light sleepers do not differ much in dream recall when awakened from REM sleep, they show marked differences when awakened from stage 2. Awakening thresholds of delta sleep are generally quite high and dream recall is extremely poor. Thus, if we base our operational definitions on behavior and cognition, delta sleep is "deep" sleep.

Patterns that are characteristic of REM sleep have been given a great deal of attention. The flat EMG seems rather paradoxical given other signs of activation in the physiology of REM sleep. Perhaps this lack of tonus in the head and neck area explains the fact that snoring is infrequent and minimal during REM. There is relaxation of the oropharyngeal cavity, including the geniglossi muscles of the tongue. Snoring during REM may be a sign of respiratory disturbance that could have effects on cardiovascular efficiency (Sauerland and Harper, 1976). Diminished EMG is not the only paradoxical characteristic of REM sleep. Cat data reveal a paradoxical dilation of the blood vessels of the ear at lowered ambient temperatures. This may be related to poikilothermic (ectothermic) characteristics of REM: (a) positive correlation between ambient temperature and body temperature and (b) absence of shivering response to lowered ambient temperature and absence of polypnea to increased ambient temperature. Another peculiarity of REM is the increase in hypothalamic temperature regardless of relative ambient temperature (see Parmeggiani, Franzini, and Lenzi, 1976). These and many other kinds of evidence strongly suggest that REM, NREM, and wakefulness are qualitatively different states.

While awakening thresholds from REM sleep are relatively high in animals, the evidence in human subjects is rather mixed. Some investigators (Williams, 1967) have reported high awakening thresholds. However, much of the evidence suggests that REM sleep in humans is associated with low awakening thresholds, compared to delta sleep (Rechtschaffen, Hauri, and Zeitlin, 1966; Wilson and Zung, 1966; Zimmerman, 1970). REM awakening thresholds are influenced by factors such as attention to dreaming rather than to external stimuli, the nature of the stimulus (e.g., meaningful vs. unimportant, visual vs. auditory vs. tactual, etc.), and individual differences. Thus, it is an oversimplification to describe REM sleep as "light" or "deep" only in terms of awakening thresholds.

Dream recall after REM awakening is typically plentiful and elaborate. While it is perhaps another oversimplification to describe REM sleep as dreaming sleep (Cohen, 1970), we will concentrate on REM sleep in exploring the nature and function of dreaming.

Temporal characteristics of sleep stages

Typically, throughout the night, NREM and REM stages follow each other in roughly 90-100 minute cycles so that by the end of a 7-8 hour night there will be about 3-6 REM periods. Again, typically, the proportion of REM to NREM sleep will increase during each successive cycle: the REM portion of the first 90 minute cycle may last only a few minutes while the REM portion of the last cycle may last as long as 45-60 minutes or more. Delta sleep is largely confined to the first third of the night so that the NREM portion of later cycles is largely stage 2. A statistically reliable relationship between log duration of a REM period and log duration of preceding NREM sleep has been suggested (Vogel, personal communication, June, 1976). The temporal sequence of events typical of an adult individual is illustrated in Figure 1-4.

It is important to note that there are wide individual differences in the dynamics of stage cycling. This is particularly noticeable for individuals with sleep disorders or significant emotional disturbance, and for subjects newly admitted to laboratory experiments. These latter subjects may, for example, miss their first and possibly their second REM periods. This kind of disturbed pattern has been labelled "first night effect". It should be taken into consideration in studies which require stable baseline sleep characteristics against which to

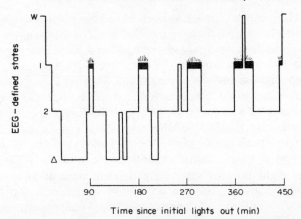

Figure 1-4   The spatio-temporal architecture of sleep throughout a 7.5 hour night (idealized). The dark horizontal bars indicate stage 1-REM as opposed to stage 1-NREM. The lines above the bars indicate eye movement activity which tends to be less marked at the beginning of the REM period. If one accepts the convention of ordering stages according to EEG-defined "depth", then there tends to be a "lightening" of sleep as the night progresses. This is indicated by (a) gradual loss of delta sleep, (b) increase of REM stage duration (with its accompanying physiological "turmoil", and (c) momentary awakening (during the fourth REM period).

judge the effect of experimental manipulations. It is of some theoretical interest because of its implication for hypotheses regarding the capacity of the sleeping individual to retain a certain degree of vigilance.

Let me dwell briefly on one implication of the missed REM period phenomenon of the "first night effect". Strictly speaking, what may be missed are some observable electro-physiological characteristics (e.g., eye movement) from which we typically infer a central organismic state. A state like REM sleep represents a temporal convergence of phenomena (e.g., low voltage fast EEG, EOG, PGO spiking, EMG suppressions, etc.) each of which is regulated by different though clearly interdependent neural structures or areas, and each of which may be dissociated (elicited in other states). In addition, while standard recordings may suggest that a REM period has been "skipped", measurements that typically are not utilized (e.g., middle ear muscle activity or MEMA) may show the usual REM pattern (Lamstein, Roffwarg, and Herman, 1975). In fact, ambiguity may occur in the measures that are typically utilized. For example, at a point where one expects a REM period to emerge out of stage 2, we may observe certain changes. The background EEG activity may become quiescent (e.g., few spindles, K-complexes) while there is an increase in body movement activity. The subject may awaken at this time. These patterns suggest a kind of organismic uncertainty with regard to commitment to one stage or another.

These observations bring up two troublesome problems: (a) How many sleep characteristics are required to define REM sleep, and are they of equal weight? For example, during the early part of sleep on the first night, does the presence of MEMA, despite the absence of EMG diminution or EOG activity, permit one to assume the presence of the REM state? After all, "had Roffwarg's middle-ear muscle activity been observed before the eye movements we would have had a definition which included MEMA as fundamental and possibly we would have talked of MEMA sleep. Similarly, we could equally easily have had PGO (or PIP) sleep or even scrotal sleep" (Lewis, 1975, p. 352).

Related to these questions is the question of how to define the central state, the deep structure of REM sleep. If electrophysiological characteristics are merely signs of surface structure, their absence is not equivalent to the absence of the central state. The distinction between central states and peripheral signs raises all kinds of difficult questions. For example, the distinction between "real sleep" (inferred from slow waves easily observed in mammals and birds) and "inactivity" of fish (inferred from behaviors and EEG recordings not clearly comparable to those seen in mammals) may refer more to surface structure than central state. Thus, the evolution of sleep may involve changes in the *articulation* of the state more than the state itself (and its function).

The cyclic nature of sleep is a fundamental characteristic. This roughly 90 minute cycling emerges by about eight months after birth when a number of EEG, autonomic, and behavioral characteristics, each with an approximately 60 minute cycle, are more neatly convergent in time (Petre-Quadens and Schlag, 1974). Across mammalian species, cycle length is correlated with life span (positive relationship), metabolic rate (negative), brain weight (positive) and gestation period (positive). According to Zepelin and Rechtschaffen (1974), brain weight seems to be the crucial determinant of cycle length. The significance of individual differences in cycle length within species is unknown.

A number of investigators believe that the 90 minute cycle is a manifestation of a general "basic rest activity cycle" or BRAC (Kleitman, 1969) which is superimposed on the circadian rhythm. Thus, under ideal circumstances, the BRAC should be observable during the day. The demands of waking events presumably mask the endogenous BRAC. Thus, Globus suggests that the kinds of electrophysiological signs which are used by sleep researchers "are not the essential process itself, but only signs by which the process can be recognized. Because of the ongoing state of the waking organism, it would be extremely difficult to pick up such signs; it is apparent that if the [REM] state were to be present during wakefulness, current techniques could not demonstrate it. The identification of [the REM] state with sleep may not only be inaccurate, but may also lead to a lack of appreciation of the wider ramifications of [REM] phenomena" (1966, p. 657). In other words, REM sleep is perhaps a clearer manifestation, an exaggerated expression, of a cyclic phenomenon which occurs throughout the 24 hours of each circadian cycle. Recent laboratory work suggests that individuals isolated from normal external distractors display a roughly 100 minute cycling of eating and daydreaming, and that these behaviors are correlated with cycling of EEG and autonomic characteristics (Lavie and Kripke, 1975). Lavie, Levy, and Coolidge (1975) predicted, on the basis of earlier results showing longer spiral after-effect (SAE) duration after REM than after NREM (delta) awakenings (Lavie and Giora, 1973), that SAE durations would show a diurnal cyclicity patterned after the BRAC. Seven subjects were given the Archimedes spiral twice every five minutes from 8:00 a.m. to 4:00 p.m. Six out of the seven subjects demonstrated ultradian rhythms, some of which were remarkably consistent with expectation according to the BRAC concept, and despite the relatively uncontrolled and demanding nature of the task.

There is evidence that subjects with elevated scores on psychiatric scales have irregular, diminished, and dissociated BRAC or circadian cycles when they are placed in experimental environments which isolate them from *Zeitgebers* (external circadian cues, e.g., clocks, lighting, noise, etc.) (Hiatt and Kripke, 1975; Lund, 1974).

It is tempting to interpret these observations as evidence that "REM-NREM" cycling occurs throughout the 24-hour circadian cycle. However, an unpublished study by Vogel and Rechtschaffen (cited in Vogel, 1974) suggests caution. They gave amphetamine late in the morning to a group of normal subjects. They reasoned as follows. Amphetamine is a REM sleep suppressant, which, like other REM suppressants, tends to elicit REM "rebound" (higher than normal amounts of REM sleep) after the drug has dissipated. If a REM sleep equivalent occurs during wakefulness, then there should be a slight elevation of REM sleep during the night following amphetamine. This effect was not observed. The problem with such a finding is that low dosage, acute administration of amphetamine, like other catecholaminergic facilitators (e.g., imipramine), is not necessarily followed by REM rebound (as is the case of chronic administration) (Stern and Morgane, 1974). However, there is additional evidence against the hypothesis that waking experience which is *similar* to REM mentation is functionally *equivalent* to (i.e., can substitute for) REM sleep. Halper, Pivik, and Dement (1969) gave subjects with high hypnotic susceptibility scores a chance to engage in hypnotically induced "hallucinations" and "dreams" during a period of REM deprivation. This treatment did not appear to prevent REM rebound, i.e., did not reduce the need for REM sleep. I take up the question of REM substitution in Chapter 4.

A difference in the *timing* of diurnal and nocturnal phases of the BRAC is suggested by the findings from an ingenious study of polyphasic sleep (multiple naps) during a 40 hour period (Moses, Hord, Lubin, Johnson, and Naitoh, 1975a). The data suggested that "the clock governing the REM cycle is sleep-dependent — it stops upon awakening and resumes at the next sleep onset. This suggests that the 90-110 minute cycle found in the awake subject are not expressions of the 90-110 minute cycle found during sleep" (p. 632). This conclusion derives from the finding of a roughly 90 minute REM cycle for the nap data when nap time was collapsed (ignoring intervening wakefulness). However, to argue that the timing of the sleep BRAC is discontinuous with the timing of the wake BRAC is not necessarily to argue against a similarity in the properties and functional significance of these two phenomena.

That there is a certain psychophysiological parallelism during wakefulness and sleep seems to be a reasonable hypothesis. Changes in CNS activation (estimated by SAE duration), eye movement activity, and alpha enhancement seem to coincide with changes in cognition (fantasy enhancement) during wakefulness. Likewise, changes in CNS activation (measured by sleep electrophysiography) are clearly related to changes in cognition (dreaming enhancement) during the nocturnal phase. These circadian changes in psycho-physiological activity appear to be adequately modeled by a BRAC hypothesis. This suggests an endogenous periodicity that is superimposed on the circadian rhythm, highly influenced by external distractors, and characterized by large individual differences in magnitude, frequency, and clarity or definition. What has not been satisfactorily established is the degree that waking "REM" patterns are functionally equivalent to REM processes. We will take up this question when we look at data on the substitutability of waking fantasy for lost REM, i.e., under conditions of REM deprivation.

Apparently, there exists a roughly 90 minute cycle for a number of psychological and physiological characteristics during wakefulness: gastric activity, eating and drinking (*ad lib.* or requiring instrumental responding), heart rate, body temperature, alpha activity, spiral after-effect, dreamlike fantasy. (See Broughton, 1975, for a review of these kinds of data.) It is also quite obvious that there is a periodic, roughly 90 minute cycling of psychological and physiological characteristics during sleep. What is not entirely clear is the relationship between the activity and rest aspects of these wake and sleep cycles. Indeed, descriptions by Kleitman (1969) and Broughton (1975) of the waking cycle suggest oscillation between an active and an inactive phase. The active phase is characterized by work, high energy expenditure, "advanced wakefulness", and increased attention to what

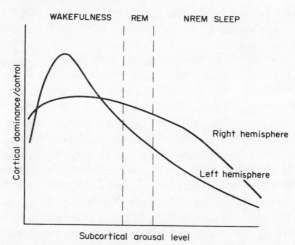

Figure 1-5   Hypothetical model of a relationship between cortical influence as a function of arousal.

might be called neocortical intellective activity. The rest phase, what Hobson has described as "an endogenous trough in an ultradian alertness cycle" (1975, p. 388), is characterized by play, rest (e.g., coffee break,[3] nap, etc.), "primitive wakefulness", and increased attention to what might be called telediencephalic catering and consumatory activity associated with individual and species survival. In fact, Broughton (1975) has suggested that what is involved is basically a shift from left (active) to right (rest) hemispheric domination, or more metaphorically, from ego (verbal-intellectual) to id (fantasy-irrational) tendencies. Of course, it should be remembered that what is being suggested is a relatively subtle endogenous rhythm that is easily masked by exogenous distractions.

Compare this theoretical description of the oscillation of two kinds of psychobiological "styles" during wakefulness with descriptions of the NREM-REM cycle. According to theorists like Shapiro (1967) and Fisher (1965), NREM sleep presents a kind of secondary process while REM sleep represents a kind of primary process. On the basis of the two sets of characteristics, the "activity" phase of the waking BRAC corresponds to the "rest" (NREM) phase of the sleeping BRAC while the "rest" phase of the waking BRAC corresponds to the "activity" (REM) phase of the sleeping BRAC.

Consider the following admittedly speculative idea regarding the relationship between circadian and BRAC type periodicities. Figure 1-5 represents the basic wake-sleep dimension along the abscissa which, for simplicity, is related to the relative degree of subcortically-mediated arousal levels in the cortex. High levels of subcortical activation associated with wakefulness are repesented on the left side of the figure, while low levels are associated with sleep. Relative arousal or influence of the left and right hemispheres is represented by different functions of subcortical activation. Thus, within wakefulness or sleep, a basic rest-activity periodicity would occur. Higher or lower levels of subcortical activation within each level defining wakefulness or sleep would be associated with shifts in the relative influence of left or right hemisphere-mediated behaviors and experiences. Thus, the more relaxed phase of the waking BRAC would be associated with psychological

---

[3] Hobson (1975) suggests that caffeine may be used to counteract the "endogenous trough". "By drinking at periodic intervals, could we be paying homage to an archaic force, a kind of physiological appendix no longer necessary to assure our survival?" (1975, p. 388).

characteristics that are relatively more saturated with right hemisphere-mediated qualities while the rest phase of the sleep BRAC (NREM) would be associated with relatively fewer of these qualities.

These speculations regarding the influence of subcortical arousal on the relative dominance of one cerebral hemisphere over the other are consonant with those of Budzynski (1976). "Perhaps the decrease in critical, analytical, logical linear-functioning that occurs with lowering arousal level is the gradual, functional disabling of the major hemisphere. We might also speculate that the minor hemisphere is not as quickly disabled as is the major hemisphere with decreasing arousal." Budzynski goes on to say that "at a still lower point on the arousal continuum (deeper sleep stages), even the minor hemisphere's efficiency drops off sharply." Then, as if to anticipate questions discussed in this book regarding the REM dream as a "window" to cortical processes (Bertini, 1973; Hartmann, 1973), Budzynski says, "it is the region between those two points, or what we might call the 'window' in which the major hemisphere would appear to relinquish control, thus allowing uncritical absorption by the minor hemisphere of external material or the emergence of internally generated material" (p. 381).

The hypothesis that there is a left hemisphere (NREM) vs. right hemisphere (REM) shift and an early REM period (right) to late REM period (left) shift is taken up later in the book (see Chapters 5 and 7). Needless to say these shifts should be considered subtle alterations rather than clear-cut changes. No assumptions are made regarding the degree to which subcortical arousal induces a cortical BRAC or vice versa. In all likelihood, the influences are concurrent and interactive.

Some interesting questions follow from such generalizations. For example, are there individual differences in the tendency to suppress this rhythmicity (e.g., unwillingness to relax and "unwind")? And what are the effects of such individual differences in the rhythmic and motivational characteristics of sleep? For instance, are individuals who suppress a strong endogenous rest component of the waking BRAC more resistant to REM deprivation? That is, is the REM sleep of such individuals particularly important in the compensation (e.g., by otherwise suppressed right hemisphere functioning) for a suppressed biological process? Which components would best "substitute" for lost REM? Implications of the relationship between waking and sleeping aspects of the BRAC are just now attracting the kind of research attention required for a more general theory of sleep and wakefulness.

REM vs. NREM sleep

Our focus will largely be on the biological and psychological characteristics of REM sleep. Whatever we say about the nature and function of dreaming must be compatible with those characteristics. That is to say, while much of what is said about dreams may not be derivable from the biology of REM sleep, it must at least be compatible with the physical facts of the event. For example, Adler (1927) speculated that dreaming is a form of self-deception. When the individual outgrows the self-deceptive life style, dreaming is less frequent or ceases altogether. We know that this inference about dreaming from the data of dream recall is fundamentally wrong. Dreaming is a natural and continuous part of REM sleep which occurs regardless of attitudes, affects, or behaviors that can affect our recall of dreaming. Psychological speculation about dreaming must be compatible with such information.

Some people believe that eating certain foods prior to sleep affects dreams. My stockbroker believes that a presleep snack including chocolate cake can make him dream more intensely. In fact there may be something in this observation. There is evidence that a diet rich in carbohydrates tends to increase REM percent (Phillips, Chen, Crisp, Koval, McGuinness, Kalucy, Kalucy and Lacey, 1975). In addition, there is evidence that such a diet tends to increase brain serotonin (which is associated with an increase in REM percentages) at the expense of brain catecholamine, while a diet rich in protein may have the opposite effect (Fernstrom and Wurtman, 1974; Wurtman and Fernstrom, 1975). It has been speculated that one role of REM sleep is catecholaminergic "restoration" (Hartmann, 1973: Stern and Morgane, 1974). It is quite possible that variation in diet may affect the intensity (and quality) of the REM process with concomitant changes in correlated characteristics of dreaming. Individual differences in susceptibility to such changes may in turn affect the probability of dream recall. These possibilities will be discussed in more detail later. Suffice

TABLE 1-1. Comparison of NREM and REM Sleep

Characteristic, event	NREM	REM
Occurs primarily in	first half of night (delta)	second half of night
Circadian entrainment	relatively low (more affected by amount of prior wakefulness)	relatively high (tends to occur in morning in humans)
Thermoregulation	homoiothermic	poikilothermic
Neural sites of origin	raphe, preoptic area?	FTG, locus coeruleus?
Neural firing rate in telencephalon	relatively diminished	relatively enhanced
Neural firing rates in certain diencephalic areas	relatively high	relatively low
DC potential shifts in brain	positive	negative
CNS temperature	decreases	increases
Cerebral blood flow	lower	higher
Oxygen consumption in brain	lower	higher
Major neurotransmitters	serotonin?	acetylcholine, noradrenalin?
Hormone secretion rate:		
prolactin, growth hormone, parathyroid hormone	relatively high	low
lutenizing hormone, 17-OH	relatively low	high
Variability in autonomic nervous system (except GSR)	low	high
GSR variability	high	low
Evoked potentials	large	small
Knee jerk reflex	normal	suppressed
Eye movement	rare, slow, nonconjugate	frequent, rapid, conjugate
Eye position	above midline	at or below midline
Correlation with IQ (in aged, retarded, organic groups only)	low	relatively high
Effect of drugs:		
antidepressants (e.g., amitriptyline)	increase	decrease
antipsychotic (e.g., chlorpromazine)	increase	increase
stimulants (e.g., amphetamine/ caffein)	decrease (stage 2)/increase (delta)	decrease
Mentation:		
content	thoughtlike, poorly organized	dreamlike, affective, well organized
amount/clarity of recall	relatively poor	relatively good

Note: The differences are maximal for comparisons of REM and delta.

it to say here that theories about the phenomena and phenomenology of dreaming will gain much from deeper understanding of the biology of REM sleep.

Table 1-1 shows how REM and NREM sleep differ on a number of characteristics. The pattern suggests two qualitatively different states with possibly different functions. Note that the data base for these comparisons is derived from animal and human studies and that the research is a mix of observation, correlation, and experiment. Also note that in many cases, a distinction among the various stages of NREM sleep ("delta" vs. "spindle" or stage 2 sleep) is often not explicit.[4] Some of these characteristics of REM sleep, which have some implication for hypotheses regarding dreaming, will be developed in more detail in later chapters. To set the stage for this exploration, let me quote from Rechtschaffen:

> If sleep does not serve an absolutely vital function, then it is the biggest mistake the evolutionary process has ever made. Sleep precludes hunting for and consuming food. It is incompatible with procreation. It produces vulnerability to attack from enemies. Sleep interferes with every voluntary, adaptive motor act in the repertoire of coping mechanisms. How could natural selection with its irrevocable logic have "permitted" the animal kingdom to pay the price of sleep for no good reason? In fact, the behavior of sleep is so apparently maladaptive that one can only wonder why some other condition did not evolve to satisfy whatever need it is that sleep satisfies.
>
> Is sleep only a vestigial remain which has outlived its functional usefulness? Probably not. How could sleep have remained virtually unchanged as a monstrously useless, maladaptive vestige throughout the whole of mammalian evolution while selection has during the same period of time been able to achieve all kinds of delicate, finely-tuned adjustments in the shape of fingers and toes?
>
> It may not be too extravagant to describe the function of sleep as one of the major unsolved biological puzzles of our age (Rechtschaffen, 1971, p. 88).

2. NEUROPHYSIOLOGICAL MECHANISMS OF REM AND NREM SLEEP

Much of modern sleep research is devoted to the question of how areas of the brain initiate and control REM and NREM sleep. Analyses may be done at the level of relatively large structures (e.g., reticular formation, hypothalamus), specific nuclei (e.g., locus coeruleus), or single cells. In addition, consideration must be given to their activity and rhythmicity, their interactions, and the transmitter substances (e.g., serotonin, noradrenalin) that are more or less specific to these structures. Different techniques, each with its advantages and disadvantages, are utilized: recording, stimulation, lesioning, as well as bioamine facilitation or depletion. Despite the elegant research findings and theorizing of Jouvet that have dominated the neurophysiology of sleep there is much disagreement regarding the regulation and control of sleep. About 15 years ago, Jasper (1961) stated: "No one has yet explained in positive and unequivocal terms the nature of sleep" (p. 307). Few would disagree that this is still a timely statement.

Neurophysiological processes

In order to appreciate the work on the neurophysiology of REM sleep one needs to have some idea about what goes on at the synaptic level. Figure 1-6 provides a simplified schematic of synaptic dynamics. These include (a) the enzymatically regulated synthesis of

---

[4] It is particularly disturbing to note the curious dearth of theorizing regarding stage 2 ("spindle") sleep despite the fact that it comprises at least 50% of total human sleep.

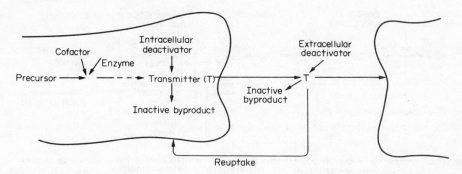

Figure 1-6 A version of the NIMH neuron. Experimenters can gain a measure of control over transmitter regulation in order to test hypotheses about neurochemical mediation of states such as REM and NREM. One can *increase* synaptic transmitter by (a) facilitating the synthesis process (e.g., electroconvulsive treatment), (b) inhibiting the intracellular inactivator (e.g., with MAO inhibitors), (c) facilitating the contraction of storage granules (e.g., with amphetamine) which results in release of transmitter into the synapse, and (d) retarding the re-uptake process (e.g., with tricyclic drugs). On the other hand, one can affect a *decrease* of synaptic transmitter by (a) inhibiting synthesis (e.g., using the rate limiting enzyme retardant PCPA), (b) interfering with the storage of transmitter (e.g., reserpine), (c) facilitating re-uptake (lithium). One can utilize a different strategy, that of affecting the functional effectiveness of the transmitter at the postsynaptic site of action. For example, chlorpromazine is thought to compete with dopamine for receptor surface sites, thereby making available dopamine less effective. Finally, one can use drugs that destroy neuronal pathways. For example, 6-OHDA can be used to "burn" dopaminergic neurons. Along with stimulation and lesion (as well as recording) methods, these biochemical methods can be used to assess specific pathways with their particular transmitters.

neurotransmitters from precursors, (b) intraneuronal regulation of amounts of amine substances (e.g., serotonin) by regulator substances (e.g., monoamine oxidase or MAO), (c) regulation of re-uptake processes, (d) "neutralization" of transmitter substances by intersynaptic regulators (e.g., catechol-*o*-methyltransferase or COMT), and (e) facilitation or diminution of transmitter effects at the postsynaptic site.

Figure 1-7 shows the metabolic steps in the production and elimination of three classes of neurotransmitter. Such a figure can be useful to clarify results from studies whose methodology includes the facilitation or inhibition of a specific transmitter at any one of a number of steps in the metabolic cycle. This information is provided to give the reader an appreciation of some of the techniques that investigators can use to evaluate the mechanisms of sleep. If, for example, it is hypothesized that serotonin, an indolamine neuro-transmitter, plays an especially important role in the regulation of NREM sleep, then a number of predictions can be made. It would be predicted that substances (e.g., para-chlorophenylalanine or PCPA) that prevent the synthesis of serotonin from tryptophan should retard sleep onset. Likewise, lesions in serotonin-rich nuclei should have similar, perhaps more profound and lasting effects. On the other hand, preloading with tryptophan (serotonin itself does not cross the blood-brain barrier) should have the opposite effects. These examples illustrate the importance of combining evidence at the structural (neural), functional, and biochemical levels for a comprehensive neurophysiological picture of sleep mechanisms.

Neurophysiological research has utilized lesion, transection, and stimulation techniques in conjunction with pharmacological strategies in an attempt to specify both neurostruc-tural and neurohumoral action underlying the initiation, control, and modification of sleep stages. In fact, the history of research on the physiology of sleep has moved from an

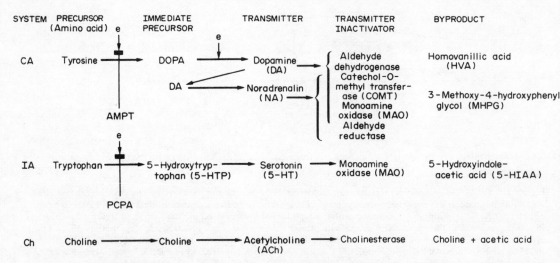

Figure 1-7 Metabolic pathway for three major neurotransmitters: catecholaminergic (CA), indolaminergic (IA) and cholinergic (Ch). Rate limiting enzymes (e) which control synthesis are not shown. However, agents which inhibit the action of such enzymes at the first stage of CA synthesis (AMPT) and IA synthesis (PCPA) are shown.

emphasis on structural aspects to an emphasis on integrating information about both structural and humoral aspects.

Both phases of this research suggest that there is a stratification of inhibiting and arousing areas. The general outline of this "vertical model of counterbalanced elements" (see Chase, 1972, p. 82) is shown in Figure 1-8. The lower brain stem (caudally from roughly the midpontine region) appears to be mainly inhibitory or sleep inducing. This area (indicated by I in the figure) includes the caudal part of the raphe system. The rostral pons

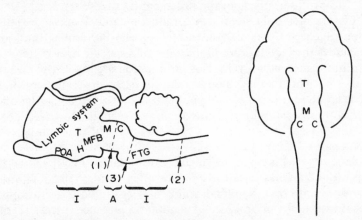

Figure 1-8 Sagittal view of a cat brain shown on the left. Dotted line (1) represents a mesencephalic transection which elicits a synchronous (sleeping) EEG pattern in front of the cut (cerveau isolé). Transection (2) at the caudal end of the medulla leaves more or less intact the synchronous-desynchronous (sleep-wake) rhythm recorded ahead of the cut (encephalé isolé). However, midpontine transection (3) yields EEG activation in front of the cut, suggesting the elimination of active, inhibitory influences from areas behind the cut. This finding is one of the major sources of evidence against a simple passive theory of sleep. T: thalamus. POA: preoptic area. H: hypothalamus. MFB: median forebrain bundle. C: Locus coeruleus. M: mesencephalic reticular formation. FTG: giant cells of the pontine reticular formation.

(including raphe, and parts of the FTG and coeruleal areas) and mesencephalon (indicated by M in the figure) appear to be largely excitatory or arousal-inducing (indicated by A). Rostral to this is a relatively large area including preoptic area, median forebrain bundle, parts of the hypothalamus and thalamus — generally what may be called the basal forebrain inhibitory area.

A stratification of arousing and inhibiting areas was first clearly suggested by the two major disturbances of sleep/wakefulness caused by encephalitis which swept through Europe after World War I. Von Encomo noted that the insomnia pattern was associated with lesions in the basal forebrain, while lethargy was associated with lesions in the mesencephalic areas. Subsequent experimental research has expanded upon these initial observations.

Determination of inhibitory or excitatory areas is largely based on results of unit recordings, electrical stimulation, chemical stimulation, lesions, and transections. For example, bulbar transection (encephalé isolé) has relatively little effect on sleep-wake cycles that are recorded in front of the cut. Midpontine transection facilitates desynchronization (arousal) patterns. The effect is probably induced by the isolation of caudal inhibitory centers (raphe and medullary solitary tract) from the rest of the brain. This is an extremely important finding. It directly contradicts the idea that sleep is merely the absence of sensory information flow to the cortex. It suggests, rather, that there are active, sleep-inducing areas of the brain. That caudal pontine and bulbar areas have an actively inhibitory influence on mesencephalic activating structures is also supported by evidence that the CNS can be activated by introducing thiopental directly to presumably inhibitory (pontine) areas. Deactivation of these areas appears to release more rostral areas (Magni, Moruzzi, Rossi and Zanchetti, 1959). The solitary tract is richly endowed with fibers that provide feedback from gastrointestinal activity. This process may be the physiological basis for postprandial sleepiness (Carlson, 1977, pp. 425-426).

There is converging evidence (e.g., Bremer, 1975) for the hypothesis that the preoptic area (POA in Figure 1-8) is sleep inducing. Introducing serotonin directly to the POA can induce NREM sleep. Stimulation here reduces evoked discharges in the simultaneously stimulated reticular formation and induces EEG synchrony (sleep pattern). This effect can be eliminated by presleep treatment with PCPA. In addition, POA units show a low rate of firing during wakefulness, an accelerated rate of firing at sleep onset, and then a reduction of firing once sleep has become established. Finally, heating the POA induces drowsiness. This may serve as an experimental analogue of the effect of high fever to induce sleepiness — a biologically useful mechanism by which homoiothermic organisms are forced into inactivity to reduce endogenous sources of heating (normally produced by activity) (see Roberts and Robinson, 1969).

One of the interesting things about these general findings is that the preoptic area is also important in thermoregulation (Heller, Colliver, and Anand, 1974; Milner, 1970). For example, there is evidence that preoptic heating increases respiratory rate during wakefulness and NREM (but not REM) sleep (Parmeggiani, Franzini, and Lenzi, 1975). Glotzbach and Heller (1976) have recently reported that in contrast to wakefulness and NREM sleep, REM sleep in the kangaroo rat is characterized by an independence of metabolic rate and experimentally induced changes in temperature in the preoptic area of the hypothalamus. This rather elegant study again demonstrates both the thermoregulatory insensitivity of REM sleep as well as its qualitative distinctiveness. In addition, "good sleep" (including ability to fall and stay asleep) appears to be related to (low) body temperature (Monroe,

1967; Moses *et al.*, 1975a). According to Sterman (in Chase, 1972, p. 91), "By virtue of its documented influences upon somatic, visceral, endocrine and nonspecific reticulo-thalamic functions, the preoptic area of the hypothalamus is particularly well-suited for an integrative role." Here is further evidence for speculations from ontogenetic and phylogenetic perspectives about the fundamental role of NREM sleep in the metabolic regulation of homoiothermic organisms. These ideas are discussed in the following chapter on the origin and development of sleep.

Mesencephalic transection rostral to the pons (cerveau isolé) elicits synchronization (probably because the connection between forebrain and reticular circuits and the midbrain activating areas are interfered with). However, it is especially important to note that the EEG synchrony of the cerveau isolé is not permanent: it is periodically interrupted by EEG arousal which has been determined to be an indication of wakefulness rather than REM sleep (see Moruzzi, 1974, p. 24). This observation suggests that there is at least a potential rest-activity cycle intrinsic to the cerebrum. "It is an experimental fact that the mechanisms underlying some basic aspects of the sleep-waking cycle are potentially present in the cerebrum. Of course we have no right to assume that rhythmicity arises within the cerebrum also when neural connections with the brain stem have not been interrupted. At any event, even if it is conceded that a sleep cycle arises in the cerebrum, when all ascending and descending connections are intact, this rhythm is likely to be modified by the brain stem" (Moruzzi in Petre-Quadens and Schlag, 1974, p. 21). In fact, the dynamic interrelationship between brain stem and cerebral activity underlying the sleep and wakefulness cycle, and the relationship between this interaction and both intrinsic circadian periodicity and situational events (e.g., increased blood pressure or CO_2, copulation or feeding, hypothetical exercise-inducing "hypnotoxins", etc.) are a complete mystery.

Undoubtedly, there are many factors that initiate sleep onset. One of the most reasonable candidates is the hypnogenic substance(s) thought to build up during wakefulness. A typical finding is that cerebrospinal fluid or blood from a sleep-deprived animal can induce sleep in a waking animal. It has been demonstrated that infusion of cerebrospinal fluid (CSF), taken from rats during their dark (active) cycle, into rats in their light (inactivity) cycle increases mean activity in the recipients; conversely, light phase CSF decreases activity of rats in their dark phase (Sachs, Ungar, Waser, and Borbély, 1976). Progress in isolating and identifying such a hypnogenic factor has been made (Pappenheimer, 1976; Pappenheimer, Koski, Fencl, Karnovsky, and Krueger, 1975; Schoenberger and Monnier, 1974). However, the effect of such a factor would be difficult to explain in the light of observations made on craniopagus twins (joined at the head and sharing brain tissue and blood circulation). Lenard and Schulte (1972) reported that both the wakefulness-sleep and REM-NREM cycles of such a pair of twins were completely independent. In addition, a Spanish group has reported evidence of sleep-wake cycle independence between a canine host and an implanted head (an encephalé isolé transplant) (de Andres, Nava, Gutierrez-Rivas, and Reinoso-Suarez, 1975). Finally, Anders and Roffwarg (1973) have reported evidence that maternal and fetal REM cycles (estimated from fetal kicking activity) are totally independent as are maternal and neonatal REM cycles. They suggest that the data do not support the hypothesis that fetal REM cycles are regulated by circulating maternal hormones. De Andres *et al.* similarly conclude that "the possible influence of humoral factors [on the sleep and wakefulness states] would be secondary to that of the central nervous system" (1975, p. 16).

Some conclusions have emerged from neurophysiological research. First, sleep is not a passive condition. There are areas of the brain which actively suppress wakefulness. This conclusion is well documented by stimulation and mesencephalic transection studies. Second, REM and NREM are qualitatively different states whose initiation is largely mediated by subcortical areas. Third, during sleep, many parts of the brain are metabolically and electrically highly active. In fact, Jouvet (1974) has referred to REM sleep as a period of "brain storming". Fourth, the notion of a single sleep center is still suspect, though as we shall see, there is good evidence for a REM sleep center. Fifth, there are endogenous, circadian sleep-wake rhythms that involve interacting areas of the brain. Sixth, sleep onset is the product of the confluence of a number of events which influence active sleep-inducing areas such as POA, raphe, solitary tract. These include reduced or monotonous stimulation which can be maximized by instrumental behavior, high temperature, gastrointestinal activity, increased blood pressure or blood CO_2, active dampening of the reticular formation, etc. Seventh, telencephalon is necessary for the slow wave or delta phase of NREM sleep but not for REM sleep. Finally, there are conditions (both naturally occurring and artificially induced) under which signs of electrophysiological arousal (low voltage fast EEG) are not correlated with behavioral alertness. Thus, from a neurophysiological perspective, a distinction among terms like "wake", "aroused", and "conscious" needs to be made. Kleitman (1963) was one of the first to emphasize this point.

Jouvet's hypothesis

Jouvet has been the most influential investigator of the neurophysiology of sleep. His work on cats strongly implicated the serotonin-rich raphe system of the brain stem in the regulation of NREM sleep. For example, he found that lesioning the raphe caused arousal patterns that were correlated with both the size of the lesion and the degree of serotonergic depletion. Likewise he found that raphe stimulation increased NREM sleep. Similar techniques have been used to assess the mechanisms of REM sleep.

Jouvet found that transections at the mesencephalon-pons border did not eliminate REM sleep (assessed by observing periodic signs of muscular atonia, high amplitude phasic discharges, eye movement), while caudal pontine transections eliminated REM. There are no signs of REM in front of a rostral pontine transection but there are behind it. On the basis of results from more specific pontine lesions, Jouvet hypothesized that REM sleep is controlled by catecholaminergically active midpontine sites such as the n. reticular pontis oralis and caudalis, locus coeruleus, and subcoeruleus. Caudal coeruleus structures supposedly control inhibitory characteristics of REM while the middle section activates telediencephalic structures. These influence the lateral geniculate which affects eye movement, and limbic structures (e.g., hippocampus) which mediate paleocortical motivation and probably affect the emotional quality of the dream experience. Routtenberg (1966) has reinforced Jouvet's idea of the importance of limbic activation ("Arousal II"), rather than reticular activation ("Arousal I"), during REM sleep. Likewise the role of the limbic system in coding information from short term memory is consistent with ideas about the importance of REM dreaming in establishing long term memories that mediate adaptive behavior (McGrath and Cohen, 1978).

Lesions in the pontine area, or application of 6-hydroxydopamine or alphamethyldopa (which inhibit catecholamine synthesis selectively) eliminate both tonic and phasic activity of REM sleep. Also, there is evidence that limbic lesions are associated with a decline in

REM sleep while electrical or chemical (acetylcholine) stimulation of limbic (hippocampal) areas facilitate REM sleep. There is evidence that to some extent the serotonergic raphe system implicated in NREM sleep also regulates some of the process of REM sleep. (For a detailed analysis, see Stern and Morgane, 1974, pp. 83 ff.) For example, lesions in certain areas of the raphe system cause discharge during NREM sleep and even wakefulness of phasic events (pontine-geniculate-occipital or PGO spikes) that are normally confined to REM. This effect can be produced by using PCPA which blocks serotonergic synthesis. Conversely, 5-HTP (serotonin precursor) or MAO inhibitor increases available serotonin and inhibits PGO discharge. In addition, there are certain groups of serotonergically rich raphe cells that are most active during REM and least active during NREM. Data on the interaction of raphe and locus coeruleus areas suggest to Jouvet that the caudal raphe is involved in "priming" REM while rostral raphe areas are involved in NREM phenomena (Stern and Morgane, 1974).

Jouvet (1975) believes that empirical evidence favors a significant role for cholinergic activity in the REM sleep process. He cites the following kinds of evidence. Injections of ACh into the central grey matter induces a transition from wakefulness to REM (i.e., bypassing the NREM phase that usually precedes the onset of REM sleep). The locus coeruleus and subcoeruleus, both implicated in the induction of REM sleep characteristics, have AChE-containing perikarya. Atropine (an ACh blocker) does not suppress NREM sleep but does suppress REM sleep and increases REM latency. Cortical release of ACh is higher during REM than NREM sleep. Pompeiano and Valentinuzzi (1976) review evidence that cataplexy (postural atonia) and rapid eye movements are induced by cholinergic facilitation by anticholinesterase, and they have developed a mathematical model to describe the phenomenon in the decerebrate cat. There is additional evidence from a recent study (Sitaram, Wyatt, Dawson, and Gillin, 1976) indicating that injected physostigmine (an anticholinesterase agent which facilitates synaptic acetylcholine) promotes a transition from NREM to REM sleep in humans. (See also Sitaram, Mendelson, Dawson, Wyatt, and Gillin, 1976.) There is a recent study by Amatruda, Black, McKenna, McCarley, and Hobson (1975) which strongly implicates cholinergically mediated brain stem processes. Also, there is evidence that eserine and neostigmine (cholinergic facilitators) suppress the REM blocking effects of imipramine. ACh release at the cortex is even greater during REM than during wakefulness. This finding, combined with evidence that ACh may elicit EEG desynchronization in the absence of behavioral arousal, provides further evidence that REM sleep is a cholinergic process.

Certain aspects of Jouvet's theory have been called into question by recent findings. Treatments which alter serotonin processes should have a corresponding effect on NREM sleep while treatments which alter noradrenergic processes should have a corresponding effect on REM sleep. For example, there is relatively consistent evidence that the serotonin precursor, tryptophan, does shorten the latency and increase the duration of NREM sleep. However, there is also evidence that the sedative properties of tryptophan may not necessarily be due to the enhancement of serotonin (Wyatt and Gillin, 1976). The Jouvet model generates the prediction that 5-HTP (the immediate precursor of serotonin) should facilitate NREM sleep. The evidence to date does not unequivocally support the prediction. Rather, the evidence suggests that there is a positive relationship between serotonin levels and *REM* sleep (except for very high levels or serotonin which inhibit REM). In humans, PCPA and methysergide, two agents that block the normal metabolic action of enzymes that act on serotonin precursors, depress REM while having little effect on human total sleep time (Mendelson, Reichman, and Othmer, 1975; Naquet, 1975; Wyatt, 1972). Discontinuation of PCPA is not associated with REM rebound. These results seem more consistent with Jouvet's hypothesis that serotonin has a priming function for REM than the hypothesis that serotonin mechanisms actively control NREM sleep.

Other problems with the Jouvet model exist. A recent report (Adrien, Bourgoin, and Hamon, 1975) described a failure of subtotal lesions of the anterior raphe of rat pups to reduce NREM sleep percentages despite a reduction of brain serotonin by 75-90%. In addition, it is known that cat insomnia, induced by administering PCPA, eventually diminishes in spite of continued low levels of brain serotonin (Dement, Cohen, Ferguson, and Zarcone, 1970). Could this be due to the action of nonserotonergic NREM-inducing centers (e.g., POA) that are normally under serotonergic influence, but which can "take over" under such artificial conditions? This would suggest that the drive or deep structure of sleep onset can be articulated by alternative means. Flexibility through redundancy of function is a well known property of the brain. Good evidence for this comes from clinical observation of compensation of function after brain damage, as well as from empirical research on compensation after single- vs. multiple-stage lesions. For example, if animals are permitted visual-motor practice between subtotal lesioning of performance-related brain areas, the loss of ability to perform is much less (or prevented) when compared to the situation where lesions are total or where no performance between multiple-stage lesioning is permitted (Walker and Walker, 1975). Thus, flexibility in the nervous system could account for compensation after a period of lesion or drug-induced diminution of sleep.

However, it should be noted that another explanation of the temporary effect of PCPA is that there is a gradual habituation to the PCPA phenomena (e.g., hallucination) which are presumably highly arousing (McGinty, Harper, and Fairbanks, 1974). PCPA could be thought of as inducing something comparable to, though more effective than, continued bombardment of a person with highly arousing, fear-inducing internal information which prevents sleep onset until either sleep motivation or habituation or both occur. The McGinty *et al.* hypothesis, that eventual diminution of PCPA insomnia represents a gradual habituation makes sense in the light of much evidence that, initially, PCPA hypersensitizes organisms. It seems to lower gustatory, auditory, olfactory and self-stimulation thresholds, increases sexual drives and both hostile and predatory aggression. It is unlikely that a nervous system characterized by adaptability through flexibility could sustain for long such a state of reduced inhibitory capacity without making some internal adjustments.

There are other kinds of observations which also are difficult to square with the Jouvet model. Alphamethylparatyrosine (AMPT) interferes with the synthesis of noradrenalin but does not interfere with REM sleep in cats (Wyatt, 1972). Stimulation of the locus coeruleus does not reliably elicit increases in REM sleep. L-Dopa, which is the precursor of noradrenalin, does not increase (rather, it may decrease) REM sleep (Wyatt, 1972) or decrease duration of REM periods (Nakazawa, Tachibana, Kotorii, and Ogata, 1973). The transitory decrease in REM sleep induced by L-Dopa is followed by REM rebound. However, L-Dopa (1000 mg) given prior to recovery sleep after one night of REM deprivation eliminated the REM rebound observed under placebo. Subtotal lesions of the locus coeruleus of newborn kittens do not necessarily disrupt normal REM-NREM patterns (Adrien, 1975).

In short, the evidence reviewed here does not provide unambiguous support for the hypothesis that NREM sleep is largely under active serotonergic control while REM sleep is largely under active noradrenergic control. However in all fairness, it should be added that the results of stimulation studies are inherently ambiguous because they introduce grossly artificial and often nonspecific conditions. In addition, pharmacological effects are often nonspecifiable (e.g., PCPA influences more than just the serotonin system), are dependent on dosage and tolerance, and are influenced by complex, reciprocal relationships among biochemical systems in the central nervous system. As Wyatt and Gillin say, "Our knowledge about the biochemistry of human sleep is based on data which are inconsistent, tertiary, and open to multiple interpretations" (p. 261). Further, they add: "It is conceivable but unlikely that the serotonergic, adrenergic, and cholinergic systems are sufficient to produce all the facets of sleep. If this is true, we shall consider ourselves lucky because they make up less than one percent of the synaptic connections of the brain and to stumble on them so early in our exploration of the brain would seem like a rare and unlikely coincidence" (1976, p. 267).

Evidence most damaging to Jouvet's hypothesis of *active* serotonin control of NREM sleep comes from the research of McGinty and his colleagues (McGinty *et al.*, 1974). They report a *decrease* in raphe unit activity after transition from wake to NREM sleep. Depression is even greater in REM than NREM. The investigations suggest that this decrease implies a *reduction* of serotonin release during NREM. Note, too, that the finding of a depression of NA (noradrenalin) activity in the subcoeruleus during REM controverts the hypothesis that NA actively facilitates REM sleep. Rather, these findings, along with lesion work, suggest that loss of REM "could be the result of a removal of a system which facilitates REM by cessation of activity rather than augmentation of activity" (McGinty *et al.*, 1974, p. 207). Changes in raphe unit activity are consistent with the idea that serotonergic systems confine certain events (e.g., pontine-geniculate-occipital spiking, hallucination) to REM sleep while suppressing these in other states.

An alternative hypothesis for REM control

Hobson, McCarley, and Wyzinski (1975) have also noted some of the difficulties with Jouvet's classical model of sleep. On the basis of recent findings, they have suggested that a better candidate for the neurological basis of REM is the collection of giant cells of the tegmental field (FTG cells, see Figure 1-8) of the pontine reticular formation. This area is located near the locus coeruleus. FTG cells selectively fire during REM sleep, and increase their firing rate exponentially just at the onset of REM (and prior to the cortical firing that indicates REM). In addition, FTG (and neighboring) cells demonstrate rather tight phase locking with phasic events of REM, with PGO bursting occurring just prior to the onset of eye movement bursts. Additionally, the activity of the FTG cells is negatively correlated with locus coeruleus and dorsal raphe cell bursting during NREM and REM stage changes. The finding that some locus coeruleus neurones actually shut off during FTG activation in REM strongly suggests that the former "play a permissive, not an executive role" in REM sleep (J.A. Hobson, personal communication, 1976). Finally, Amatruda *et al.* (1975) found that carbachol (cholinergic facilitator) injections into the FTG enhances REM sleep while carbachol injections in the locus coeruleus is associated with relatively less REM sleep. FTG effects were found to be dose dependent, and graded with respect to the centrality of the FTG location. These investigators consider FTG and locus coeruleus sites to be reciprocally interactive, the former cholinergic, the latter noradrenergic. These findings are entirely

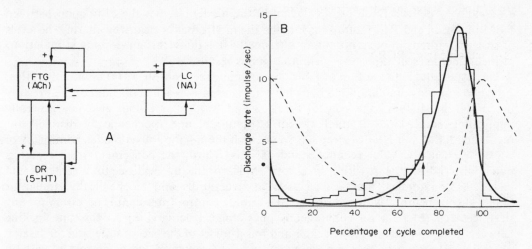

Figure 1-9   The Hobson-McCarley model of pontine control of REM sleep. (A) FTG: Giant cells of the pontine reticular formation (see Figure 1-8). DR: dorsal raphe cells. LC: locus coeruleus (adapted from Hobson, 1975). (B) The solid line histogram gives the average time course of discharge activity of an FTG unit over 12 sleep-waking cycles, each normalized to a constant duration. A cycle begins and ends with the end of desynchronized sleep. The solid curve describes the FTG time course and the dotted line the inhibitory population as predicted from the model. There is a good correspondence between the theoretical and actual FTG time course curve data; further, as the model predicts, the average time of the desynchronized sleep onset (arrow) occurs at about the same point as the equilibrium values for the two populations (dot on ordinate) is crossed (from McCarley and Hobson, 1975).

consistent with predictions based on single cell research (Hobson, 1974, p. 245) and illustrate the usefulness of such research in understanding neurobiological phenomena, e.g., effects of lesions, neurohumoral manipulations, stimulation.

The reciprocal inhibition hypothesis modeled in Figure 1-9 shows a spontaneously active cholinergic REM generator (FTG). This group of cells has excitatory effects of self and on a reciprocally inhibitory population of REM suppressing noradrenergic (locus coeruleus) and serotonergic (dorsal raphe) cell groups. Since these latter centers are also self inhibiting, they eventually reduce their own activity such that FTG cells are released from inhibition. Activity of FTG then gradually increases the activity of the other two centers. The result is a temporally displaced set of sinusoidal rhythms resulting in a sequence of NREM and REM sleep.

There are many reasons for considering this empirically founded model to be a conceptual advance over the pioneering work of Jouvet. First, it can be expressed in mathematical form. McCarley and Hobson (1975) have suggested that various assumptions about the excitatory, inhibitory (pictured in Figure 1-9), and potency characteristics of the nonlinear interaction can be handled by Volterra-Lotka equations[5] to yield curves which closely fit observed patterns of cellular rates. Second, the model yields testable predictions about the effects of nonphysiological treatments such as lesioning or stimulation. Third, the model provides support for the felicitous idea of a sleep center. Fourth, the model provides strong support for the view, largely developed on the basis of electrophysiological data, that REM sleep is a qualitatively different state with qualitatively different phenomenological (dream) concomitants (Johnson, 1973a, 1973b) and psychological functions,

---

[5] These equations were originally developed to define mathematically the reciprocal interaction effects of preditor-prey population sizes.

e.g., memory deficits (Hobson, 1977). Fifth, the model clarifies the distinction between REM initiation and REM duration. Finally, the model makes clear why altering the levels of either noradrenalin or serotonin, or altering the functions (through lesions, stimulation) of locus coeruleus or raphe can yield ambiguous results.

The argument for the notion of REM sleep center (see Hobson, 1974) essentially is this. First, "lesion and stimulation methods have in many cases reached the limit of their resolving power in studying the control of sleep and waking". Second, evidence generally implicating some kind of dual system (structurally and biochemically distinct) for regulating REM and NREM sleep has some merit though the Jouvet model, admittedly of enormous heuristic value, cannot stand as it is. Third, the concept of sleep center is potentially viable, at least with respect to REM sleep. Ideally, evidence for a center would include (a) anatomical data, e.g., cluster of structurally and biochemically similar or homogeneous neurons with widespread and remote control (presumably necessary for any sleep center), (b) data on spontaneous physiological activity, e.g., tight time locking between firing of neurons of the center and onset-offset of the (sleep) state, and (c) data on physiological responsiveness, e.g., stimulation of the center should be correlated with an increase in the state, lesions with a decrease. Fourth, the FTG cells, as a group, appear to satisfy these kinds of criteria and thus may be at least tentatively assumed to be a REM center, that is, responsible for initiation and control. Hoshino and Pompeiano (1976) have recently found an increase in FTG discharge rates concomitant with postural atonia induced by cholinergic facilitation. Cataleptic flaccidity, cholinergic activation, and high rates of FTG cell activity are consistent with the model proposed by Hobson for REM control.

Despite competing hypotheses regarding specific cell groups, there is little argument that REM sleep is initiated in the pons. This seems especially clear with respect to both PGO activity and EMG reduction. That the pons should play so important a role in the initiation of what otherwise appears to be a "higher" (cortical) function makes sense in the light of what is now becoming known about its role as a major relay station for the eventual integration of sensory information that guides motor movement. This function has recently been clarified by Glickstein and Gibson (1976). These investigators describe how visual information, which reaches the visual cortex via the lateral geniculate bodies, is relayed to the pons. The pons, in turn, relays the information to the cerebellar cortex which then relays it through the thalamus to the motor cortex which in turn has the final control over motor output. The information from other sensory sources (e.g., auditory, tactile) follow a similar course from sensory cortex to pons, etc. Thus, the pons is a major route between sensory and motor analysis. Therefore, it should not be surprising that during REM it might have both inhibitory (e.g., muscle tonus) and enhancing (e.g., sensory aspects) functions with respect to these kinds of information. (The role of the other pontine cell groups, i.e., vestibular nuclei which influence eye movement, is discussed in Chapter 2, Section 1.)

These investigations support the view that the "higher" centers responsible for information processing have a substantial influence on primitive, sleep-related centers of the brain stem. Thus, there is scientific evidence of a mechanism by which experimental manipulations of psychological variables (e.g., asking subjects to engage in fantasy or arithmetic thinking) could affect the timing or duration of REM sleep. For example, any psychological manipulation that induced significant diminution in REM onset latency might be hypothesized to involve a cholinergic process that has an effect on pontine centers such as FTG. I will raise this possibility in the context of a discussion of sex differences in REM sleep latency that we have just discovered.

The importance of the pons in controlling both the REM phenomena of sleep and sensorimotor information flow during wakefulness is generally consistent with an interesting idea about the role of REM dreaming proposed by Lerner (1967). She suggested that dreaming contributes to personality functioning by reactivating body image schemata through kinesthetic fantasy, thereby maintaining or restoring personality integrity. Expanding on this idea, we can think of the REM process as providing compensatory emphasis during sleep of that sensorimotor aspect of intelligence which is so prominent during infancy and childhood. At the risk of abusing the privilege of speculation, I would like to suggest that these neurophysiological data on pontine control of REM sleep are also consistent with some of Freud's views on "topographic regression". This quasineurological concept refers to the tendency during dreaming sleep for information flow to reverse its normal sensory-to-motor direction under conditions of motor paralysis. During dreaming, ideas (latent content) cannot be realized in motor behavior. Could it be that the role of the pons is to redirect information flow *back through* the lateral geniculate structures to the occipital cortex rather than out through the cerebellum, through thalamus to motor cortex? Could this be partially represented by PGO spiking? Can the pons be thought of as the controlling agent for the "topographic regression"? These are clearly speculative, perhaps fanciful, ideas, but they do fit rather nicely the view that dreaming is a regressive as well as a creative process.

Relatively little is known about the role of neural circuits and their respective neurotransmitters in the regulation of, and influence over, dreaming and dream content. A number of investigators have suggested that the hallucinatory quality of REM experience is largely determined by suppression of the inhibitory influence of serotonergic circuitry. However, this hypothesis is undoubtedly insufficient because it tends to make too many oversimplifying assumptions and because it rests on an incomplete view of complex and correlated neurophysiological events in other neural circuits. Some of the untenable assumptions referred to above are (a) the synonomy of REM sleep and dreaming, (b) a parallel between REM dreaming and LSD type hallucinatory experience, (c) assuming that nonvisual sensory experience during REM dreaming is sufficiently trivial to justify ignoring it.

Even more, the yield of pharmacological research to the problem of REM phenomena and phenomenology has been disappointing (though it should be pointed out that the magnitude of the research effort in the area of drugs of REM sleep has been smaller and suffers from the absence of broad, organizing theoretical perspective). Further, it is complicated by problems related to dosage level, nonspecific and uncontrollable (and unknown) effects, individual differences, and other problems related to experimental control. Four points should be noted. First, a distinction needs to be maintained between background spontaneous neural activity which is the consequence of a sleep stage, and neural activity which controls the onset and offset of stages. Second, research on neurohumoral aspects is complicated by feedback and homeostatic dynamics. Attempts to increase or decrease monoamines, for example, induce adjustments that counteract and therefore minimize such treatments. Third, inferences about the neurohumoral role in controlling sleep are complicated by the fact that monoamines play a role in all sorts of basic survival functions including arousal, feeding, sexual, and agonistic behavior. How does one separate the effects of altering monoaminergic activity on these vs. sleep *per se*? Fourth, the "meaning" of rates and rate changes in neural unit activity associated with REM and NREM sleep requires behavioral correlates. For example, while most cortical and many limbic areas are associated with higher activity during wake and REM than during NREM, some limbic areas show the opposite pattern. That increased activity is probably inhibitory (and therefore consistent with a view that NREM is a biologically quiescent state compared to wakefulness and REM sleep) is suggested by evidence that activity in these sites is associated with inhibition of "catering" behaviors (e.g., feeding) while lesions in such areas are associated with exaggerations of such behaviors.

It is not immediately evident what kinds of conclusions about REM phenomenology one can draw from results showing that bioamine facilitators (e.g., imipramine) and bioamine inhibitors (e.g., chlorpromazine) tend to diminish REM time (though relative differences in these effects may be of some importance). The problem is further complicated when one realizes that the effects of different drugs within a similar class (e.g., antidepressive) may have a similar effect on REM sleep (e.g., diminution) yet operate in quite different a manner (e.g., one on noradrenergic sites, another on serotonergic sites). For example, imipramine tends to increase hostility in REM dreams (Kramer, Whitman, Baldridge, and Ornstein, 1966). In order to determine the relevance of such a finding to hypotheses about the psychobiology of REM phenomena we need additional information. It would be useful to know how other antidepressives, that act in different ways, differentially affect REM dreams. Nevertheless, a biological explanation of drug induced disinhibition of "the blocked self-directed aggression, so commonly observed in the depressed" (Kramer *et al.*, 1966) would surely not indicate why the aggression was expressed in a particular way in each subject. Clearly, the symbolic meaning of the dream is not (yet?) amenable to neurophysiological explanation.

Neurophysiologically based hypotheses about NREM and REM function

Needless to say, we are far from a comprehensive and satisfactory theory of neurophysiological regulation of sleep. However, investigators have speculated on the basis of comparative and physiological data about the possible role of REM sleep. These speculations have much in common with psychological theorizing about dreaming and thus are of special importance to us.

Physiologically based theories of the function of sleep (i.e., what sleep does) have often distinguished between brain and bodily restoration. REM sleep presumably has something to do with the former while NREM sleep presumably has something to do with the latter. Consider the following observations. Delta sleep tends to increase after starvation, or circumcision, under conditions of hyperthyroidism, and during enforced gradual reduction of sleep time to about 5 hours (Oswald, 1973; Webb and Agnew, 1974). In normal subjects, a positive correlation between presleep thyroxine levels and delta sleep time, and a negative correlation between presleep thyroxine level and REM time has been reported (Johns, Masterson, Paddle-Ledinek, Winikoff, and Malinek, 1975). This finding clearly implicates delta sleep in the metabolic economy of the organism. Delta sleep seems less entrained to the circadian rhythm than is REM. That is, delta sleep appears to be more dependent on number of hours of prior wakefulness than time of day (Hume and Mills, 1975), and delta sleep can more readily be induced to shift to later parts of the night than can REM sleep be induced to shift to earlier parts of the night (Agnew and Webb, 1968). In addition, growth hormone secretion is most active during delta sleep even when sleep is inverted 180 degrees. Finally, after complete sleep deprivation, NREM sleep predominates over REM prior to REM rebound. On the basis of these kinds of data, Oswald (1973, 1974) and others (e.g., Hartmann, 1973) have concluded that NREM sleep, especially the delta component, is functionally related to basic bodily (vegetative) restoration/conservation.

There are other sources of evidence that NREM sleep, especially delta sleep, has a special relationship to vegetative maintenance, or more specifically, to the metabolic processes that underlie homoiothermic regulation. First, amount of delta sleep seems more clearly to be a function of amount of prior wake time rather than what goes on during wakefulness. (Evidence that delta sleep is enhanced by exercise is mixed [Bouhuys and Van den Hoofdakker, 1975; Horne and Porter, 1976; Shapiro, Griesel, Bartel, and Jooste, 1975; Webb and Friedman, 1971]. Also note that *total* sleep time, unlike delta time, is *inversely* related to prior wake time.) There seems to be a built-in (instinctive?) regulator that promotes metabolic levels around those observed during relaxed wakefulness (Kleitman, 1963). This would represent a relatively fail-safe system that insures that an otherwise intrinsically active and reactive, metabolically demanding, organism is forced to shut down. Second, there is evidence from Feinberg, Koresko, Heller, and Steinberg (1973) of the declining quality of NREM parameters (e.g., lower EEG amplitude) with age. This can be contrasted with more clearly defined relationships between REM and adequacy of brain function. Third, there is the provocative finding of less delta sleep in aged males compared to aged females; and males on the average live about eight years fewer than do females. Could it be that a subtle decline in the metabolic machinery underlying the thermoregu-latory process, a decline most clearly reflected in parameters of delta sleep, is fundamentally related to physical survival in homoiotherms?[6] Fourth, the preoptic area of the basal forebrain is a center for both NREM sleep onset and thermoregulation [something which fits nicely with recent thermoregulation data reported by Parmeggiani, Franzini, and Lenzi (1975) and with the Allison *et al.* theory of NREM evolution which is discussed in the next chapter]. Fifth, consider Hartmann's (1973) data on the sleep of habitually long (8 hours plus) vs. short (less than 6 hours) sleepers. The only stage of sleep which is not shorter for the short sleepers is delta sleep — all other stages (1, 2, REM) are shorter. A recent study of extremely short (less than 4 hours) sleepers (Stuss, Healey, and Broughton, 1975) indicated that almost 50% of sleep was devoted to delta! Delta percentage was even higher when sleep was curtailed (over 80%). Sixth, there is evidence that reduction of total sleep time from 7-8 hours to 5.5 hours initially enhances delta sleep time (and decreases REM time) and elicits shorter delta onset latency (Webb and Agnew, 1974). In fact, it does not seem to matter whether sleep restriction is imposed by having subjects go to sleep progressively later (while holding awakening time constant) or by having subjects awaken progressively earlier (holding time to sleep constant). Delta time does not diminish though REM time does (Weitzman, Pollack and McGregor, 1975). This is exactly what one would expect on the

---

[6] It is equally likely that a decline in the "quality" of NREM sleep (loss of delta waves) is a loss only of the surface structure of NREM sleep, not the deep structure. If this is so, then the loss of delta sleep may have little implication about thermoregulatory efficiency in old age. Still, the loss of delta sleep may indicate something about the metabolic efficiency or energy conservation ability of older people. Only direct measurements of these activities in groups that differ in amount of delta sleep *diminution*, in conjunction with information on longevity, would provide the evidence needed to assess the meaning of delta sleep decline in the aged.

basis of a hypothesis that delta sleep has a special, instinctively regulated relationship to prior wakefulness and the metabolic thermoregulatory demands that wakefulness makes on homoiothermic organisms.

On the other hand, the primary function of REM sleep, again following Oswald (1973, 1974), seems more clearly related to brain "restoration" and growth. Presumably, this is facilitated through the process of protein synthesis during REM sleep. Emphasis on brain functioning during REM sleep is based on the following kinds of data. Feinberg and Evarts (1969) present evidence that the pattern of firing of cortical neurons is different from that of both NREM sleep and wakefulness. REM sleep patterns are characterized by "brief burst of intense, almost convulsive, neuronal discharge" which "appears less highly organized" compared to that of wakefulness (p. 334). They also point out that this patterning of discharge is "consistent with a role in either engram consolidation or decay" (p. 341). Thus, the as yet unexploited technique of correlating neuronal firing patterns with psychological data (e.g., learning and memory, dreaming patterns) might be quite useful to test hypotheses about the active, information processing role of REM sleep (Dewan, 1969; Shapiro, 1967).

Also, there are differences in the pattern of REM rebound after different kinds of REM deprivation carried out for a week. When REM deprivation is affected by repeated awakenings (during which REM percentages are uniformly low), post deprivation REM rebound curves are characterized by relatively steep and short-lasting shapes that represent about 50% compensation. That is, about 50% of the lost REM (estimated from baseline) is made up. On the other hand, when REM deprivation is affected through drugs (e.g., antidepressives such as imipramine), there is a gradual increase in REM time (though still far below normal levels) during treatment. Upon withdrawal of the drug, there is a REM rebound characterized by a more gradual increase of REM sleep across nights. It lasts for a longer time and dissipates more slowly so that from 100 to 150% of lost REM is made up. Oswald suggests that the latter curve is consistent with what is known about the time constant of protein turnover in the brain. These speculations about the role of protein synthesis are consistent with what is known about the high blood flow, temperature, and metabolic rate in the brain during REM, as well as with experimental observations of low REM time in the retarded, the aged, and the organic-aged (Feinberg et al., 1973). There is now some preliminary evidence that total protein content of cat midbrain perfusates obtained during REM sleep is even higher than that obtained during wakefulness (Drucker-Colin, Spanis, Cotman, and McGaugh, 1975).

In the light of research on protein synthesis in memory (Hyden, 1970) and the hypothesis that REM dreaming integrates recent and more remote information into new (possibly creative) patterns (Breger, 1967; Dewan, 1969), Oswald's speculations are of particular relevance to hypotheses about the biological basis of dreaming. For example, Rossi (1973) suggests that "dreaming is a process of psychophysiological growth whereby dramas played out on a phenomenological level involve the corresponding synthesis and/or modification of proteins in the brain; this synthesis serves as the organic basis for new developments in the personality" (p. 1094).

In addition, Stern and Morgane (1974) make the following important distinction between REM process or mechanism and REM function. If administration of a REM suppressing drug is followed by little or no REM rebound, this implies that the drug has superseded the REM function to satisfy the need that REM normally fulfills. On the other hand, if a REM suppressant effect is followed by a significant rebound, this suggests that the REM mechanism, not the need, has been affected. Once the REM mechanism is freed from the inhibitory effect of the drug, it rebounds in the context of a continuing (and building) need. This distinction holds for *acute* (short-term) treatments only: after chronic treatment, adaptation by the CNS to new levels of aminergic functioning would leave the drug-free organism in a state of relative deprivation, and would be followed by significant REM rebound. It is pointed out that the only *acute* treatments that induce REM suppression followed by little or no REM rebound are administration of tricyclic antidepressants, MAO inhibitors, and ECT, all of which have been implicated in significant catecholaminergic facil-itation. They go on to suggest that there is a relationship between REM function, catecholaminergic restoration, and protein synthesis. There is evidence, for example, of increased rates of protein synthesis during elevated levels of REM sleep. It is possible that one relationship between protein synthesis and catecholaminergic activity is via metabolic rate-limiting enzymes derived from protein synthesis and which are implicated in the synthesis of bioamines. For example, there is evidence that learning deficits caused by the protein synthesis blocker puromycin can be reversed by catecholaminergic facilitators (e.g., imipramine, amphetamine).

Starting from the general premise that REM sleep has something to do with brain restoration, Hartmann (1973) proposes that REM sleep helps to restore worn out or depleted catecholamine systems. There is some ambiguity with regard to the deficit — whether it is simply low levels of catecholamines, insensitivity of neurons to catecholamine activity, etc. — and this ambiguity affects the precision of its predictions and *post hoc* explanations. Nevertheless, the theory can account for a number of observations.

For example, antidepressives markedly increase catecholamine activity and markedly decrease REM sleep, i.e., the need for REM sleep is reduced. In addition there is evidence that short term treatment with catecholamine facilitators is not associated with REM rebound. This is consistent with the idea that the drug-induced process reduces the need for REM rather than that it disrupts the mechanism of REM. Alphamethylparatryptamine (AMPT) and 6-hydroxydopamine (6-OHDA), which interfere with catecholamine synthesis, increase REM sleep. Manics (who are believed to be too high in catecholamine function) tend to have less REM, while psychotic depressives tend to have more REM (though the results for the latter are mixed). REM deprivation reduces amphetamine lethality in rats. This would be consistent with the idea that low levels of catecholamine due to REM deprivation make the animal more tolerant of drugs that elevate catecholamine levels. In addition, there is evidence that learning deficits produced by REM deprivation can be reduced by amphetamine, pargyline, and L-Dopa (catecholamine facilitators), but not by cholinergic regulators such as scopolamine and eserine (Stern and Morgane, 1974).

At the psychological level, Hartmann provides evidence that emotional dysphoria in nonpsychotics is associated with longer REM time. This finding is interpreted as supporting the idea that dysphoria is largely catecholaminergically mediated, "wears out" the catechol-aminergic system, and increases the need for REM sleep to restore the system.

Hartmann's theory is impressive in its breadth, explanatory power, and capacity to generate hypotheses. However, there are some observations that do not seem readily explained on the basis of the hypothesis. For example, Oswald (1974) has pointed out that some antidepressives (imipramine) selectively accelerate catecholaminergic activity while others (amitriptyline) selectively accelerate serotonergic activity, yet both types have a similar depressing effect on REM sleep. It should be noted that tricyclic antidepressants, those with (amitriptyline) and without (imipramine, desipramine) sedative effects have significant anticholinergic properties beyond their primary effects on catechol or indole amine systems. Evidence of excessive cholinergic activity in depression (Davis, 1975), along with evidence of cholinergic factors in REM onset (review above), is consistent with what is known about the effect of tricyclics on both REM sleep and endogenous depression. In addition, Vogel's work clearly indicates that REM deprivation by forced awakenings is therapeutic for psychotic depressives (Vogel, McAbee, Barker, and Thurmond, 1977). Surely a disease that is supposed to involve catecholamine depression should not respond favorably to a procedure that prevents a process whose assigned function is to restore catecholamine function.

In my view, the hypothesis is least impressive with respect to its application to psychological phenomena such as dysphoria and tiredness. Hartmann cites evidence of a correlation between dysphoria and sleep (especially REM) time. Does this correlation indicate a greater *need* for REM? The following observations suggest that it may not be so. First, the longer one sleeps, the higher will be one's REM percentage. This follows from the fact that REM sleep tends to occur in the latter half of the night. Regardless of need, longer sleep time will be associated with more REM time and higher REM percentages. At a minimum, it is not clear that the long sleepers *who were elevated in presleep dysphoria or trait anxiety* were the ones with relatively high REM percentages.

Recall that duration of sleep is multiply determined. For some individuals, it reflects natural variation in the nocturnal phase of the circadian cycle, while in others, it may reflect dysphoria. In other words, the overall difference between long and short sleepers in REM time may be as much, or more, related to natural variations in circadian and ultradian cycles of the sleep instinct than to the need for REM. There is evidence that predominantly aggressive individuals do not differ from predominantly anxious individuals in catecholamine output. Shouldn't we predict that they have as great a need for REM sleep? Yet the aggressive, highly active individual tends to be a short sleeper and tends to get less REM sleep. And there is evidence that neurotic children have *less* REM sleep (measured either in time or percentage) than controls (Leygonie, Houzel, Guilhaume, and Benoit, 1975). This finding directly contradicts the hypothesis unless we assume that dysphoria in children is not primarily catecholaminergic while dysphoria in adults is primarily catecholaminergic.

What is required is an *experimental* rather than a correlational approach. If variation in REM time reflects variation in a need for REM, then REM deprivation might be used to assess individual differences in REM need, e.g., to assess REM rebound. For example, it would be expected that dysphoric individuals, or individuals with high levels of trait anxiety, should show greater REM rebound than relaxed, low trait anxiety individuals. However, if anything, just the opposite seems to be true. Sensitizers show *less* REM rebound than do repressors. These data will be discussed in full detail in subsequent chapters. Suffice it here to say that there is no experimental evidence that state anxiety (e.g., experimental manipulation of ego threat) or trait anxiety (preselection of subjects) is associated with greater REM rebound (i.e., REM need).

Hartmann (1973) has some interesting things to say about different kinds of sleep motive. A corollary of his theory is that a need for REM is experienced as a mental fatigue (tiredness 2) while a need for NREM sleep is experienced as a physical fatigue (tiredness 1). The former is associated with dysphoria, strain, tension, "regressive" behavior; the latter is a more pleasant condition without neurotic-like features. On the basis of individual differences in REM need that I will discuss later, I would like to suggest that there may be three types of sleep motive. One would be the tiredness 1 proposed by Hartmann, a requirement for inactivity after extraordinary levels of concentrated physical activity, and requiring relatively little total sleep time. (It might be an instinctive, brain stem-mediated, mechanism to reduce the probability of overheating.) There would be no special requirement for increased amounts of REM. The second type would be associated with manifest dysphoria, high neuroticism, etc. It would be associated with longer, less refreshing total sleep time (perhaps because the ensuing sleep would be fragmentary, light, inefficient). No special need for *relatively* increased amounts of REM sleep would be associated with this condition. A third type would be associated with excessive defensiveness (denial, repression) especially under conditions of ego threat. This type would not be associated with longer sleep time but perhaps higher REM percentages. However, let me emphasize that under normal sleep conditions, REM time might not be increased. The key to demonstrating greater need specifically for REM might require REM deprivation and subsequent REM rebound measures. I say this because under normal conditions, a small amount of REM sleep might be sufficient to accommodate different levels of induced need.

The credibility of the distinction between physical and mental types of fatigue would be strengthened were it possible to demonstrate that they are mediated selectively by activity in different areas of the central nervous system. It would seem reasonable that physical fatigue might be handled mainly by brain stem mechanisms (raphe system?) while mental fatigue might bring basal forebrain inhibitory (POA?) and cerebral processes into play. This supposition has intuitive appeal because it suggests a relationship between neurological and psychological phenomena from a phylogenetic perspective. It is consistent with the view that phylogenetic advances do not eliminate earlier accommodations, but rather produce novel, supplementary mechanisms. Thus, the mechanism by which organisms are forced into periodic inactivity (sleep in more advanced vertebrates) because of circadian and consummatory events may be mediated by hindbrain mechanisms. Fatigue induced by excessive motion and emotion may be mediated largely by hypothalamic and basal forebrain centers that are functionally a part of the telediencephalic systems which control individual- and species-survival behaviors. Finally, fatigue, induced by stress, conflict, ego threat, might be more readily influenced by basal forebrain and cerebral inhibitory mechanisms.

Implications for hypotheses about the dreaming process

It is unfortunate that so little research has aimed at clarifying the physiological and psychological "bridge". Perhaps this state of affairs is a joint function of mutual distrust between two kinds of investigators (e.g., simple-minded reductionists vs. muddle-headed phenomenologists?) and the relatively poor yield of psychophysiological correlate research on dream content (Rechtschaffen, 1973). Occasionally the best of both camps is expressed in the research and writings of a major investigator whose interests and competence spans both areas of research. Consider the following almost lyrical passage from Jouvet (1973, p. 31): "Perhaps paradoxical sleep represents some form of genotypic pattern of stimulation (possibly effectuated through the process of the PGO spikes) which remodels our brain during sleep. If this is true, nature is prevalent over nurture and [REM sleep] serves to reorganize our higher nervous center according to some genotypic blueprint." Note that much of this is based on observations of inordinate amounts of REM sleep in neonates obviously prior to the modulating effects of experience. Jouvet goes on: "According to this hypothesis our brains are submitted during dreaming to some coding during which archaic (or genotypic), primarily inherited programming serves to reorganize a kind of basic circuitry responsible for the inner core of so-called personality or character." To test this hypothesis, Jouvet suggests the use of cats either isolated from or subjected to normal environmental programming (including fight and flight), and later given lesions in the pontine motor inhibitor of REM sleep. Similarities in the "acting out" behavior of these two sets of cats during REM "dreaming" would be useful to evaluate the validity of the hypothesis. That endogenous, genetically programmed neural activity largely independent of (at least visual) experience characterizes the early ontogeny of REM sleep is supported by a study by Fishbein, Schaumburg, and Weitzman (1966). These investigators reported that dark- and light-reared kittens up to two months of age showed similar REM characteristics (percentages, eye movement patterning).

Regardless of the logic of this argument, it is important because it illustrates the biological roots of the dreaming experience that are so often overlooked by investigators who are committed to meaning divorced from matter. I find such a position unpalatable since it is just as reasonable to assume that dream symbolism expresses bodily conditions as social or psychological conditions. Clinicians are fond of premonition dreams. For example, a woman dreams of seeing herself disappear inside a large box situated in an otherwise desolate and colorless environment. A few days later she becomes psychotically depressed. Is this kind of dream an example of the potential sensitivity of the dreaming process to physiological events? Observations of epileptics (who often can feel a seizure coming on prior to overt signs), biofeedback research (which has demonstrated how extraordinarily sensitive to internal events we can become), and research on psychoses (which establishes beyond a doubt the role of biological factors) all indicate that dreaming, whatever else it symbolizes, must be "in touch" with biological processes. It is not unreasonable to suggest that under certain conditions, and for certain individuals, dreaming may provide a sensitive indication of such internal biological events.[7]

In the interest of pursuing such a lead, we are currently collecting home dream data on pregnant women. We hope to show a correlation between the sex of the fetus and differences in dream content. Differences, for example in the masculinity or femininity of the dream content (Cohen, 1973b) of women who eventually give birth to male or female offspring would go a long way to reinforce the relevance of the biological substrate to dreaming and dream content.

The late Hernandez-Peon offered (1967) a general outline of the neurological basis underlying the formation of dream experiences. According to the model, the sequence of events begins with the heightened activation of a brain stem "sleep system". This system reduces the influence of the mesodiencephalic "vigilance system". Release of paleocortical (e.g., entorhinal cortex) and neocortical ("mnesic") processes contributes to the activation of manifest content, while release of limbic ("emotional and motivational") processes contributes to latent content. Manifest content refers to recent and relevant remote memories rather than subjective experience. The latter is produced by "a highly specialized integrating system in the rostral part of the brain stem" (1967, p. 112). Thus, the model postulates separate but integrated systems (interpretable at the neuronal or the psychic

---

[7] Epstein and Collie (1976) suggest that certain patterns of dream content may be facilitated by specifiable and genetically transmitted disturbances of the CNS. Their clinical report draws attention to a familial pattern of repetitive negative content ("bad dreams") and abnormal spiking from bilateral temporal and occipital areas during wake, stage 1, and REM.

level) for recent and remote memory, affect and impulse, and consciousness, all released by the active dampening of the vigilance system by the sleep system.

An important feature of the model is its recognition of the importance of limbic and paleocortical activity which some might interpret as consistent with an emphasis in some psychological theories on ontogenetically old (id) processes, what Brown (1977) calls "a limbic level of semantic realization (distortion, displacement, condensation)" (p. 95). On the basis of research available at the time, and following the logic of his own model, Hernandez-Peon suggested that the Freudian theory of dream formation was consistent with the neurophysiological speculation that "daily disinhibition of the emotional and motivational limbic systems during sleep may prevent an interfering overflowing of their excessive neural discharges into extraneous brain pathways during waking behavior" (1967, p. 124).

The idea that the dream, like the hallucination, is a disinhibitory phenomenon has a long history. It is consistent with both Jacksonian and Freudian as well as modern variants of neurophysiological theory. A basic component of this view is that a diminution of the influence of those functions which mediate the processing of information originating in the real world is associated with the release of normally inhibited personal information, i.e., somatic, affective, and otherwise subjective. West (1962, pp. 280–281) has offered a compelling analogy of a person standing at a window watching a sunset while a fire burns in a fireplace opposite the window. As the brightness of the external scene diminishes, the presence of the fire, reflected by the window, becomes progressively more apparent. Finally, it becomes the most salient property of consciousness. The implication is that a diminution of the influence of those (ego) functions which normally mediate the processing of external information ("reality") is associated with two correlated phenomena: a hallucinatory intensification and a deterioration of information processing. It seems to me that this assumption cannot account for certain conventional REM dreams which have an organized and realistic quality. That is, those principles which operate in the formation of waking or sleep onset hallucinations do not provide sufficient explanation for many REM phenomena. The latter strongly suggest that a significant influence of secondary process may exist along with the hallucinatory experience associated with isolation from the influence of the external world.

The distribution of weightings suggested by Table 1-2 illustrates the point I wish to make about the unique property of REM sleep. The REM dream is not merely a psychedelic concatenation of hallucinatory nonsense released by defective processes operating in isolation from external reality. It is not merely another example of cognitive processes like those induced by drugs, fatigue, or transitional states (stage 1-NREM). Ironically, it is the more conventional, realistic, and pedestrian of REM dreams (see Snyder, 1970 and Chapter 6 of this book) that seem most remarkable. They challenge the facile view that prolonged isolation from the influence of external reality, especially in the context of volitional passivity, autonomic activation, and diminished capacity for reality testing is inevitably associated with a degradation of cognition. Even if we accept, for argument's sake, the view that REM dreams tend to be symbolically, cognitively, and instrumentally limited in comparison with waking thought, they remain marvels of constructional invention and reproduction for which theories of hallucination cannot account. Indeed one of the paradoxes of paradoxical (REM) sleep is how it is capable of producing such veridical experiences despite the suspension of reality testing, volition, and self-consciousness.

Considering the traditional interest shown by sleep researchers in psychophysiological correlates, it is surprising how little has been said about the relationship between dreaming

TABLE 1-2.   Hypothetical Influences Characteristic of Six Biological States

Characteristic	Relative influence during:					
	W	1	2	Delta	REM	Drug
External influences[a]	+++	+	0	0	0	+++(+)
Personal influences[b]	+	++	+	0	+++	+++
Secondary process[c]	+++	+(0)	+(0)	0	++	++(+)
Reality testing[d]	+++	+	0	0	0	++(+)
Hallucinatory elaboration of thought	0(+)	++(+)	+(0)	0	+++	+++

The + and 0 symbols refer to the usual degree of influence in one state relative to that in others. The symbols in parentheses suggest alternative weightings that reflect situational or individual differences. Delta sleep is thus described as a more or less apsychic and unconscious state. The pattern of weightings for REM is different from that of either transitional (stage 1-NREM) or drug induced patterns, the latter two of which may turn out to be more similar. It is the concurrence of a modest degree of secondary process (especially during later REM periods, see Ch. 7) in the absence of reality testing which is one of the paradoxes of REM sleep.
[a]Tendency to pay attention to and be influenced by the external environment (reality).
[b]Influence of somatic-affective and mnesic information that is unrelated, or personally rather than logically related, to current external demands.
[c]Rational or at least conventional thought, i.e., concrete and formal operations.
[d]Capacity to distinguish between external and personal sources of information, reality from fantasy (hallucination).

and the right cerebral hemisphere. In Chapter 7, I will discuss some data that suggest that there may be a change in the relative dominance of left vs. right hemisphere during the night. Here, I want to summarize briefly an integration of data offered by Paul Bakan suggesting that the right hemisphere has a dominant role in the organization of REM experience. Bakan's unpublished paper ("Dreaming, REM Sleep, and the Right Hemisphere: A Theoretical Integration") suggests that REM dreaming is a relatively primitive kind of experience mediated by the right hemisphere. Bakan ranges far and wide through psychological, neurological, and psychiatric literature. The following are some of his more basic points.

First, REM experience (e.g., perceptual, fantasy, "primary process") is similar to experience thought to be mediated by right hemisphere, experience that is in fact elicited when the right hemisphere is stimulated artificially or during epileptic discharges. (It should be noted, however, that such a description of REM experiences is statistical in nature, a generalization that does not hold for many REM experiences. For example, there is a world of difference between the dreamy auras of epilepsy, the hallucinations of acute schizophrenia, and many rather pedestrian, thoughtful, secondary process REM experiences.) Second, there is evidence of a relatively greater EEG activation of right compared to left hemisphere during REM than during NREM sleep. (However, it should be noted that this has been found in animals for whom the lateralization of function is still in doubt; but see Corballis and Beale, 1976.) Third, there is evidence of reduced interhemispheric communication during REM sleep of animals. In addition, there is evidence of reduced correlation in right vs. left EEG variability in humans. In the light of structural differences in corpus callosum and interhemispheric information transfer observed between schizophrenics and normals (Beaumont and Dimond, 1973), and in the light of traditional assumptions about the comparability of schizophrenic and dream experience, these kinds of findings support the contention that during REM sleep the right hemisphere enjoys a special status due to its relative independence from left dominance. Fourth, there is clinical evidence that damage to right (occipital and parietal) hemisphere is associated with a loss of both dream recall and imagery capacity. (This is strong evidence for right hemisphere mediation of dream experience though it may indicate the relatively greater importance of the right hemisphere in the translation of thought [deep structure] to imagery [surface structure], that is, the *experience* of the dream more than the processes underlying the dream. However, this line of reasoning needs to be squared with the evidence reported by Jus, Jus, Villeneuve, Pires, Lachance, Fortier, and Villeneuve [1973] that damage to the frontal lobes is associated with the absence of REM dream reports.)

One of the more interesting implications of Bakan's analysis is the degree of individual differences in brain functioning. Presumably, the dreamier and more "primitive" the REM experience, the more the right hemisphere may play a dominant role. Is it possible that individuals whose waking experiences are relatively more right hemisphere dominant (or, more poorly integrated by left hemisphere functioning), e.g., schizotypes, have REM experiences which will be characterized by similar qualities? This supposition would make sense from a dispositional view that requires continuity from wake to sleep in certain personality related characteristics.

In addition, it is possible that individual differences in the *need* for REM are in part a function of the degree of right hemisphere "suppression" during wakefulness. In the light of this speculation, it is interesting to note that schizophrenics generally have little REM rebound while male repressors show relatively high levels of REM rebound under conditions of REM deprivation. Galin (1974) has suggested that repression may involve a functional isolation of material from the left hemisphere; that there is a "parallel between the functioning of the isolated right hemisphere and mental processes that are repressed, unconscious and unable to directly control behavior" (p. 574). Thus, there may be a rough association among the following: the ability to isolate (repress) experiences during wakefulness, degree of hemispheric specialization, clearer "boundaries" between psychobiological states, psychological differentiation, and the need for REM sleep. If this hypothesis is essentially true, then the following characteristics should be associated with relatively greater REM rebound under conditions of REM deprivation: repression, field-independence, convergent thinking. The following should be associated with relatively little REM rebound: infancy, split-brain conditions (right hemisphere free of left dominance), schizophrenia, divergent cognitive style. There is some evidence, both published and unpublished but largely preliminary, that some of these predictions are empirically supportable. This situation or compensatory view is taken up and discussed in Chapter 5.

In Chapter 7, I will discuss evidence that Bakan's characterization of the REM experiences is more applicable for earlier than for later REM periods. It is possible that for normal individuals, the early phase of sleep is associated with right hemisphere "compensation" during which information processing of a qualitatively different kind takes place. The question of changes in lateral specialization during sleep is potentially one of the most exciting yet one of the least explored issues in sleep research.

I have focused on the evidence that there is, relative to wakefulness, a shift during REM sleep toward right hemispheric domination in cortical activity. Now there is evidence that the same may be true for NREM sleep as well. Myslobodsky, Ben-Mayor, Yedid-Levy and Minz (1976) have reported that spindle activity is more prominent over the right hemisphere, especially during the early part of the night. In addition, they reported a reversal in a slow component of the visually evoked potential which was, during sleep, most prominent over the left side. These observations are consistent with the hypothesis that sleep in general, though perhaps REM in particular, constitutes at least a partial reversal of hemispheric dominance relationships, and that this reversal is most pronounced during the early part of the night. I will return to this question in Chapter 7 where I will discuss the change in dream content across REM periods which is consistent with the concomitant change in underlying cortical changes.

CHAPTER 2

ORIGIN AND DEVELOPMENT OF REM SLEEP

1. ONTOGENETIC ASPECTS OF REM SLEEP

Infant sleep

In their classic paper on the ontogeny of REM sleep, Roffwarg, Muzio, and Dement (1966) state: "There can no longer be any doubt that a dream, far from being merely a diaphanous and elusive creature of mind, is the sensate expression of a fundamental and rhythmically repetitive, and enormously active neurophysiological state" (p. 3). According to Roffwarg *et al.* (1966), REM sleep constitutes up to 50%, or about eight hours, of total sleep time for the newborn. This figure declines steadily through infancy (30-40%) and childhood (up to 25%), thereafter stabilizing (about 22%) until late adulthood when it declines to less than 15%. Almost all of the decrease in the high REM% observed at birth occurs during the first two years, during the period of maximal brain growth and development. However, the REM% figures given for infancy depend on the criteria used to score REM sleep, and these vary across studies. Each experimenter is free to decide how many and which physiological/behavioral characteristics must be observed simultaneously to call a given sleep pattern "REM". Ontogenetic changes in REM sleep include increasing temporal congruence of the activity phases of many variables. If we require too many of these variables to be at peak activity at the same time then low REM percentages will obtain even for the neonate. Thus, some investigators have reported an increase in REM percentage with age, but obviously the increase reflects consolidation of REM characteristics (Anders, 1975). In short, the changes in REM percentage are determined in part by real physiological changes and in part by scoring conventions. However, most investigators use EEG, EOG, and EMG criteria. On the basis of more or less independent work, they have arrived at a fairly reliable range of 45-55% for the percentage of total sleep devoted to REM in the full term newborn. It is thus necessary to distinguish between REM sleep and the maturation of REM sleep.

On the basis of more recent observation, Petre-Quadens (1974) suggests that REM sleep or "active sleep" in infants be divided into two categories: Stage *a* is characterized by an EEG that is slower but equal in amplitude to that of wakefulness, *isolated* eye movements (primarily vertical), moderately irregular respiration, strong sucking, an active EMG, and a low arousal threshold characterized by crying. Stage *d* (or "paradoxical sleep") is characterized by very low EEG amplitude, no sucking, eye movement bursting with accompanying increases in respiration, a virtually flat EMG with movement in the extremities, irregular and superficial respiration,[1] and relatively high waking threshold. Stage *d* is also notably characterized by facial grimacing and smiling about which Roffwarg *et al.* have this to say: It "gives the appearance of sophisticated expression of emotion or thought such as perplexity, disdain, skepticism, and mild amusement", characteristics which are not observed in these infants while they are awake (p. 6). Perhaps motoric articulation of the neonatal physiognomy can be placed in the ontogenetic-developmental sequence suggested by data reviewed by Sroufe and Waters (1976). With respect to smiling, they suggest a general trend from (a) reaction to intense cutaneous stimulation to (b) reaction to visual change, to (c) reaction to the specific (especially social) content of stimulation, and finally, to (d) active production of information which then elicits the behavior. Gottlieb (1976) has suggested that motoric patterns observable in the fetus are produced by endogenous (nonreflexive) programs rather than being reactions to sensory stimulation. (The fetus is capable of sensory reception, but experiments using neural transections that eliminate such information do not eliminate the endogenous motor output patterns.) Perhaps the grimacing observed during the REM sleep of the neonate is part of the transition from endogenous control to external sensory (and later social informational) control of motor patterns. The interesting idea is that to a large extent it is the stimulus control rather than the motor output of affective behavior which is acquired during socialization. The work of Freedman (1974) on the smiling behavior of the congenitally blind infant is consistent with this idea. Unfortunately there are no data on affective expressiveness during the sleep of congenitally blind infants.

Observations of infant sleep suggest that REM characteristics include capacities that mature at varying rates (e.g., limbic and brain stem capacities early, cortical — including dreaming — capacities late). Although there is no experimental evidence, it is likely that dreaming is a psychological capacity that evolves well after a significant degree of maturation of REM physiology has taken place. In fact, Metcalf (in Petre-Quadens and Schlag, 1974, ch. 20) speculates that the capacity to experience dreams develops about 6 months after birth when K-complexes that evolve out of background EEG noise can be elicited by external stimulation. This would take place roughly about the time that "stranger anxiety" begins to develop. However, he admits that "this speculation may not be researchable".

Categories of sleep that are defined by Petre-Quadens appear to have a temporal organization which is statistically regular. For example, stage *a* usually follows wakefulness while stage *d* usually follows NREM or stage *a*. Wakefulness usually follows either type of REM sleep (*a* or *d*). Petre-Quadens interprets stage *a* as a relatively "primitive" form of sleep since it disappears after about one month,[2] and since it is virtually the entire sleep of the premature. While it is possible that cortical immaturity may account for the relative prominence of stage *a* relative to stage *d*, there is evidence that vestibular dysfunction (or

[1] Respiratory irregularity associated with REM sleep has inspired the hypothesis that an exaggeration of the phenomenon may underlie sudden infant death or "crib death" syndrome (SIDS). In addition, the association between respiratory pauses, especially those which are prolonged beyond 9 seconds (apneas), and snoring (including increased blood pressure) has stimulated interest in REM respiration (Lugaresi, Coccagna, Farneti, Mantovani, and Cirignotta, 1975). The fact of the matter is that sleep apneas tend to occur during the NREM rather than the REM sleep of infants who are at risk for SIDS (near miss and premature infants) (Guilleminault, Peraita, Souquet, and Dement, 1975).
[2] Metcalf (in Petre-Quadens and Schlag, 1974, p. 406) suggests that the onset of behavioral "fussiness" at about 4-5 weeks is an indication of the dissipation of a "stimulus barrier" inherent in the immature CNS of the newborn. It would be interesting to assess the correlation between the timing of the dissipation of stage *a* ("primitive" sleep) and the onset of fussiness, and finally, the waning of fussiness and increase in other characteristics of sleep. Some attempts at this sort of research goal are described in Chapter 20 of Petre-Quadens and Schlag (1974).

immaturity) may play a role in at least the eye movement parameters of REM sleep. On the basis of lesion work, Pompeiano and Morrison (1965) have suggested a regulatory role for vestibular nuclei with respect to eye movement activity. This hypothesis is supported by observations that autistic children (presumed to have a vestibular disfunction) have REM period eye movement bursts whose duration is markedly short (Ornitz, Ritvo, Brown, LaFranchi, Parmelee, and Walter, 1969). Ornitz, Forsythe, and de la Peña (1973) demonstrated that vestibular stimulation during REM sleep induced a decrease in eye movement per eye movement burst in autistic compared to normal children. This deficit was not observed during control REM periods. These observations are consistent with evidence of suppressed nystagmus observed in autistic children during wakefulness and support the hypothesis regarding maturational lag that can affect eye movement patterns in both wakefulness and sleep. These findings might also be construed as further evidence, albeit indirect, for the potential role of REM sleep in the integration of sensory motor information.

During the first year, there are changes in the frequency of discrete EEG signs, differentiation of sleep stages, amount of sleep devoted to each sleep period, and in the sleep-wake cycle. With respect to discrete signs, the following changes occur: (a) Stage *a* sleep disappears by the end of the fourth to fifth week at which time (b) adult-like spindles appear. The latter are initially of large amplitude and long duration, but these qualities are reduced during the first five months (with the exception of certain kinds of mental retardation which are characterized by the continued presence of "extreme spindles" [Gibbs and Weir, 1973]). At about five months (c) K-complexes are clearly indicated. (d) Phasic events increase, e.g., there is an increase in REMs per unit of REM sleep. Finally, during the first year, (e) there is a diminution in the frequency of 10.5-15 cps activity (not spindles in form but overlapping in spindle range) during REM sleep (again with the exception of certain pathological conditions such as infantile autism [Ornitz *et al.*, 1969]).

During the first year there is a gradual differentiation of sleep into the familiar REM and NREM stages. Various parameters of sleep (eye movement, EEG, EMG, body movement) show increasing temporal concordance such that the stages of sleep are more easily (and reliably) observed. Anders (1975) has suggested that this process be conceptualized in the framework of the comparative-developmental theory of Heinz Werner.

> Separate systems develop intrinsic patterns of serial and spatial regulation which become integrated with other systems into higher levels of organization as they become more complex and interdependent. Hierarchial organization leads to integration which in turn proceeds to more complex organization. Sleep physiology in the developing organism offers a unique opportunity for investigation of these sequences. First individual physiologic measures become regulated into patterns of alternating quiescence and activity. Next, as several separate physiological measures become phase related, sleep stages appear as a new level of organization. A fundamental reason for studying sleep in the developing organism, therefore, is to better understand the basic mechanisms and correlates of the maturational process *per se* (pp. 60-61).

In addition, there are concomitant changes in both the proportion of time devoted to the different stages and changes in the patterns of sleep/wake cycling. These include (a) a precipitous decline in the percentage of sleep devoted to REM; (b) relatively little change in percentage of delta sleep during childhood followed by a decline during adulthood, more marked during old age, especially in males; (c) a reduction of total sleep time (from about 16 or more hours in infancy to 8 or fewer hours in adults and the aged); (d) an increase during the first 8 months of life in the duration of the REM/NREM BRAC from 50-60 to

90-100 minutes; (e) a coalescence of diurnal and nocturnal sleep periods ("polysleep") into one single nocturnal sleep period; and (f) an increase (during the fourth to fifth month of life) in the probability of NREM (rather than REM) sleep onset. It should be noted that there are enormous individual differences in the onset, latency, duration, and reliability characteristics of these developmental changes.

Aging and sleep

A point needs to be made about so-called changes in sleep characteristics with age. The fact is that with few exceptions representing short term observation, all developmental sleep data are in the form of comparisons of different age cohorts (cross-sectional method). Thus, as in the other ontogenetic research areas such as those concerned with development and decline of IQ, the characteristic of change is inferred from group differences. It is not directly observed. Therefore great caution is required lest we make erroneous assumptions about stability or decline. For example, consider the evidence from Roffwarg *et al.* (1966) that there is a decline in REM time in the aged. Jovanović (1976) has argued that the data from oldest subjects are unreliable, and that REM sleep may be quite high. Examples are given of an 85- and a 96-year-old with REM percentages of 29 and 26 respectively. The problem with this argument is that these data may be atypical, coming as they do from individuals whose ages are well beyond life expectancy. The presence of significant amounts of both REM and delta sleep may be a clinical sign of extraordinary viability and therefore may not be readily generalizable to the normal population. For example one study obtained near normal REM percentages and only slightly reduced delta sleep percentages (but highly reduced stage 4 components) for 10 male and female subjects aged 64-87 years (Kales, Wilson, Kales, Jacobson, Paulson, Kollar, and Walter, 1967). However, these were highly selected subjects who were "in good general health, and were mentally alert and active for their age".

We are still left with the question of how sleep characteristics actually do change in different kinds of people. It is my guess that were it possible to acquire long range longitudinal data, the *average* person would show a decline of both REM and delta sleep, while those individuals who are genetically related to individuals with extraordinary longevity would not show these declines. Preliminary test of this hypothesis could be done with the usual cross-sectional methods by comparing the sleep stage percentages of individuals who have not reached life expectancy limits (e.g., 50-65) but whose first degree relatives differ significantly in longevity. The major point is that the older the cohort, the less likely the resulting sleep data can be used to make inferences about ontogenetic changes in the *normal* population

An additional point is that cross-sectional methods tend to confound four kinds of influences each of which may affect total sleep time and possibly sleep staging: (a) maturational *changes*, (b) generation *differences* that are primarily biological (e.g., differences in activity, nutrition, etc., (c) generation *differences* that are primarily social or cultural, and finally (d) historical changes to which each generation is exposed (e.g., *changes* in cultural or physical conditions, values, etc.).

Compared to research on REM sleep in infancy, work on aging populations has been sparse. Generally, the effects of aging on sleep appear to be in the reduction of REM and delta (but especially stage 4) sleep. Also, there is reduction of the latency to the first REM period, possibly due to loss of stage 4. In addition, the following characteristics are observed in the sleep of the aged: (a) more awakenings, (b) poorer "quality" of spindles, sometimes of less than normal frequency, (c) relatively similar durations of REM periods across the night (e.g., relatively long initial REM periods). These and other characteristics are described in some detail by Kahn and Fisher (1969).

One important example of research in this area is that of Feinberg *et al.* (1973). Recordings of sleep over four to five consecutive nights were made of young normals (mean age 27 years), aged normals (77 years) and chronic brain syndrome (CBS) aged (78 years), each group composed of 15 subjects. Results regarding REM sleep characteristics are of particular interest. While there was no difference in number of REM periods for the three groups, the CBS group had the shortest (43 minutes) REM onset latency and the lowest REM percent (17%). The REM onset latency finding is important since short onset latencies have been reported for psychotic depressives. But more interesting were the findings regarding the relationship between REM sleep time and performance on the Wechsler Adult Intelligence Scale. For the normal aged group REM time correlated .72 with performance. But REM time also correlated negatively with age (—.67), and age correlated negatively (—.58) with performance. What is the significance of the correlation of REM time and performance? Results from the CBS group suggest that this correlation is important aside from the factor of age. For the CBS group, age was *not* correlated significantly with performance but REM time was highly correlated (.72) with performance. This finding gains support from a recent report that REM time correlated .84 with *change* in WAIS performance over 18 years in a group of 75-90 years old healthy subjects (Prinz, Obrist, and Wang, 1975). The Feinberg *et al.* (1973) results are confirmed by other research showing positive correlations between various measures of amount of REM and various IQ measures (Kahn and Fisher, 1969).

These results are also compatible with others suggesting a positive relationship between IQ measures and REM time for populations of limited intelligence (organics, retardates). Feinberg *et al.* (1973) interpret their findings in the form of a hypothesis which distinguishes between capacity (circuitry) and efficiency (circuitry relative to metabolic rate). That is, for most individuals, regardless of their intellectual endowment, when they are functioning efficiently (i.e., up to capacity), there should be little difference among them in REM sleep characteristics. With age, deficiencies in metabolic activity would bring those differences into sharper focus and the result would more clearly be evident in REM characteristics.[3] In this regard, it is interesting that despite the lightening of sleep (more awakenings periodically throughout the night, less delta sleep), there is also less dream recall in normal and CBS aged (Kahn and Fisher, 1969; Kramer and Roth, 1975). Consider that the "salience" of dreams affects their recall, that brain metabolic rates are higher in REM than in NREM sleep, and that dream recall is more extensive after REM than after NREM awakenings. These observations suggest that metabolic activity in general, and brain amine activity in particular, are relevant to an understanding of dreaming and dream recall. In addition, there is evidence that short term memory for visual information declines more sharply in aged populations than does short term memory for auditory information (Boyle, Aparicio, Kaye, and Acker, 1975). Decrement in dream recall in the aged makes sense in the

---

[3] This type of hypothesis is similar to one I offer throughout this book. The idea is basically that individual differences are often most readily observed under conditions of psychological (e.g. threat, insult) or organismic (e.g., fatigue, old age) "challenge" rather than under ideal or relaxed "baseline" conditions. I have found this to be so repeatedly in my research on individual differences.

light of evidence that visual short term memory correlates with individual differences in dream recall (Cory, Ormiston, Simmel, and Dainoff, 1975).

Other developmental sleep data, suggesting differential patterns between the sexes, provide additional evidence for the hypothesis that sleep is an expression of metabolic "efficiency" in humans. If, within a homoiothermic species, longevity is tied up with metabolic efficiency, and if we agree with a number of investigators that NREM sleep in particular evolved to promote metabolic conservation, then we should expect to find: (a) negative correlations between aging and NREM (especially delta), (b) significant differences in NREM (especially delta) for the longer vs. shorter living members of the same species, and (c) similar differences in NREM (especially delta) sleep between short vs. long living species which have roughly comparable metabolic rates. There is some evidence supporting the first two expectations. The third is not supported.

First, there is evidence that aging is associated with a diminution of delta sleep. Second, there are cross-sectional longitudinal normative sleep data indicating that aging men (who have a shorter life expectancy than women)[4] show a relatively greater decline in delta sleep than do aging women (Williams, Karacan, and Hursch, 1974). Since aging women sleep longer, with fewer intervals of wakefulness, the net result is more delta sleep.[5] Does "efficient" sleep *promote* longer life by facilitating the metabolic efficiency of homoiotherms, or does better sleep merely *reflect* a metabolically more efficient organism? All we can say is that, within the human species, normal levels of delta sleep (and REM sleep) appear to be correlated with healthy psychobiological functioning.

The difference in delta sleep between aged but not young males and females suggests the importance of *organismic challenge* to revealing individual differences in certain basic biological processes and their interrelationships. Aging may be considered one form of organismic challenge (Feinberg *et al.*, 1973). Sleep or delta deprivation may be considered another type of organismic challenge. Let us consider the possibility that sex differences in delta sleep might be demonstrable in younger subjects under conditions of organismic challenge, i.e. sleep deprivation. This would support the hypothesis that the indirect connection between delta and longevity, represented by the finding that females (who, on the average, live longer) show more delta sleep during old age, might be revealed under appropriate experimental conditions. There is no report in the literature, *based on experimental manipulations*, either that long living individuals or females in particular have more delta rebound (after sleep deprivation). What follows is a description of some new data that I have obtained from a study which was carried out for entirely different reasons, but which are pertinent to the question of sex differences in delta (and thus indirectly, to the question of latent differences in indications of longevity).

The study is described in more detail at the end of Chapter 4. Briefly, both male and female college students underwent REM deprivation or NREM control awakenings during the first six hours of sleep on a single night. They were permitted uninterrupted sleep during

---

[4] In the 65 years and older group there are roughly 70 males for every 100 females (Money and Tucker, 1975, p. 48).
[5] That there may be a larger number of females than males, especially in the elderly age groups, who have problems with insomnia (Rechtschaffen and Monroe, 1969) would not necessarily invalidate the argument developed here. First, not all insomnias involve significant alterations of sleep staging, i.e., many are sleep onset rather than sleep maintenance problems. In fact, differences between insomniacs and normals or poor sleepers and good sleepers have often not been manifested as a difference in delta sleep (Monroe, 1967). Second, even if such a difference were observed, the group with *significant* insomnia compared to the population would be too small to affect the kind of general sex difference in delta sleep effect discussed above. Finally, the data base for the belief that there are substantial sex differences in insomnia is not truly adequate.

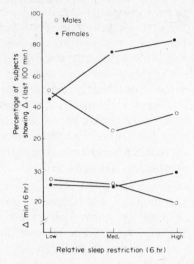

Figure 2-1   Amount and presence of delta sleep in males and females as a function of level of sleep restriction during the first six hours of a night. For each sex at each level of sleep restriction, Ns vary from 11 to 12.

the last 100 minutes of the night. Depending upon a number of factors, including pressure to get back into the REM period after each experimental awakening, these individuals differed with respect to the total amount of sleep time that they attained. Thus, it should be kept in mind that (a) sleep restriction was not experimentally manipulated in an independent fashion, but (b) there were, for each level of sleep restriction, no sex differences in number of awakenings, REM pressure, or total sleep time. Figure 2-1 shows (a) mean delta minutes attained during the first six hours, and (b) the percentage of subjects with some delta sleep during recovery sleep. Note that while there were no sex differences in delta measures under conditions of least sleep restriction during the first six hours (total sleep time roughly more than five hours), there were significant sex differences under moderate and especially under high sleep restriction (total sleep time roughly less than 4.5 hours).

While these findings are certainly not confirmatory, they are consistent with the hypothesis that the connection between delta and longevity (decline of stage 4 in the aged, and especially in the male aged) may well represent a significant biological relationship.

Regarding between-species differences in sleep time and longevity there turns out to be a *negative* correlation across mammalian species (for whom data are available) between longevity and sleep time (—.45 for either REM or NREM sleep) (Zepelin and Rechtschaffen, 1974). Even if we control for metabolic rate (correlated +.64 with total sleeping time), the longer sleeping organism is not the longer living organism. This fact has not always been obvious. For example, it has often been pointed out that the shrew, which sleeps very little, lives only about two years while the bat, which gets about 20 hours of sleep a day, lives about 18 years. Clearly, factors such as degree of metabolic slow-down and security during sleep can explain this *exception* to the rule. However, there is no reason to assume that there is a negative correlation between sleep time (or quality) and longevity *within* a species. Neither do these comparative data argue against the hypothesis that sleep develops (and probably evolved) to support as well as to reflect the biological integrity of the homoiothermic organism. (I will deal more extensively with this issue in the phylogeny section of this chapter.)

S.D.   1

Let us return momentarily to the longevity and delta sleep characteristics of aging males and females. If delta sleep (rather than total sleep time) is directly related to, or reflective of, longevity, then a rather straightforward hypothesis is suggested. The males or females aged 50 and over who spend the most time in delta sleep will live the longest. This is a particularly interesting prediction because it suggests that years *left*, rather than years *old*, may be as useful or more useful an indication of age. Surely one can question the logic that a 60-year-old about to die of natural causes ought to be placed in the same category denoting age as a 60-year-old who will live an additional 30 years. Establishing a strong, positive correlation between delta time and years of life remaining to the individual would not only be of theoretical interest. It might serve the practical needs of older but fitter individuals (good "delta types"), e.g., to obtain better life insurance rates![6]

The work of Feinberg and others clearly implicates a number of sleep parameters in the metabolic activity underlying the life process of homoiotherms. I will return in more detail to this issue shortly. However, it might not be overly speculative to suggest at this point that there may be at least a superficial connection between aging and certain forms of depression. Both are viewed as expressions of change (usually temporary in depression) in metabolic characteristics, certainly in physiological activity. While the data base for my suggestion is still rather slim, and while it does not apply to all forms of depression, there are certain sleep characteristics that the aged and the depressed seem to have in common. For example, both tend to have short REM onset latencies, relatively small amounts of delta sleep, and shortened or fragmented sleep. In addition both may involve dissociation of biological cycles, disturbance of catecholamine functioning, and both appear to include deficits in short rather than long term memory. There is a danger in making too much of these kinds of similarities. Not all of the above-mentioned characteristics have been established conclusively. Some of the above characteristics have been seen in acute and chronic conditions other than depression and aging (e.g., schizophrenia). Sleep studies often do not provide adequate distinctions between subtypes of depression (e.g., endogenous-exogenous, unipolar-bipolar) that appear to be etiologically distinct. Aging and depression in the same individuals are not always separated statistically. (Depressives tend to be older than other groups, and there is much depression in clinical groups of aged individuals.) Nevertheless, a more direct assessment of sleep characteristics associated with aging and depression would be useful.

Development of sleep cycles and abnormal sleep

The ontogeny of sleep can be described in terms of the development of circadian, ultradian, and state characteristics. Polyphasic sleep-wakefulness gradually shifts to a single wake-sleep circadian cycle. Fifty to 60 minute cycles of varying arousal and behavioral dimensions gradually lengthen to the 90-100 minutes cycle characteristic of the adult. Finally, there is a coalescence of parameters within a more or less time locked pattern that reveals more clearly the qualitatively different states of REM and NREM. Normal variation among individuals as well as many sleep disorders that develop in childhood and adulthood can be thought of as reflections of, or disturbances in, one or a number of these

---

[6] After writing this I came across a paper by Williams, Karacan, Salis, Thornby, and Anch (1975) which, less explicitly, also suggests that there may be a relationship between delta sleep measures and longevity, and which also suggests a similarity between the sleep of the aged and that of depressives (and schizophrenics).

three characteristics. For example, differences in circadian periodicity may account for some of the differences between "good" and "poor" sleepers, long and short sleepers. Consider an individual whose circadian cycle is 30 rather than 24 or 25 hours, and whose cycle is relatively refractory to entrainment. (I am suggesting that there are some individuals who are more responsive to their ultradian, circadian, infradian cycles than are others; these are the people who really "got rhythm" in the biological sense.) Such an individual will have trouble falling asleep (because he has a longer activity phase) and awakening (because he hasn't had sufficient time to sleep). Thus, we have an example of primary insomnia caused by variation in an instinctive pattern that is in constant clash with periodicities of social demands, and which may cause secondary psychological disturbances.

Consider another individual. He has a 24 hour cycle but a very short nocturnal phase. This individual will be one of those rare extra short sleepers capable of doing well on two or three hours plus perhaps a couple of hours in bed reading. No psychopathology is implied in this pattern. In fact, there is evidence (see Hartmann, 1973) that such individuals are most successful, highly productive, and happy. The term "insomniac" is inappropriate for these individuals; rather they should be considered hyposomniacs, more fortunate cousins of hypersomniacs who appear to have the opposite kind of circadian disturbance, i.e., an extremely long nocturnal phase of the circadian cycle. Some of the primary as well as secondary (e.g., neurosis-induced) insomnias probably reflect disturbances in circadian patterns with "shallow" or "unreliable" nocturnal phases.

Now consider some of the individual differences that might be manifestations of BRAC characteristics. Frequent awakenings (sleep maintenance insomnia) may be an indication of faulty mechanisms underlying the activity phase of the BRAC. Some forms of postsleep fatigue ("poor sleep") may be the result of "shallow" sleep, that is, sleep with little or no delta time. This pattern is seen more readily in aging and severe depression.

Finally, consider some of the individual differences in sleep patterns that might arise from faulty mechanisms in the timing of some or all of the components of sleep states. Narcolepsy is a condition marked by REM sleep "attacks": catalepsy (muscular atonia and collapse of posture), and sleep onset hallucinations. This condition tends to be induced by emotion, and, because it tends to run in families, appears to have a genetic basis (Kessler, 1976). Perhaps it is arbitrary to consider narcolepsy as a mixture of aroused wakefulness shifting to active (REM) sleep rather than a failure of the circadian cycle. In any case, this surprisingly prevalent pattern is a primary disturbance of sleep-wake mechanisms rather than a secondary expression of psychopathology. Related to narcolepsy is sleep paralysis, occurring during transition to wakefulness. It is probably due to a disassociation of the muscle atonia of REM which carries over into the wake state. If so, it would represent a failure of processes necessary for smooth transition from one to another state. Another example is suggested by the work of Dement (see Dement et al., 1970). His argument is that hallucinations in schizophrenia represent the breakthrough of a process normally confined to sleep. A mixture of sleep and wake processes constitutes a blurring of state boundaries. Another example may be the so-called "night terror", a disorder of arousal from delta sleep more terrifying to both sleeper and researcher than the nightmare of REM sleep. It is as though there is a confluence of two events that are usually disassociated; organismic inactivity of delta sleep and a (sudden) full consciousness of that organismic condition. Perhaps the panic associated with such awareness is similar to the feelings of impending disintegration and insanity that affect some individuals who are on some drugs: awareness of an organismic state (relative disorganization) normally associated with unconsciousness.

Thus, if we take a broad ontogenetic view, we see disorders of biorhythmic and state maintenance functions that develop relatively early during the maturation and consolidation of sleep (e.g., narcolepsy) and during old age (sleep onset and maintenance insomnia). These can be interpreted as the failure of sleep mechanisms. Other patterns of individual differences in sleep characteristics (e.g., length of sleep time) are normal expressions of the maturation and development of instinctive variation during the life cycle of the human being. The relationship between these patterns and dreaming is virtually unexplored.

Ontogenetically based hypotheses about REM function and dreaming

Research on the cyclic, ontogenetic, and comparative aspects of REM sleep lends itself to hypotheses about the function of REM. These hypotheses in turn must eventually be taken into consideration in formulating hypotheses about the nature and importance of the dreaming process. Roffwarg et al. (1966) have suggested that REM sleep provides endogenous stimulation to the immature oculomotor nervous system when a good deal of time is spent out of contact with exogenous visual stimulation. Organisms with highly developed visual capacities (cats, subhuman primates) require visual motor exercise for healthy development and functioning of wired-in capacities. The work of Held and Hein (1963) and others clearly indicates that reduced visual stimulation not only decreases capacity, but may lead to degeneration of neural fibers. Not even REM sleep can prevent such dysfunction. (It is not known if REM deprivation can enhance the neural degeneration and/or behavioral deficits caused by deprivation of visual and visual/motor experience.) There is no requirement in the Roffwarg et al. hypothesis that the endogenous stimulation of REM be organized or conscious, i.e., there is no requirement that dreaming be a part of the process. What is suggested is that during infancy, there is a relatively greater source of stimulation from endogenous compared to exogenous sources. What we are learning about the neurophysiology of REM strongly suggests that the origin of such endogenous stimulation is subcortical.

Recent work on vestibular mechanisms in autism may be consistent with the Roffwarg et al. hypothesis. I have already mentioned the importance of the pons in the initiation and organization of REM phenomena. The work of Pompeiano (Pompeiano and Morrison, 1965) has clearly implicated the vestibular nuclei of the pons in generating or modifying at least the eye movement characteristic of REM sleep. These nuclei are intimately involved in the integration of sensory and motor information. Indirect evidence that such mechanisms may be defective or immature in autistic children comes from the work of Ornitz (Ornitz et al., 1969; Ornitz et al., 1973). While general sleep patterns (e.g., REM percentages, sequencing of REM periods, etc.) are similar in autistic and normal children, there are certain differences that imply a vestibular dysfunction. The duration (not the number) of eye movement bursts is lower in the autistic child. The number of eye movements per eye movement burst is lower for the autistic child during vestibular stimulation (accomplished by bed movement during REM). This finding is consistent with evidence that during wakefulness, vestibular stimulation induces less eye movement (nystagmus) in these children. Thus, autism may be an "experiment of nature" which is consistent with the general view that REM mechanisms, or at least some components of the REM state, facilitate normal maturation of the central nervous system during early fetal and neonatal development. But this interpretation would require evidence that vestibular dysfunction affects neural mechanisms in oculomotor centers in other parts of the brain (e.g., oculomotor cortex).

While the Roffwarg et al. hypothesis has intuitive appeal, it is not without its critics. Feinberg (1969) argues that at least one prediction that could be made on the basis of the hypothesis is not supported by observations: prematures do not have less REM sleep than do full term neonates of comparable conceptional age. Nevertheless, one could argue that REM percentages in the immature organism are influenced far more by endogenous factors determined by evolution than by the exigencies of birth. There are two other points that Feinberg raises. First, let us interpret the Roffwarg et al. hypothesis to require that the activity of the oculomotor system be structured or highly organized under conditions of REM. This assumption comes from evidence that it is *pattern* rather than intensity *per se* which facilitates sensorimotor development. Feinberg argues that the unorganized, "almost convulsive" neural activity of REM is a poor candidate for the kind of function suggested by the hypothesis. However, Roffwarg believes that while the discharges of REM may not be *predictably* patterned, they are patterned (H. Roffwarg, personal communication, October, 1977). Second, let us interpret the hypothesis to require only increased *amounts* of endogenous stimulation. However, the high level of neurological/physiological/ metabolic activation typical of post-infancy REM is *not* characteristic of neonate REM. This is not a serious challenge to the hypothesis because there is no *a priori* way to determine how much activation is sufficient for a given level of cortical immaturity. However, it does raise interesting questions about the maturation of REM sleep and its relationship to NREM sleep. For example, we know that neonatal REM is to some extent an artifact of a scoring convention that determines how many of the components of REM must be present to satisfy scoring criteria. Initially these components are poorly time-locked with respect to each other. Then which component, or combination of components, performs the best job in satisfying the hypothesized function of oculomotor stimulation? Is stage *a* just as good as stage *d*?

Feinberg argues that it is the immaturity of higher centers of the brain rather than a requirement for endogenous stimulation which explains the high levels of (immature) REM sleep observed at birth. This is an interesting point which, on the basis of unpublished data, Roffwarg et al. believed was of minimal importance. It is, however, consistent with the idea that initially NREM sleep is controlled largely from caudal pontine inhibitory areas without benefit of the still immature basal forebrain and cerebral areas which will eventually transform neonate sleep into adult sleep. Thermoregulatory mechanisms are poorly developed in mammalian neonates (Satinoff, McEwen, and Williams, 1976), and a major candidate for homoiothermic (endothermic) regulation is the preoptic area which, as we have seen, is also implicated in NREM sleep control. Therefore, Feinberg's suggestion is also consistent with the speculation that true mammalian NREM sleep is the product of the phylogenetic (as well as ontogenetic) achievement of homoiothermy. This latter idea is discussed in detail in the next section of the chapter.

Ephron and Carrington (1966) have offered a hypothesis that is in many ways compatible with that of Roffwarg et al. (1966). They suggest that during NREM sleep cortical deafferentation periodically elicits "reafferentation" through REM processes that tone up the system. Clearly, the brain is characterized by continuous activity which may be modified and lowered because of other biological requirements. However, a high degree of activation seems required at least on a periodical basis. Whatever else we may be able to say about dreaming (e.g., whatever its particular meaning and effect), it is certainly a product of a largely autonomous increase in endogenous activity initiated in the brain stem. Thus, regardless of the content and organization of the dream elements, it is clear that the REM dream is initiated and modifed by biological processes that are largely remote from and antedate variation in social and interpersonal events.

The Roffwarg et al. (1966) and Ephron and Carrington (1966) hypotheses have at least two more specific theoretical implications. One is that the function of REM is especially related in some way to the encephalization characteristic of mammals: that organisms with relatively large brain/body weight ratios have a greater need for endogenous stimulation especially paranatally when the requirement for sleep predominates over the opportunity for environmental stimulation. The second implication is that REM is *not* especially suited to satisfy the requirements of highly telencephalized organisms, but rather facilitates maturation during gestation of either the CNS as a whole or the oculomotor systems in particular. I will have more to say about these two (not necessarily exclusive) hypotheses when I discuss some of the comparative data and phylogenetic speculations on sleep in the next section of this chapter.

Observations on the ontogeny of REM sleep have some implications for hypotheses regarding the relationship between dream experience and biological events. It should be noted at this point, however, that there is an intimate and mutual interrelationship between dream characteristics and physiological activity. While variation in dream content is *to some degree* correlated with variation in physiological characteristics such as eye or middle ear muscle activity, two points should be kept in mind. First, the direction of causality is far from clear. Second, REM characteristics (especially eye movement patterns which have been given most attention in the psychophysiological literature) differ depending on (a) whether or not the organism is intact, (b) level of maturity, and (c) whether it is reasonable to infer that the organism is capable of dreaming. For example, although decerebrated cats, dark-reared kittens, congenitally blind humans, and neonates have eye movements during REM, the patterns of these eye movements are different from those observed in healthy mature organisms. Thus, REM dreaming of the adult human is the product of the mutual influence of the maturation of the central nervous system and the acquisition (and reprogramming) of experience.

I have been speaking about the ontogeny of REM sleep. What is the origin of dreaming? Clearly, infants cannot report private experience. They, like animals, provide nonverbal behavioral evidence from which inferences about cognitive capacity can be made. However, inferences about the phenomenology of REM from the behavioral events of REM are inherently risky. For example, the presence of eye movement during REM does not constitute *a priori* evidence for the presence of visual imagery. Aside from the data on eye movement in the congenitally blind, there is evidence of normal eye movement patterns in dark-reared kittens (Fishbein et al., 1966). If we define dreaming as incentive-related information processing during REM sleep regardless of whether or not there is concomitant imagery (consciousness), then it may be possible to adapt conditioning procedures from neonate experimental psychology to provide a tentative answer. Lipsitt (1972) has reviewed a number of paradigms that have been employed to assess the learning capacity of infants. For example, it has been demonstrated that operant learning, say of a head turning gesture, can be increased in frequency when followed by the introduction of a pacifier. In one study, the frequency of right leg movements could be increased if the response caused the movement of a mobile. Clearly, infants are interested by a wide variety of stimulus variation; in the terminology of White (1959) they are "neurocentrically" as well as "viscerocentrically" motivated.

I would suggest the following kind of experimental approach to the question of the dreaming capacity of neonates. First, the subjects would be trained to make a right leg movement in the presence of a particular visual stimulus in order to get some kind of reinforcement. Left leg movement would be ineffective. Right leg movement in the absence of the discriminative stimulus would likewise fail to produce the reinforcement. Other infants could be trained to move the left leg to the same discriminative stimulus. Baseline, experimental, and extinction measures of leg movements during REM sleep could be assessed for evidence of sensorimotor information processing (dreaming). Presumably, if it could be demonstrated that the required movement were visual stimulus-specific, its presence during REM could be assumed to indicate the processing of visual stimulus information. It is possible that while infants could spontaneously demonstrate behavioral evidence of information processing, neonates might need a "reminder". For example, some subjects might learn to produce the response-to-visual stimulus after a tactile cue is given. The cue would provide a set to attend to the appropriate visual information. During REM sleep, the neonate might require the tactile cue to initiate the sequence. That is, REM information processing (dreaming) of the neonate, compared to the infant, may be more passive-dependent on immediate and proximate sensory information.

The experimental behavioral paradigm that I have just suggested might be used to explore the role of REM sleep in learning (adaptation). Let us suppose that an infant has learned to produce a response (say, to a tactile cue) that produces novel visual information. If such a response can be cued off repeatedly during REM sleep, would the infant demonstrate a change in responsiveness *the next day* compared to appropriate control condition infants? Would the change be toward less responding (habituation) or toward more responding (greater interest out of increased sensorimotor skill with the information)? In either case, it could be argued that some kind of learning took place during REM, an adaptation with respect to one aspect of the environment.

2. PHYLOGENY AND EVOLUTIONARY SIGNIFICANCE OF REM SLEEP

REM sleep has been observed in all the placental and marsupial species that have been studied. It is a brief but detectable characteristic of avian sleep, and has even been reported to exist, albeit in somewhat modified form, in the sleep of some reptilian species (Tauber, 1974). Why has REM sleep persisted so long in so many species? What were the forces that shaped out such a "paradoxical" state within sleep, and to what extent do such forces continue to modify the instinct? Does REM sleep continue to function in a similar manner in existing species (whatever other functions REM sleep may have acquired), or, less optimistically, is REM sleep an elaborate behavioral vestige that is in the process of devolving? Is sleep itself unimportant in the modern world even though, through its instinctive operation each 24 hours, we are forced to comply with its program? Finally, does speculation on the phylogenetic origins of REM sleep provide any perspective on the evolution of the dreaming phenomenon?

Speculation about the evolutionary significance of sleep is based on data from living organisms rather than from fossil remains. A working assumption is that clues regarding phylogenetic origins of sleep in long-extinct species can be derived from analyses of living representatives at different levels of the phylogenetic spectrum. However, one cannot be sure that sleep patterns in primitive animals are unchanged versions of patterns of sleep in extinct species such that the present patterns can be taken as "living fossils". In fact, it is likely that to some unknown extent, sleep evolved and is still evolving differently in each species. There is no harm in speculating about the evolution of sleep on the basis of comparative data if we recognize its limitations. And yet, having said this, I should add that such speculations have raised some of the most interesting questions to be found in sleep/dream research.

As we have seen, sleep is defined in terms of EEG and behavioral characteristics that are typically derived from more advanced, usually mammalian, organisms. At what phylogenetic level activity-inactivity gives way to "true" wakefulness-sleep is unknown. In fact, the distinction may be somewhat arbitrary and circular if one defines sleep in terms of mammalian electrophysiological characteristics. Nevertheless, from a purely descriptive perspective some general differences across classes of animals can be discerned. All animals from insect to primate show periods of inactivity. These are associated with raised response thresholds and characteristic postures, and, along with periods of activity, have a circadian organization. Only birds and mammals appear to have relatively high voltage slow wave sleep. Only marsupial and placental mammals have NREM sleep spindles, and only primates have K-complexes. The presence of REM sleep in reptiles is debatable, as is the significance of the miniscule amounts of REM sleep observed in birds (Meddis, 1975).

Because the characteristics we usually recognize as REM and NREM sleep appear unambiguously only in birds and mammals, and because the REM sleep of birds comprises only a tiny fraction of total sleep, I will focus on the phylogenetic significance of REM sleep in mammals. However, before proceeding, I should again reiterate the possibility that what we call sleep in higher species is different from inactivity of lower species only or largely in its overt expression rather than in its basic function.

Neurophysiological and phenomenological properties of REM suggest the hypothesis that its evolution is closely tied up with the "intellectual" needs and capacity of organisms. This in turn would suggest that REM time is related in some way to intelligence, brain power, or brain weight. Evidence for such a hypothesis could be obtained by looking at the correlation between degree of encephalization or brain/body weight ratios and REM time. Evidence that NREM sleep has something to do with physiological restoration suggests that its evolution may be tied up with homoiothermic requirements or with the metabolic characteristics peculiar to homoiothermic organisms. We will deal with these and other possibilities from the perspective of comparative data.

There are four major biological processes that will be relevant to questions about the original and current function(s) of sleep: (a) *Encephalization* (both in the sense of neocortical relative to subcortical development and in the sense of brain weight relative to body weight); (b) *Metabolic rate* (rate at which structure is broken down or built up by living organisms); (c) *Viviparity* (live bearing); (d) *Homoiothermy* (physiological ability to maintain a relatively constant internal temperature despite variations in ambient temperature).

Encephalization and sleep

First, there is no obvious relationship across mammalian species between REM sleep time and neocortical endowment. Consider the following "primitive" exemplars of the three broad classes of mammals. The echidna (a monotreme or egg-laying mammal) has no REM sleep. The opossum (a marsupial) has a REM time of about 5.5 hours or about 30% of total sleep time, yet the opossum has a *lower* encephalization quotient than does the echidna (Jerison, 1973). The mole (a placental) has a REM time of about 2 hours which represents about 23% of total sleep time. This latter set of figures is not very different from those of the typical adult human. The fact that human sleep is not extraordinarily endowed with REM time despite high brain/body weight ratio (and presumably high intelligence) contradicts the hypothesis that REM sleep has a special evolutionary significance with respect to neocortical "brain power". This is not to deny that REM sleep in intelligent organisms may provide special advantages (e.g., mediating learning, memory, information reorganization, etc.). It should be noted that REM time is probably determined by factors that determine NREM time and therefore total sleep time. In addition, REM time is a rather crude measure in the sense that time *per se* may not be highly correlated with importance. Cross-species comparisons are even more tenuous. Conceivably, whatever REM does can be carried out as well in 10 minutes as in 30 minutes. Just as brain size is an ambiguous indication of brain power, REM time may be an ambiguous indication of function or importance or need. Much the same could be said for sleep time. For example, Taub, Tanguay, and Clarkson (1976) reported that afternoon naps of one half hour or two hours had a roughly equivalent restorative effect. Both improved performance on an auditory reaction time task.

Let us look more closely at the evidence which contradicts the hypothesis that REM duration is a direct function of the encephalization of organisms. The comparative data indicate that there is a *negative* cross-species correlation between brain weight and REM time. On the basis of primary data reported by Zepelin and Rechtschaffen (1974) and shown in Table 2-1, I calculated cross-mammalian species correlations between brain (grams)/body (kilogram) ratios and both REM time and REM%. (The importance of

TABLE 2-1. Correlation Coefficients Among Sleep Parameters and Other Constitutional Variables (from Zepelin and Rechtschaffen, 1974)

	SWS time	PS time	PS%	Cycle length	Life span	Metabolic rate	Brain weight	Gestation period
TST	0.96** (39)	0.76** (38)	0.06 (38)	-0.66** (23)	-0.52** (43)	0.64** (49)	-0.71** (38)	-0.69** (41)
SWS time		0.58** (38)	-0.17 (38)	-68.0** (23)	-0.45* (34)	0.67** (39)	-0.70** (30)	-0.58** (33)
PS time			0.67** (38)	-0.39 (23)	-0.45* (35)	0.48* (40)	-0.54* (31)	-0.64** (35)
PS%				0.27 (24)	-0.05 (35)	-0.12 (40)	0.10 (31)	-0.09 (35)
Cycle length					0.81** (24)	-0.83** (24)	0.92** (22)	0.79** (24)
Life span						-0.68** (46)	0.85** (37)	0.73** (41)
Metabolic rate							-0.96** (40)	-0.77** (45)
Brain weight								0.85** (38)

The number of cases for each coefficient is in parentheses. Logarithmic transformations were used for all variables except TST and SWS time. Metabolic rate was derived from body weight.
$*p < 0.01$. $**p < 0.001$.

such a ratio will become evident later in the chapter.) These two correlations were .13 and —.16 respectively. In fact, selecting brain/body ratios from a group of species of roughly comparable body weight (1-5 kg) yields more clearly negative correlations between degree of encephalization and REM time (—.44) and REM% (—.29).

Next, consider the fact that while birds show the same degree of brain to body weight relationships as do mammals, their REM time is minuscule. On the other hand, as I noted before, the echidna has no REM sleep yet it is mammalian with respect to encephalization. Thus, whatever REM may do, it does not seem to have evolved specifically to promote postreptilian encephalization. However, this conclusion does not contradict the hypothesis that, within species, a developmental *change* in REM may indicate something important about both telencephalic integrity and psychological competence.

Metabolic rate and sleep

It is intuitively obvious that sleep time is related to the metabolic regulatory process. On the basis of their correlational analysis of cross-species data, Zepelin and Rechtschaffen (1974) develop the following argument. Energy expenditure for thermoregulation is significant in homoiothermic organisms. Physical activity, especially in smaller animals, is extremely expensive in that it requires a metabolic cost many times that of basal metabolism. Sleep can be thought of as an effective method of insuring that a highly responsive organism will maintain low metabolic expenditures during those times when energy-acquiring or species-perpetuating activity would be inefficient (i.e., energy output required for a given amount of energy attainment). This view of sleep as *enforced rest* is consistent with the hypothesis, discussed shortly, that NREM sleep evolved as a mechanism to ensure the survival of early mammalian forms with high metabolic requirements determined by their novel thermoregulatory characteristics. The cross-species data evaluated by Zepelin and Rechtschaffen are consistent with this idea. However, these data do not indicate a special function for REM sleep.

Homoiothermy, viviparity, and sleep states

The echidna is an egg-laying mammal (monotreme) which shows no evidence of REM sleep. On the basis of this observation Allison, van Twyver, and Goff (1972) developed a speculative hypothesis about the differential evolution of REM and NREM sleep. They begin with the basic assumptions that the monotreme is a living model of therian (marsupial and placental) precursors, and that NREM sleep is predominantly a postreptilian development. They then suggest that REM and NREM sleep appeared at different periods during evolution and that they provided different functions. They suggest that NREM sleep first evolved during the evolution of homoiothermy. This would put the origin of NREM sleep about 180 million years ago. At this time, oviparous poikilotherms (mammal-like reptiles or therapsids) were evolving into oviparous homoiotherms (reptile-like mammals or monotremes).

On the other hand, REM sleep is hypothesized to make its appearance with the evolution of viviparity, about 130 million years ago. REM sleep would have provided a mechanism to facilitate brain development during the short gestation periods that characterized these early therians.

Let us consider these speculations by Allison *et al.* (1972), first about the origin of NREM sleep and then about the differential function of NREM and REM sleep. The Allison *et al.* hypothesis regarding the origins of NREM sleep is particularly interesting in the light of two recent contributions to evolution theory (Bakker, 1975; Jerison, 1976). First, consider Jerison's (1977) analysis of brain/body weight ratios across the following groups: extinct reptiles, living reptiles, birds, extinct mammals, and living mammals. When available encephalization data points are plotted on log:log (brain weight in grams/body weight in kilograms) coordinates, they form elongated polygonal distributions with slopes of 2/3 (see Figure 2-2). The 2/3 slope obtains regardless of the group of species, and regardless of

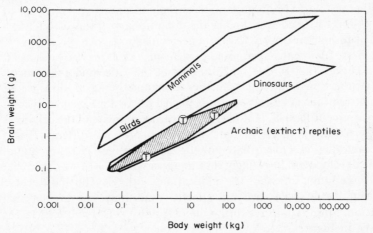

Figure 2-2   Relationship between brain and body weight (from Jerison, 1976). Note that about 80% of the cross-species variance in brain weight can be accounted for by knowing body weight (but the within-species association is trivial when age is controlled). The roughly linear relationship is determined by the requirement that body surface and sensorimotor apparatus be "abstracted" in brain structure. However, cross-species variability in brain weight occurs at any point along the body weight scale. This variability, i.e., that which is not merely related to body "mapping", is one way to define "encephalization". Jerison has proposed an encephalization quotient (EQ) to represent the ratio of observed to expected encephalization for a given body weight. The EQ is roughly correlated with a species' "intelligence level". The *T*s in the reptilian polygon refer to therapsids. These are called "mammal-like reptiles" because they are similar to or close to mammals in tooth differentiation, skull, jaw (therapsid means "dog jaw") and palatal structure, skeletal structure (which permitted mammal-like locomotion), and number of joints and length of digits in hands and feet. There is some evidence that they were homoiothermic. On the other hand, they were clearly reptilian in encephalization.

whether the group is living or extinct. However, relative to the overlapped distributions of extinct and living reptiles, the distributions of birds and mammals are *displaced upward* with virtually no overlap with reptilian distributions. (The distribution for extinct mammals, not shown in the figure, is midway between those of the reptiles and living mammals.) Thus, evolutionary change from reptilian to mammalian form appears to involve two major events: development of homoiothermy and acceleration of encephalization.[7] If accelerated encephalization and homoiothermy evolved together, which one

[7] According to Jerison (1976), progressively greater encephalization was the joint function of the following: (a) Evolution of species that were active at night, correlated with (b) evolution in these species of a dependency on rod (night) vision along with audition and olfaction, the latter two of which require more extensive neural elaboration within the brain than does vision. "And so we see that the first expansion of the vertebrate brain may have been primarily a solution to a packaging problem and that it may only incidentally have resulted in the evolution of

characteristic was more crucial to the evolution of NREM sleep? If there were living examples of a homoiothermic species with reptilian encephalization, we might have a more definitive answer. There is evidence that such species once existed.

Bakker (1975) reviews three sources of evidence that dinosaurs (and their reptilian-like ancestors, the thecodonts) were actually homoiothermic. The evidence includes (a) histological characteristics preserved in fossil bones from which inferences about homoiothermic metabolism can be made, (b) geographical distribution of extinct species with corresponding evidence about climate, and (c) predator/prey ratios. Bakker's analyses, together with those of Jerison, suggest the following rather novel conclusion. The ancestors of dinosaurs (thecodonts), the ancestors of birds (dinosaurs), and the ancestors of mammals (therapsids) were "reptilian" in encephalization but "mammalian" in thermo-regulation. If Bakker is correct, and if the evolutionary origin of NREM sleep is more closely related to homoiothermy than to encephalization, then the origin of NREM sleep may be even more remote than proposed by Allison *et al.* It may go back as far as the end of the Permian period, that is, the last third part of the Paleozoic Era (roughly 250 million years ago). At this time homoiothermic thecodont and therapsid forms were evolving from poikilothermic reptilian ancestors, a drama played out on the vast geological stage provided by the protocontinent Pangia. However, if the earlier estimate of the origin of NREM sleep is correct, it is likely that the form that NREM sleep took was different from that observed in living homoiotherms. Given that slow (delta) waves require some minimum degree of telencephalic development, it is likely that therapsidian NREM was more like stage 2 than delta sleep. In addition, following the implications of the Zepelin and Rechtschaffen (1974) analysis, sleep would have become shorter (and longevity greater) with increasing encephalization. Speculations regarding the origin of NREM and REM sleep are graphic-ally portrayed in Figure 2-3.

An interesting study commensurate with the hypothesis of NREM function proposed by Allison *et al.* has been reported by Walker and Berger (1974). They found that at the point where suckling opossums began to show evidence of homoiothermic regulation they began to show signs of NREM sleep. Prior to this point, which occurred about 65 days after birth, REM sleep predominated. Of course, neither the Allison *et al.* hypothesis nor the Walker and Berger data clarify the exact relationship between homoiothermy and NREM sleep, either in young or adult living organisms or during the evolution of ancestors of living organisms. For example, NREM sleep may facilitate homoiothermy, or homoiothermic ability may be mediated by brain structures that determine that the inactivity phase of the circadian cycle has the form of NREM sleep. In addition, it would be necessary to distinguish between the motivational and instrumental components of homoiothermic regulation. Mammalian neonates apparently have the drive to compensate for externally imposed temperature variations but have not yet developed the ability to affect internal regulatory changes (Satinoff *et al.*, 1976). Does NREM sleep in some way relate to the drive, or more likely, the ability to respond effectively to the drive, toward internal regulation of temperature?

Consider the speculations by Allison *et al.* on the relationship between the evolution of viviparity and the origin of REM sleep. There is the negative correlation across mammalian species between REM time and duration of gestation obtained by Zepelin and

intelligence" (1976, p. 99). (c) Resolving those three sense modalities into a single, integrating model or code to locate relevant objects in space and time, a code that is the presumed evolutionary precursor of human conscious-ness.

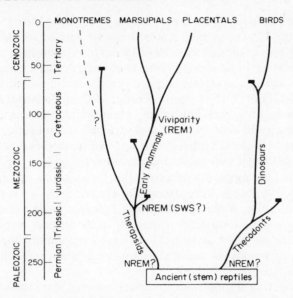

Figure 2-3   Possible evolution of NREM and REM sleep. The figure is an integration of the evolutionary schemes suggested by Allison *et al.* (1972) and by Bakker (1975). The Allison *et al.* scheme for mammalian evolution (on the left side of the figure) is largely, though not entirely, retained. Reptilian evolution is left out, and the Bakker (1975) scheme, shown on the right, is tentatively accepted. Thus, if NREM is essentially an expression of homoiothermy, and if the Bakker scheme is essentially correct, then NREM sleep may have evolved at two points shown by "NREM?" on the figure (about 250 million years ago). REM sleep would have evolved 120 million years after NREM (around 130 million years ago) when early oviparous homoiothermic mammals gave rise to the two parallel mammalian viviparous groups, the marsupials and the placentals.

Rechtschaffen (1974). In fact, this —.64 correlation is the largest one between REM time and any of the biological measures (gestation, metabolic rate, brain weight, life span) that they obtain. However, the high correlation between REM and NREM time, and the fact that the REM time-gestation correlation is not significantly different from other correlations involving REM time suggests caution in interpreting such a result as supporting the hypothesized function for REM sleep. It might be interesting to evaluate the difference in REM time across bird species which differ in incubation durations. Birds have minuscule amounts of REM sleep (which is consistent with the idea that REM is relevant to viviparity rather than oviparity). If such a study could demonstrate that, other things (metabolic rates) being equated, birds which have longer periods of incubation had less REM than birds with shorter incubation time, this would support the Allison *et al.* hypothesis. The problem then would be to explain why oviparous organisms might require at least small amounts of REM.

   A recent analysis of mammalian sleep data (Allison and Cicchetti, 1976) provides supplemental information to the Zepelin and Rechtschaffen (1974) analysis. It lends support to the Allison *et al.* hypothesis regarding the relationship between REM sleep and viviparity, and furthers the distinction between REM and NREM function. Allison and Cicchetti applied correlational methods to three kinds of information on 39 mammalian species: REM and NREM sleep time, biological characteristics (i.e., body and brain weight, life span, gestation time), and ecological ratings (i.e., of predation threat, sleep exposure, and overall danger). A factor analysis yielded two general and statistically independent factors. The first or "size" factor showed more negative loading for NREM than for REM sleep time. The second or "danger" factor showed a more negative loading for REM than for NREM sleep. While this analysis suggested that NREM sleep time seems to be related to organismic characteristics while REM time seems to be related to ecological characteristics, a stepwise multiple regression analysis suggested a more specific and more interesting relationship. The two best predictors of NREM sleep, in order of their statistical strength, were *body weight* (one can substitute metabolic rate, brain weight, etc. since these are highly intercorrelated) and *overall danger*. These two variables accounted for 58% of the variance in NREM sleep time. On the other hand, the best two predictors of REM sleep time were *overall danger* and *gestation time* together accounting for 66% of the REM time variance. That is, biological and ecological characteristics are rather highly negatively correlated with both REM and NREM time but the strength of the relationships is reversed for the two kinds of sleep. In addition, while overall danger is highly predictive of both NREM and REM time, the body weight variable of the size factor is more important to predicting NREM time while the gestation variable of the size factor is more important in predicting REM time. The authors point out that the negative correlation between REM and gestation time is independent of other influences.

Two interesting theoretical points are tentatively derived from these data. First, Allison and Cicchetti suggest that the Zepelin and Rechtschaffen hypothesis be modified. Rather than considering NREM sleep a mechanism by which animals are forced to inactivity to conserve energy, NREM sleep may be the *effect* of size (e.g., large herbivores need more wake time to feed) and danger (e.g., large herbivores are more subject to predation). Second, the low correlation between gestation time and danger, the two best predictors of REM time, reinforces the importance of the gestation variable and its theoretical significance to the hypothesis of the evolution of REM sleep in conjunction with the origins of viviparity in mammals. In addition, as the two investigators point out, these findings support the hypothesis proposed by Roffwarg *et al.* (1966) that REM sleep is particularly important in the maturation of the central nervous system.

Unresolved questions

Speculation that REM sleep appeared during the evolution of viviparity must deal with some unresolved questions. First, there is the question of the relationship between adult and neonate REM time. Can we infer something about the function of REM in fetal and neonatal maturation from cross-species correlations between gestation time and *adult* REM time, and then go on to speculate about the evolutionary significance of these relationships? Neonate REM time is positively correlated with immaturity (Anders, 1975). If immaturity is roughly correlated with gestation time, then the neonate REM time is positively correlated with gestation time. How does this fit with the idea that REM time facilitates brain development for species with *short* gestation periods? What does this say about the relevance of the negative cross-species correlation between adult REM time and gestation time?

Second, if REM is so important to gestation (e.g., speeding up CNS maturation during short gestation periods), why is it that the REM sleep in the human fetus and newborn is more of the stage *a* than stage *d* (paradoxical or normal REM) type of sleep? Clearly, if Petre-Quadens' classificatory scheme is valid (see Petre-Quadens and Schlag, 1974, Ch. 18), then paradoxical sleep (PS) as we know it requires a degree of CNS maturation not seen until roughly the time of birth. Unless stage *a* is *functionally* similar to stage *d*, or unless stage *a* is similar to the kind of REM which first appeared during viviparous evolution, it is hard to understand how stage *d* (which is not observed in the premature or expected in the fetus) can serve the biological requirements of gestation in viviparous organisms. Perhaps this stage, and its fetal precursor, give way to a more mature form (namely stage *d* or paradoxical sleep) whose *expression* is determined, in part, by maturational factors (telencephalization) underlying the expression of NREM sleep. Perhaps, after all, the "rhombencephalic sleep" of the neonate is a crude expression of the evolutionary precursors of more evolved mammalian sleep. Perhaps it is a poikilothermic remnant that was entirely suppressed during early homoiothermic evolution (*viz.* echidna) but reacquired, first, in the service of gestational maturation and, later, in the service of telencephalic toning and tuning.

Third, although the REM-viviparity hypothesis would not necessarily be contradicted by observations of REM in birds (and establishment of REM in reptiles), it certainly does not explain the REM-like phenomenon observed in these species. Fourth, if the adult echidna has no REM sleep, what kind of sleep does the *neonate* echidna have? The work of Walker and Berger (1974) suggests that neonate marsupials are poikilothermic, attaining homoiothermy somewhat later in ontogeny than do the more advanced placentals. During the poikilothermic stage, their sleep is entirely REM. Assuming that the "more primitive" monotreme requires at least as much, perhaps more, ontogenetic time to develop homoiothermic capacity, and if Allison *et al.* (1972) are correct in assuming that even during infancy the monotreme has no REM sleep, what kind of sleep does it get prior to attaining homoiothermy?

There are other questions that need to be resolved. For example, it is customary to talk about "real" sleep as basically that seen in homoiotherms. However, there are some reports of either NREM or REM sleep (or both) in submammalian vertebrates, especially the reptiles (e.g., tortoise [NREM], turtle [NREM, and possibly REM], lizards [possibly REM]). Also, there is evidence of eye movement activity during the inactivity periods ("sleep") of some species of fish. Should we expect a correlation between such events and the viviparity/oviparity characteristic? What are the neurostructural differences between mammalian and submammalian vertebrates that might correlate with difference in the characteristics of sleep?[8]

In addition, there is evidence on the capacity of heterothermic fish to have NREM sleep. For example, the bluefin tuna, though more cold blooded (about 30°C) than the average landed homoiotherm, is capable of maintaining a fairly level internal temperature in its swimming muscles despite gross variation in ambient water temperature. Does this species have NREM sleep? Note that the evidence for NREM or REM sleep in fish and reptiles would not necessarily invalidate the Allison *et al.* hypothesis. These species are

---

[8] Many of these studies correlate behavioral and electrophysiological data to provide evidence of a psychophysiological state that can be compared with those of homoiotherms. It is important to recognize that physiological (e.g., EEG) and behavioral arousal are *not* necessarily correlated, or are correlated in a way that is different from that seen in homoiotherms. For example, lesions in the posterior hypothalamus induce behavioral lethargy despite low voltage fast (aroused) EEG induced by reticular formation stimulation. Likewise, reticular lesions can elicit high voltage (sleeplike) EEG in a behaviorally active organism. With regard to arousal-behavioral patterns that are different from those seen in homoiotherms, consider the fact that in a number of amphibians (e.g., frog), behavioral "sleep" is associated with low voltage fast activity while wakefulness is associated with synchronous EEG patterns (Tauber, 1974).

not uninfluenced by their own evolution and may have evolved mechanisms analogous to those of the early mammals. In fact, the NREM and REM of early mammals may have evolved from primitive, rather nondescript NREM and REM precursors common to the poikilothermic ancestors of present-day reptiles, birds and mammals. (Heterothermic fish may have evolved a kind of NREM sleep for the same reasons as did the early oviparous mammals.) Thus, it would not be surprising to find NREM and REM (or NREM-like and REM-like) sleep in some submammalian species.

Let me suggest one possible explanation for the absence of REM sleep in the echidna. In addition to being oviparous, the echidna is "almost poikilothermic" (Dawson, 1973). While there is some argument about the ability of the echidna to adjust homoiothermically to changes in ambient temperature, it is clear that its basal body temperature (about 28°C) is significantly lower than that of therians.[9] Recall the evidence presented in Chapter 1 that REM sleep is a poikilothermic state. Is it not likely that at the time that organisms were developing their capacity for homoiothermic adjustment, they could ill-afford, even periodically, to revert during sleep to a poikilothermic state? (Parenthetically, one has to wonder what possible advantage the poikilothermic REM characteristic accrues to a homoiothermic animal.) Such a state might be especially dangerous despite mitigating factors such as low metabolic rate and burrowing. A recent study provides data that are consistent with this line of reasoning. Walker, Glotzbach, Berger, and Heller (1975) reported an absence of REM in hibernating ground squirrels when brain temperature went below 27°C (80.6°F).

In addition to reproduction and thermoregulation, neuropsychological differences exist between echidna and therians. That is, unlike marsupials and placentals, monotremes have a markedly different distribution of cortical areas specialized for function. Specifically, the visual, auditory, somatic, motor cortexes are uniquely differentiated, closely interrelated, and displaced over the posterior portion of the cerebrum. Virtually all of the "association cortex" occurs rostrally to the primary areas, and "is reliably more extensive than in any other mammal, including man" (Sarnat and Netsky, 1974, p. 253). If nothing else, these ideas raise the question of the value of the echidna as an "experimental" animal. That is, since the echidna differs from therians not only in terms of oviparity but also in terms of thermoregulation and cortical differentiation, it is not clear that absence of REM can be so readily explained by one biological characteristic (oviparity).

Perhaps the most definitive approach to the enigma of REMless sleep in the echidna will come from research on differences between monotremes and therians in neurostructure. Such information would undoubtedly contribute much to our understanding of REM mechanisms beyond those occurring at the level of the pons. For example, the forebrain mechanisms of NREM sleep appear to include the POA which, consistent with the Allison *et al.* theory, is implicated in homoiothermy. Are there structures in *phylogenetically more recently developed* forebrain areas that relate both to REM and to viviparity?

A fundamental problem raised by all these questions is the very definition of REM sleep as a confluence in time of neurophysiological and psychophysiological components. If we take our cue from the parallel between ontogeny and phylogeny, we are faced with additional questions. To what extent must certain events be developed and how many of them must be present simultaneously before we define them as "REM sleep"? Do one or a few of the components of REM appear separately during evolution? If so, which of these, or combination of these, is most important to the hypothesized function of REM, or is any one

---

[9] In addition, its metabolic rate is roughly half that of placentals.

of them equally representative of some underlying activating process which itself satisfies the hypothesized function?

There have been other speculations about the phylogenetic origin and significance of REM and NREM sleep. For example, Snyder (1966) opined that REM sleep had a sentinel function: to permit periodic assessment of a potentially dangerous (dinosaur infested) environment and to prepare the organism for rapid and more effective adaptation (e.g., escape) upon awakening. While it is true that organisms behave more effectively upon awakening from REM sleep, there are certain facts which appear to compromise the sentinel hypothesis. First, why is it that the awakening threshold is usually *higher* during the REM sleep of animals? Why is it that predator sleep is characterized by much more REM than is the sleep of prey? Why is there such a large difference in the REM percentages of "fossorial" animals such as echidna, opossum and mole? Why do ungulates tend to have relatively more awakenings from NREM than from REM sleep? Why do animals (e.g., rats) sleeping in a hostile environment (i.e., in the presence of a predator) show a decrease in REM sleep? Why do humans sleeping in a novel environment such as the sleep laboratory sometimes miss their first and even their second REM periods? An equally reasonable hypothesis is that periodic awakenings represent a failure to inhibit momentary fluctuations in arousal characteristic of sleep rather than indicating a sentinel or vigilance function.

General remarks

Throughout this book I will be distinguishing between the characteristics and hypothesized functions of REM and NREM states. We should be clear, however, that both states are variants of sleep and therefore probably have much in common. For example, there is evidence that recovery sleep with large amounts of REM or delta restores psychological processes that are adversely affected by the total sleep deprivation (Johnson, 1973a). Despite the findings shown in Table 1-1, it is too early to know just how discrete are the dual nature and function of sleep. Therefore, the degree of emphasis on differences is as much a reflection of theoretical and didactic convenience as a reflection of empirically established fact. Figure 2-4 shows two kinds of emphasis assuming that there are actually three kinds of sleep: REM, "spindle" or stage 2, and delta or SWS. The Venn diagram on the left side of the Figure represents the assumption that while the three kinds of sleep have some common characteristics/function(s), they are relatively unique. "It is true that there are common

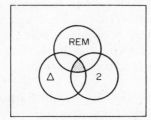 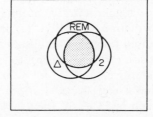

Figure 2-4   Representation of two hypothetical positions with respect to the relative distinctiveness of characteristics/functions of three kinds of sleep: that they are relatively distinct, having a small number of characteristics in common (left) or that they are relatively similar, distinctions among them being relatively few or trivial (right).

elements in the two sleep states, including the continuity of behavioral quiescence and the interruption of recall of consciousness. It is an important challenge to find the substrate of this continuity. However, since the brain sites studied thus far do not show this continuity, it appears to be most useful to separate the discussion of the two states" (McGinty et al., 1974, p. 176). Qualitative differences in the neurostructure of different stages of sleep consistent with the assumption portrayed on the left side of Figure 2-4 are described by McGinty et al., 1974, p. 182, for three brain areas: cortex-thalamic, limbic-hypothalamic, and brain stem.

The Venn diagram on the right of Figure 2-4 represents the assumption that the differences in the surface structure of sleep stages belie a largely common function. The comparative analysis of mammalian sleep data provided in the Zepelin and Rechtschaffen review (1974) tends to support such an assumption. It will be clear that my view, like that of many sleep researchers, lies somewhere between the two assumptions presented in Figure 2-4.

What is required for a full analysis of sleep from the perspective of phylogenetic theory? What were the environmental and organismic variables that influenced the evolution of the sleep (both REM and NREM) instinct?[10] These must have included temperature variation, prey availability, predator availability (danger), security of sleep conditions, metabolic rate, brain size, ability to store food, etc. It is my guess that the evolution of homoiothermy freed animals from the immediate impact of two physical conditions that control the inactivity phase of the circadian cycle in poikilotherms, and which reduced their competitive advantage against nocturnal animals: darkness and cold. Homoiothermy frees the temperature-sensitive metabolic processes from ambient thermal gradients. It therefore permits the organism to be active at night when it is colder. Thus, it extends the potential duration of the activity phase of the circadian cycle. In addition it means that the organism can be more *intensely* active for a longer period. Duration and intensity of activity are metabolically expensive, as is the homoiothermic process itself. An organism with these characteristics would appear to require a reliable *active inhibitory* mechanism (an instinct) to counteract expenditures of energy which might otherwise "wear out" the organism before it had a chance to reproduce. Did the active process of NREM sleep evolve out of reptilian inactivity, and thus represent a "solution" to a fundamental biological problem, that of increased metabolic demands?

A kind of NREM sleep may thus have *gradually* evolved to compensate for the metabolic demands of homoiothermy. However, it may have evolved further once the organism evolved a nocturnal life style. The latter would make a relatively greater metabolic demand because it would be associated with greater heat loss and increased activity to obtain energy. Thus, nocturnal life would, if Jerison (1973, 1976) is correct, encourage (a) more efficient homoiothermy, (b) a higher level of encephalization (to "package" and integrate auditory and olfactory information centrally), (c) increased responsiveness (higher intelligence) and therefore increased potential for sustained activity, and (d) increased requirement for an active mechanism (NREM sleep) to sustain inactivity when activity would be metabolically maladaptive.

How was this brain stem-based instinct modified by the influence of more recently acquired neural structures? Clearly, the REM sleep of primitive organisms, however similar

---

[10] That sleep appears to be a highly heritable instinct is demonstrated by recent work on inbred strains of mice (Valatx and Chouvet, 1975).

its surface structure, cannot be identical to that of telencephalically more sophisticated organisms. How is the instinct of sleep modified on a day to day basis by *current* environmental factors? Whatever the central tendency of the instinct of a species (e.g., sleep time, REM-NREM cycle, etc.), factors such as those referred to above (prey and predatory availability, security of sleep arrangement) must vary in such a way as to influence sleep parameters through their influence on basic biological variables such as calorie intake, energy expenditure, body weight. In what ways do psychological factors influence sleep characteristics? Is the effect of calorie intake simulated by the effect of informational intake (new learning)? Clearly, variation in the onset of sleep must include factors such as lack of information (monotony, boredom). On a speculative level, one might say that if sleep onset mechanisms operate to "shut down" the system when the ratio of energy expenditure to calorie acquisition is high, the same might be true for the ratio of attention spent on extracting information vs. low information yield. That is, other things being equal, it would be advantageous if an organism would stop responding (go to sleep) when high energy expenditures are rewarded by high entropy (low grade food or information).

A fundamental implication of a wide array of direct and indirect evidence is that sleep represents "an enforced state of rest" rather than a radical diminution of metabolic rate relative to relaxed wakefulness (Zepelin and Rechtschaffen, 1974). The origin of sleep probably related to a balance between the need for activity involving a relatively high degree of energy expenditure compared to energy consumption, and the need for enforced inactivity involving a relatively high degree of energy conservation. High metabolic rates tend to be associated with high amount of food consumption relative to body size (e.g., 25% in the mouse vs. 4.5% in the elephant) and with longer sleep time. Longevity may represent the biological "success" of the particular species' balance between energy consumption-related activity and energy conservation-related enforced inactivity (sleep). It is of course entirely possible that within-species differences in sleep time or in quality (e.g., relatively high delta sleep regardless of total sleep time) is positively correlated with longevity. The point is that the negative cross-species correlation between sleep time and longevity cannot be taken as evidence against the hypothesis that sleep evolved to promote the life process (Zepelin and Rechtschaffen, 1974).

The view that sleep enforces inactivity to promote metabolic conservation and physical protection lends itself to comparisons with the view that sleep provides the opportunity to recuperate from the wear and tear of wakefulness. Meddis (1975) has argued that the former but not the latter view is consistent with evidence of very short sleep time, and the possibility of zero sleep time, in some species and individuals. That is, for those organisms capable of efficient metabolic and effective self-protective adaptability, sleep would be of little value. Meddis (1975) reviews evidence of relative sleeplessness in the shrew, Dall's porpoise, and swift, as well as two humans studied in the laboratory who appear to require one hour or less of sleep per night with no apparent ill effects. Meddis does not rule out the possibility that sleep facilitates recuperation as well as the operation of an instinct toward immobilization. Rather, he is impressed with the ability of the immobilization hypothesis to account more readily for individual differences in sleep time. This view would be greatly strengthened were it possible to demonstrate through some neurophysiological manipulation that sleep could be eliminated without immediate or long term adverse effects. Needless to say, no such demonstration has been reported.

Implications for the dreaming process

With two notable exceptions, there has been virtually no experimental data-based speculation regarding the phylogenetic origins of dreaming as a psychological process. Vaughn (1964) conducted a sensory deprivation study of rhesus monkeys which strongly suggests that primates at least have the capacity to experience visual imagery (dreams?) during REM sleep. The technique involved training the subject to make a bar press response contingent upon a series of varying visual stimuli presented on a screen in an otherwise dark room. Once this response was well learned, and after falling asleep, the subject was observed to show periodically vigorous signs of bar pressing behavior *as though* reacting to visual stimuli. This sleep behavior was correlated with eye movement activity. To my knowledge, this study has never been replicated or extended within the context of sleep research objectives. However, because of the potential usefulness of this kind of behavioral paradigm for assessing dreaming capacity at various phylogenetic levels, I would like to suggest a method that would allow stronger inferences to be made about the specific nature of the "dreaming" experience.

Darwin argued that "as dogs, cats, horses, and probably all the higher animals, even birds have vivid dreams, and this is shown by their movements and the sounds as uttered, we must admit that they possess some power of imagination". However, the natural behaviors emitted during REM sleep (e.g., grimacing) are insufficient to establish either that the organism is dreaming (processing information) or that it is consciously experiencing some sort of hallucinated "story". The same can be said for the infant who, during certain phases of REM sleep, *appears* to be reacting to dream imagery. Recall the Roffwarg *et al.* (1966) observation that such apparently sophisticated facial gestures belie the infant's relative immaturity which can be inferred from waking behavior, EEG and brain structure, and limited experience. In addition, it is likely that some degree of ontogenetic and phylogenetic development of cortex is a likely prerequisite for cognition and consciousness. Thus, it is clear that only through a behavioral *experimental* paradigm such as that used by Vaughn will it be possible to assess the "phylogeny of dreaming" which in turn could provide an evolutionary perspective for hypotheses regarding the psychological function of dreaming. However, before I go on to suggest an extension of Vaughn's paradigm, some work done by Jouvet should be mentioned. Jouvet found that when certain pontine nuclei (caudal locus coeruleus) known to inhibit muscle tonus were lesioned in cats they seemed to "act out" their REM periods as though responding to hallucinated predators or prey. Descriptions of such post-lesion behavior cannot do justice to observations. After viewing a movie of this behavior, the hypothesis that these cats are actually dreaming (in full visual hallucinatory sense) is quite compelling. But even given such data, there remains an inference to be put to more rigorous testing.

I would suggest the following experiment to determine more precisely what it is that the nonhuman organism might be dreaming about. A chimp or monkey would make a good subject because it is phylogenetically close to man, and like man, visually oriented. A young subject (say a monkey) is brought up in isolation but with the opportunity to provide himself with a companion on a periodic basis by responding to a discriminative stimulus, e.g., light, in a morphologically unique way, e.g., making a special hand gesture. Let us call it I(s) for instrumental response: social. To establish a control gesture, the monkey could be trained to make a morphologically different response to gain access to food. Let us call it I(f). Given what we know about the importance to most primate species of social contact, the I(s) should be readily acquired and the periodic schedule of social reinforcement of an otherwise isolated monkey should make that companion an extremely salient *incentive* object. During the acquisition phase, the sleep of the subject would be monitored to establish a baseline for both I(s) and I(f). After some time, an extinction of social reinforcement phase would be carried out. That is, I(s) would not yield the companion. There is evidence that at least for certain species, a "disengagement syndrome" (Klinger, 1975) would ensue. This would be composed of at least two sequential phases beginning with protest (agitation, anxiety) and leading to depression (inactivity, "despondency").[11] If, during the REM sleep of these two phases, there is a significant increase in I(s) (compared to I(f) or other nonspecific signs of increased motor activation), we would have a strong basis for inferring something about what the monkey is dreaming about. It is clear that under conditions of loss of a significant social object, the organism is particularly preoccupied with that object and especially responsive to the return of that object (Klinger, 1975). Perhaps the increase in frequency of I(s) would be a sign of the "re-cognition" of the lost object (wish fulfillment?).[12] This kind of research design, applied to organisms at different levels of phylogenetic development, might help to document the origin of cognitive capacity during sleep, to reinforce psychological hypotheses regarding the incentive nature of dreaming, and to provide an evolutionary perspective for evaluating the adaptive significance of sleep mentation.

REM sleep is a salient biological marker for intense psychological experience in man and, in all likelihood, in all the higher species. Comparative and developmental data also suggest that REM sleep is one of those characteristics which serves to define our phylogenetic continuity with both our human ancestors, forerunners, and predecessors. That a phylogenetic perspective for psychological approaches to dreaming seems both desirable and unavoidable is suggested by recent developments in psychology and physiology. First, there is evidence of a strong genetic basis for individual differences in general intelligence, cognitive style, and temperament (Buss and Plomin, 1975; Jensen, 1972). Second, there is growing evidence for the hypothesis that there are marked differences across species in "biological preparedness" for cognitive, affective, and instrumental behaviors (Seligman, 1970). Third, it is now patently clear that we can no longer consider the nervous system merely as a passive, reflective switchboard-type mechanism. Single cell and electrophysiological recordings, as well as behavioral and cognitive studies, clearly indicate that nervous functioning, even during sleep, is spontaneously active. Together, these behavior genetic, comparative, and electrophysiological data constitute an empirical basis for the view that intellectual functions (including dreaming) are strongly influenced by endogenous characteristics of the organism. It is evident that biologically determined wiring greatly affects the rate, selectivity, permanence, and utility of what is learned and also how that learning is expressed cognitively, affectively, and instrumentally.

A number of implications follow. We must seriously question the assumption that the individual is best conceptualized as a "dependent variable" subject to the influence of environmental "independent variables". Arrangement of such relationships in the laboratory may be of questionable ecological validity (Bowers, 1973; Cohen, 1974c).

[11] A third phase, "despair", relatively refractory to the re-presentation of the lost object, is sometimes seen, and might be used as a further "experimental" condition under which I(s) during REM sleep would not be expected to occur.

[12] Chimps like the Gardiners' Washoe, with their demonstrated ability at sign language communication, would be outstanding subjects for the kind of sleep study I am proposing.

Dreaming, like other memory processes, is a *reconstructive* as much as a reproductive process (Bartlett, 1932), an expression of the organismic inventiveness of a spontaneous nervous system. Thus, an adequate theory of dreaming must go beyond an analysis of environmental opportunities and demands. In this respect, Jung's hypothesis that there is an inherited disposition toward symbolic representation of phylogenetically derived organismic characteristics is at least theoretically consistent with the argument developed here.

The treatment of dreaming in the writings of both Darwin and Jung strongly implicate phylogenetic continuity between, and communality within, species in determining similarities in the process of dreaming. Jung's hypothesis, simply stated, is that dream symbolism reflects general (phylogenetically derived) and specific (environmentally derived) *organismic* conditions. "The unconscious ... seems to be guided chiefly by instinctive trends, represented by corresponding thought forms — that is, by the archetypes. A doctor who is asked to describe the course of an illness will use such rational concepts as 'infection' or 'fever'. The dream is more poetic. It represents the diseased body as a man's earthly house, and a fever as the fire that is destroying it" (Jung, 1964, p. 78). And again, "why should one assume, then, that man is the only living being deprived of specific instincts, or that his psyche is devoid of all traces of its evolution?" (Jung, 1964, p. 75). Stripped of the misconceptions that surround it,[13] the nucleus of Jung's vaguely Lamarkian phylogenetic hypothesis of dreaming seems, in its broadest outline, compatible with modern psychobiological concepts, especially that of "biological preparedness":

Just as the human body represents a whole museum of organs, each with a long evolutionary history behind it, so we should expect to find that the mind is organized in a similar way. It can no more be a product without a history than is the body in which it exists. By "history" I do not mean the fact that mind builds itself up by conscious reference to the past through language and other cultural traditions. I am referring to the biological, prehistoric, and unconscious development of the mind in archaic man, whose psyche was still close to that of the animal. This immensely old psyche forms the basis of our mind, just as much as the structure of the body is based on the general anatomical pattern of the mammal. The trained eye of the anatomist or the biologist finds many traces of this original pattern in our bodies. The experienced investigator of mind can similarly see the analogies between the dream pictures of modern man and the products of the primitive mind, its "collective images", and its mythological motifs (Jung, 1964, p. 67).

---

[13] Jung argues that what is inherited is a *tendency* or disposition to transform acquired information in certain ways, that is, to *assimilate* experience according to tendencies that are characteristic of the information processing apparatus produced by evolution. Only the disposition ("the possibilities or germs of ideas"), not the conscious representation (the phenomenological archetype), is inherited; "it would be absurd to assume that such variable representations could be inherited" (Jung, 1964, p. 67).

CHAPTER 3

INFORMATION PROCESSING DURING REM SLEEP

1. CAPACITY TO RESPOND TO INFORMATION

There is a parallel between the hypothesis that REM sleep is a state characterized by information processing and the hypothesis that dreaming is a state which is characterized by problem solving. The former is derived from neuropsychological applications to the observations of sleep and is of relatively recent vintage; the latter is derived from clinical psychological tradition and therefore has a more venerable and luxuriant history. Both hypotheses include some basic assumptions about the adaptive properties of brain or mind. In later chapters we will dwell at some length on the question of adaptation largely from the perspective of the dream. For now, I will describe theory and research that bears upon the problem from the biopsychological approach to REM sleep. The electrophysiological, neurophysiological, developmental, and comparative data clearly imply that REM sleep is an active and nearly ubiquitous mammalian characteristic with an ancient history. These data compel us to pay special attention to brain function and, inevitably, they invite speculation about cognitive mediation.

There are many variants of the idea that information processing is a fundamental characteristic of REM sleep in the more sophisticated organism. One of the more influential of these is Dewan's p (programming) hypothesis (1969). A schematic description will suffice to provide some formal perspective for the discussion of research data that follows. REM sleep is described as one of a number of biological states which has a compensatory role in adaptation with respect to new or current needs. Information representing those needs must of course be recognized and responded to during wakefulness. However, during sleep ("off-line", as it were), this information is subject to further analyses (comparison, computation, revision, integration) and storage. In the process, information that is temporally both recent and remote is revised and transformed from a semipermanent or incompletely coded state to a permanent or completely coded state. Reprogramming can be thought of as a characteristic of mammalian information processing. Fixed action patterns and conditioning (instinctive) s-r mechanisms of reptilian "intelligence" are distinguished from true mammalian intelligence which involves learning *about* the environment and what to do *about* the environment. Presumably, the less programmed (i.e., the less biologically prepared) the organism for specific s-r connections, the more reprogramming is required. Thus, REM sleep, essentially a mammalian phenomenon, provides the opportunity for off-line reprogramming.

The importance of REM sleep to such off-line reprogramming is related to phylogenetic and ontogenetic factors which in turn are related to intrinsic flexibility and sophistication.

For example, REM sleep would be especially important to the processing of information during the infancy and childhood of higher organisms. And in revising brain function (at both the neural and cognitive levels), REM sleep is said to influence behavior. Thus, the hypothesis can be tested, not only by reference to descriptive data on brain function during REM sleep, but through experimental analysis of neurological, cognitive (including dream), and behavioral events which change in predictable fashion. Two approaches can be used. The organism can be challenged or stressed in order to assess consequent changes in REM. Or, REM sleep can be altered or prevented in order to assess consequent changes in other kinds of events. The variety of approaches that I will describe in this and the next chapter can be thought of as a collective test of the hypothesis that REM sleep serves to program information.

Despite pontine-induced inhibition of muscle tonus, there is a good deal of behavioral activity during REM sleep. This activity can be categorized as (a) *spontaneous* when it seems to occur in response to internal stimuli (e.g., sleep talking, tooth grinding, etc.), (b) *reactive* or orienting when disturbing environmental stimuli are present, and (c) *instrumental* when a goal-specific behavior is emitted in response to a cue (or instruction) either given during sleep or learned presleep. Each of these categories of behavior has implications for hypotheses regarding the psychology of dreaming. I will discuss in a subsequent chapter the psychological significance of behaviors in the spontaneous category. Therefore, I will dwell in more detail here on the other two categories of behavior. In addition, I will not emphasize what I think is an artificial (though perhaps convenient) distinction between behaviors that occur during REM sleep and the behavioral aspects of REM sleep. That is, REM sleep itself can respond to external information both non-specifically (changed patterns or the absence of REM entirely) and instrumentally (as when REM sleep changes to NREM prior to an expectable awakening stimulus). Therefore I will use examples of behaviors that occur during REM as well as REM behavior to draw implications about the psychological properties of REM sleep.

REM characteristics and the presleep environment

REM sleep is in some sense a state of vigilance. It can be thought of as a balance between external and internal orientation. Normally, the balance during REM is toward the processing of recent and remote information already in the system. However, novel or threatening information arising from external sources can induce a shift in the balance of attention. There is evidence that organisms pay a psychological price (e.g., postsleep fatigue or poor performance) when this balance is shifted toward external information (Le Vere, Morlock, and Hart, 1975). What is the evidence for this characterization of REM sleep as vigilant?

A most obvious example is the so-called "first night effect". The first time in the laboratory (or, in all likelihood, any new environment), some individuals show disturbances in a number of sleep characteristics such as stage percentages and cycling. Sometimes the first or even the second REM period does not emerge at all. Frequently, the REM dreams of subjects are replete with obvious and symbolic references to the laboratory and experimenter, though there are large individual differences that reflect type of subject and presleep condition. While these effects will be taken up in more detail later, consider the following unpublished data on incorporation of experiment-related information during REM sleep. Twenty-two male subjects, each of whom spent a single night in the laboratory, were divided

TABLE 3-1.   Percentage of "Denier" and "Non-denier" Subjects Showing Evidence of Experiment-related Material (Incorporation) During REM Periods

Group	Time since lights out (hours)		
	3–4	5–6	7
Deniers	50	83	63
Nondeniers	50	60	17

into two groups on the basis of their responses on a presleep mood questionnaire. The "denier" group was composed of 12 subjects whose ratings on the three affect scales were close to the zero (neutral) point. The "nondenier" group was composed of 10 subjects whose rating deviated from zero thus indicating that they were willing to admit (or actually were experiencing) significant affect (positive or negative). Table 3-1 shows that a high percentage of "denier" subjects continued to dream about the experimental situation even by the end of the night. The "nondeniers" showed a decrease after the first part of the night. While the within-condition comparisons only approach statistical significance, they do suggest a potentially important source of individual difference in vigilant behavior.

There is evidence that REM period characteristics continue to reflect conditions of the presleep situation. Baekeland, Koulack, and Lasky (1968) found higher eye movement activity during poststress REM periods, and Goodenough, Witkin, Lewis, Koulack, and Cohen (1974) reported a tendency for eye movement activity and shorter breath times to be associated with film-induced presleep stress and dream affect. The importance of individual differences in REM sleep reactivity are clearly documented by results from a study conducted in my laboratory (Cohen, 1975).

Thirty-one subjects with at least two REM periods were selected from a larger sample described in a different report (Cohen and Cox, 1975). There were 17 high neuroticism $N > 34$) and 14 low neuroticism ($N < 16$) subjects who were classified on the basis of the Maudsley Personality Inventory. The two groups experienced one of two types of presleep condition, one of which was designed to be ego threatening. In the stress condition, 14 subjects were given little information about the experiment, were isolated for at least 15 minutes after having "failed" an IQ test, and were treated in a rather perfunctory manner. The 17 subjects in the positive condition were given a good deal of information about sleep research in general, treated in a friendly manner, "passed" their IQ test easily, and spent a good deal of time with the experimenter while the experiment was being set up. Each subject spent a single night in the lab during which his sleep was monitored in the standard fashion (Rechtschaffen and Kales, 1968). Five minutes after the onset of each REM period (as well as during intermediate NREM [stage 2] periods) he was awakened to obtain information about any dreaming experiences.

REM density (mean eye movements per 20 second epoch) during the first five minutes of the first and second REM was used as the dependent measure.[1] Figure 3-1 shows the results. Commensurate with previous reports, there was significantly more eye movement activity in the negative condition ($p < .03$). However, the effect is almost exclusively due to the

[1] Some subjects from the parent study (Cohen and Cox, 1975) could not be used in this analysis because the relatively short, recording period (7 hours), first night effect delay of initial REM onset, and NREM awakenings conspired to prevent more than a few REM periods from occurring.

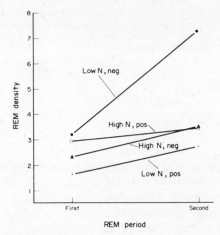

Figure 3-1   Eye movement density during two REM periods for low and high neuroticism (anxiety) groups under positive and negative presleep conditions.

contribution of the low neuroticism subjects. There was a significant interaction for groups and conditions ($p < .007$), which is more clearly marked in the second REM period. That is, compared to high neuroticism subjects who were little affected by conditions, low neuroticism subjects in the positive condition had relatively little REM density while in the negative condition they had a good deal of REM density. What is particularly noteworthy about this differential psychophysiological pattern is that it tends to be opposite to the pattern of results derived from pre-sleep mood data. This differential pattern suggesting greater variation across conditions in the *questionnaire* data of high neuroticism subjects vs. greater variation in the *psychophysiological* data of low neuroticism subjects has been noted in a number of studies (Schwartz, Krupp, and Byrne, 1971) though not always (Lazarus and Alfert, 1964).

It is tempting to speculate about the nature of information processing during REM sleep under presleep conditions that elicit denial of affective involvement (which we have seen tends to be related to laboratory incorporation). Many have speculated on the role of dreaming in working through problems that have not been given sufficient attention during the day due to distraction or defensiveness. This idea is similar to the Poetzl hypothesis which assumes that there is a tendency to become pre-occupied with those aspects of perceptions that are peripheral to the focus of waking attention. Despite failures to support the hypothesis under improved experimental conditions (Johnson and Eriksen, 1961), there is anecdotal evidence for such a phenomenon (e.g., Foulkes, 1966, pp. 149-152). The hypothesis needs to be revised with the qualification that certain individuals (deniers, repressors?) are more likely to give more dreaming emphasis to "innocent day residue" insufficiently attended to during wakefulness if that information is of relatively great emotional importance to the subject. And perhaps one psychological function of REM sleep is to provide a biological context within which to process such information.

A somewhat different approach to the functional significance of REM sleep focuses on the effect on REM characteristics (e.g., eye movements, REM time) of a novel learning situation. It has been hypothesized that REM sleep promotes the consolidation of new learning (Dewan, 1969; Fishbein and Gutwein, 1977; McGrath and Cohen, 1978; Shapiro, 1967).

This idea is similar to clinical views on the role of dreaming in the integration of recent and long term memories that are of affective significance (Breger, 1967). The programming hypothesis is readily testable once the assumption is made that certain characteristics of REM (duration, eye movement density, latency) reflect the amount or intensity of, or motivation for, information processing. However, it should be noted that the assumption is still an empirical question.

Typically, REM deprivation is used to assess the role of REM sleep in the mediation of learning. A little-used alternate technique is to study the characteristics of REM during uninterrupted sleep following learning. For example, Fishbein and Kastaniotis (1973) reported an increase in REM time over baseline in mice trained for one hour on an active avoidance task compared to yoked controls. Likewise, Lecas (1976) reported that REM but not NREM time increased during sleep subsequent to new learning in cats, an effect that was maximal just prior to reaching criterion. In a preliminary study of six 6-month-old babies it was reported that following "successful learning" (head turning response reinforced by visual stimulation), REM time but not quiet sleep time increased over control sessions (Paul and Dittrichova, 1975). In addition, there was no increase in REM time during sleep which followed "unsuccessful learning" (which required a double head turn, too difficult for the babies to learn). This effect of new learning on REM time has been supported in more recent unpublished research (reported at the 1975 meeting of the International Sleep Congress) that suggests a positive correlation between speed of learning and REM increase. There are two extensive reviews of research on the augmentation of REM by enriched, challenging environments and by novel or challenging learning (Fishbein and Gutwein, 1977, and McGrath and Cohen, 1978). Briefly, the animal data are clearly consistent with the hypothesis that REM augmentation is elicited by new learning. In fact, in nine studies using mice or rats or cats, all nine reported heightened REM time or REM% following any of a variety of learning situations. The data on REM augmentation in humans are sparser and less consistently supportive. However, it should be noted that the use of humans to test the hypothesis requires that they be sufficiently challenged by the presleep learning situation. It is now clear that simple paired-associates learning experiences are insufficient (McGrath and Cohen, 1978). One of the more intriguing preliminary observations is the positive correlation between augmentation and incomplete learning. There is evidence that augmentation is maximal during learning, and diminishes at the point where learning appears to be complete. Fishbein and Gutwein (1977) suggest that the augmentation phenomenon is consistent with theories which describe REM dreaming as a problem-solving process or at least as incentive-related information processing.

In addition there is some new (unpublished) evidence that wearing goggles which displace the visual field upside down increases REM time while decreasing eye movement activity (especially that of vertical movement). Unfortunately, the small literature on the effect of manipulations of presleep perceptual processes (as opposed to affective states) on REM characteristics has yielded rather inconsistent findings. Initially, Zimmerman, Stoyva, and Metcalf (1970) reported that wearing goggles that distort the perceptual field is associated with more, and more intense, REM sleep. However, Allen, Oswald, Lewis, and Tagney (1972) were unable to confirm these relationships in a group of subjects who wore goggles that rotated the perceived environment 90 degrees in a counterclockwise direction and which reversed the left and right visual fields. Allen *et al.* (1972), like Bowe-Anders, Herman, and Roffwarg (1974) whose subjects wore goggles that altered perceived color and illumination, found no significant alterations in normal sleep patterning and REM characteristics. These results are not clearly consistent with de la Peña's hypothesis about the relevance of eye movement to information processing (de la Peña *et al.*, 1973). Nevertheless, the *sensory control for information processing* (SCIP) hypothesis is sufficiently important to require some brief elaboration.

It postulates two interrelated aspects that are reflected in both waking and REM eye movement activity: what might be called a trait aspect and what might be called a state aspect. The trait aspect is reflected in the assumption, which is supported by correlational data reported by de la Peña *et al.* (1973), that there is a positive relationship between the intensity of waking and REM eye movement activity. This consistency in level of eye movement from wakefulness to sleep is presumed to reflect the sophistication of the brain in both states. Sophistication is defined as the ability to recognize quickly sensory and cognitive mismatches, to reduce uncertainty, to move on to new information. This ability is reflected in short fixation times, longer eye tracking lengths, etc. Thus, individual differences in these characteristics of waking eye movement and their correlated counterparts during REM will reflect physiological maturation and experience as well as innate capacity.

The situation aspect, on the other hand, is described as a homeostatic regulation of information processing rate as reflected by eye movement activity. That is, *relative to an individual's level of sophistication*, low rates of informational input in one state will encourage relatively higher rates in another state. REM serves to regulate the overall rate of information processing during the 24-hour cycle. Thus, sensory or informational deprivation, relative to the individual's requirement, will induce a compensatory shift in the endogenous flow of information during REM. Thus, combining the trait and situational aspects, the hypothesis makes the following prediction (assuming the validity of eye movement activity as an external sign of rate of information flow): there will be a positive between-subject, but a negative within-subject correlation between eye movement activity during wakefulness and during REM sleep.

The de la Peña hypothesis is particularly interesting for two reasons. First, it suggests readily testable predictions for the more general hypothesis that REM sleep makes an important contribution to the regulation of information processing required for both genotypic and external reasons. Second, it demonstrates the importance of taking into consideration individual differences in the requirement for information. For example, it makes clear why it is important that presleep conditions be defined with respect to the individual. This qualification is discussed later (Chapter 8) with respect to the meaning of "stress" manipulations which are often used to assess the role of REM sleep in emotional adaptation. For example, the SCIP hypothesis would predict that the increase in REM density expected after presleep sensory deprivation would be greater for relatively brighter individuals, while these same individuals would be relatively less likely to show diminished eye movement activity during REM after wearing perceptually distorting goggles. The SCIP hypothesis makes an additional contribution. It requires that we distinguish between the duration of the REM period and the number and organization of events that occur within the REM period. It raises the interesting question that beyond a certain minimum, duration of REM may not be particularly relevant to the testing of some hypotheses. On the other hand, it suggests that some kind of combined measure, e.g., an additive or multiplicative combination of duration and activity, might be more relevant to predictions regarding REM function.

The eye movement data shown in Figure 3-1 and de la Peña's SCIP hypothesis (de la Peña *et al.*, 1973) can be integrated within the context of one of the hypotheses proposed in this book: that there are individual differences in the importance of REM sleep. For example, the responsiveness of the REM sleep of repressors to variation in certain kinds of stressful events (e.g., ego threat, deprivation, etc.) is discussed at length in the next chapter and summarized in Figure 4-1. Suffice it to say here that one reasonable interpretation of the relatively high REM density of stressed repressors is that it represents a compensatory heightening of rate of information processing: Perhaps the "denial" of stress is, in effect, a slowing down of information processing, i.e., a tendency not to pay attention to the stressful event. If it could be demonstrated that repressors under stress show relatively less eye movement density during presleep wakefulness, their relatively greater REM density could more directly be interpreted as a compensatory process within the framework of the SCIP hypothesis. Another possibility is suggested by evidence that suppression of fantasy is associated with high levels of eye movement. Perhaps some individuals show *continuity* (rather than a compensation) between heightened information processing during wakefulness (e.g., during the process of "denial") and the heightening of information processing during REM sleep (higher eye movement density, transformation of dream content into "safe" or symbolically remote representations of the situation, etc.). The point is that, whatever the mechanism, repressors seem more dependent on the REM process to adapt to variations in stress, and the characteristics of their REM periods are more differentially responsive to variations in situations. This hypothesis is taken up in the next chapter.

Thus, if the question "Is REM sleep important?" is put to us, we need to respond with further questions: "For what species?", "Under what kinds of conditions?", "*For whom?*" A major weakness in the REM function literature is the frequent failure to pay attention to individual differences. I trust that one of the contributions of this book will be to point out this problem and to provide some data preliminary to its eventual solution.

REM characteristics and stimuli during sleep

So far, we have been preoccupied with the capacity of REM sleep to respond to information acquired during the day. Next we turn to some aspects of REM responsiveness to information impinging on the subject while he is in REM sleep. This usually involves (a) the capacity to respond to *awakening* stimuli (arousal threshold), (b) the capacity to respond *instrumentally* to cues introduced during REM, and finally (c) the capacity to respond purely *cognitively*, i.e., to dream about the stimulus.

Since animal research (in particular, research on cats) revealed relatively high awakening thresholds from REM sleep, it was considered "deep" sleep. However, the bulk of the research on humans suggests that while the auditory arousal thresholds or behavioral thresholds of responsiveness during REM and stage 2 do not differ appreciably, they are lower than those for stages 3 and 4 (Goodenough, Lewis, Shapiro, Jaret and Sleser, 1965; Rechtschaffen *et al.*, 1966; Wilson and Zung, 1966; Zimmerman, 1970). But note that the issue is complicated by a number of important variables that as yet have been given insufficient attention. First, there are marked individual differences. For example, there are light and deep sleepers, the latter tending more often to be psychologically sensitive, if not clinically disturbed. There is some evidence that women (and possibly male homosexuals) have lower REM awakening thresholds, though these differences are clearer for NREM than for REM and tend to wash out when the awakening stimulus is significant (Wilson and Zung, 1966; Wilson, Zung and Lee, 1973). There is some evidence that proximal (e.g., tactual, somatosensory) stimuli more readily elicit stimulus incorporations in the dreams of REM than do auditory and especially visual stimuli (Dement and Wolpert, 1958; Koulack, 1969). The well-known difference in arousal thresholds from REM sleep for stimuli that require awakening, e.g., a baby's cry, vs. stimuli that do not is clearly important in that it documents the capacity of the REM-sleeping individual to assess the environment continuously for significant information. Relatively little is known about individual differences in this capacity which must have had significance for both males (assessing external danger) and females (responsiveness to infants) during the early evolution of human sleep. With respect to the capacity during sleep to detect and to assess external stimuli in the context of knowledge given by instinct or acquired through experience, Rechtschaffen *et al.* (1966) have this to say: "Surely such an adaptive mechanism represents the product of 'careful' natural selection and deserves attention as a fundamental biological phenomenon. The clinical importance of malfunction of this mechanism, as in the easily disturbed sleep of insomniacs, is apparent" (p. 937).

TABLE 3-2.   Factors that Affect Estimates of "Sleep Depth" and the Capacity to Process Information During Sleep

---

A. *Operational Definition of Responsiveness:*
   1. EEG measures (e.g., alpha, K-complex, evoked potential)
   2. Manual operation (e.g., operating on a thumb switch)
   3. Speech
   4. Dream incorporation

B. *Method of Stimulus Presentation:*
   1. Method of constant stimuli (i.e., measure percentage of positive responses)
   2. Method of limits, i.e., gradual increase in intensity (measure threshold intensity)

C. *Nature of Stimulus:*
   1. Meaningful
      (a) verbal–nonverbal
      (b) awakening required vs. not required
   2. Meaningless
   3. Modality (e.g., visual, auditory, tactile)
   4. complex–simple

D. *Temporal Factors:*
   1. Time of night (e.g., real time, early vs. late REM periods, etc.)
   2. Duration of accumulated sleep time prior to stimulus presentation
   3. Time since last body movement

E. *Biological State Factors:*
   1. Stage of sleep
   2. Body temperature
   3. Phasic events (e.g., K-complex, spindle, eye movement, etc.)
   4. Need state (e.g., presleep manipulation of hunger; prior sleep or REM deprivation)

F. *Individual Differences (normal and abnormal):*
   1. Situational
   2. Dispositional
      (a) intelligence
      (b) temperament
      (c) attitudes, values, interests
      (d) sex

The problem of awakening threshold is inextricably tied to REM dreaming. Although the specifics of the process are unknown, it is clear that responsiveness to external information can be expressed by awakening and/or in dream-incorporating the information; the balance between the two kinds of response modes will depend on initial differences in reception of the information (detection), motivation (to sleep vs. to awaken) and response capacities (e.g., mental innovation that satisfies the requirement of the disturbing stimulus). According to Berger, "the lack of overt response to auditory stimulation during REM periods in humans may be a manifestation, not of elevated auditory threshold, but of a perceptual response that incorporates the stimulus into the dream" (1963, p. 793). Thus, failure to take into consideration the prominence and nature of consciously experienced information processing during REM raises a question about the value of the comparison of REM vs. NREM awakening thresholds in humans.

Beyond the simple observation that delta sleep is associated with higher auditory awakening thresholds to simple sensory stimuli than is stage 2 or REM, the concept of "sleep depth" is obscured by enormous complexity (see Table 3-2). There is no obvious or systematic correlation between various physiological or phenomenological variables and estimates of responsiveness during, or awakening from, sleep (from which we interpret "sleep depth"). Characteristics of REM that might, a priori, be taken as signs of "depth" (e.g., lowered body temperature, little GSR activity, little EMG tension, insensitivity to visual stimulation, relatively low amplitudes of the P1N1 component of the auditory evoked potential) occur simultaneously with characteristics that, a priori, would be taken as signs of "shallowness" (e.g., high neural activity, eye movement, intense dreaming, relatively low auditory awakening thresholds). Despite the large physiological differences between REM and stage 2-NREM, their awakening thresholds are similar. Nor do changes in sleep characteristics across the night provide any help in clarifying the problem. These include increases in ostensible "depth" characteristics (e.g., lower body temperature, lower level of tonic autonomic activity) and increases in ostensible "shallowness" characteristics (e.g., lower auditory awakening thresholds to simple sensory stimuli, more phasic activity in autonomic measures, more intense dreaming, more eye movement activity, more spontaneous and evokable body, limb, and digit movement, flatter recordings of background EEG during stage 2). Without the kinds of qualifications suggested by the list of factors shown in Table 3-2, the concept of "sleep depth" is, at best misleading, at worst, meaningless (Rechtschaffen et al., 1966).

The interrelationship of external information impinging on the sleeping subject and ongoing information processing can be illustrated by two kinds of research, one focusing on the instrumental capacity of the sleeping subject, the other on the capacity to incorporate information into ongoing dreaming.

The capacity of the sleeping subject to make simple responses (button press) to external or internal (dreaming) cues is well known.[2] This responsiveness is enhanced during stages 1, 2, and REM, and especially when punishment (e.g., rude awakenings) is employed (Salamy, 1970, 1971; Williams, 1973). It is also known that, if information presented to a sleeping subject is to be recalled upon awakening, the preawakening EEG must have low voltage fast

---

[2] Fiss reported some preliminary evidence that after repeated awakenings during the middle of REM periods (REM interruption) a subject might terminate a REM period by shifting into stage 2 just prior to the scheduled onset of the awakening stimulus. This suggested that the REM period itself has avoidance behavioral properties. Whether interruption of biological REM or dreaming explains the phenomenon, and whether there are individual differences with important implications is largely unknown at this point.

activity characteristics for a brief period of time (Lehmann and Koukkou, 1973). In the light of what is known about the EEG characteristics of REM sleep, it is perhaps not entirely surprising that an individual can respond instrumentally to cues presented during REM even though the subject does not wake up or show signs of electrophysiological wakefulness (e.g., alpha).

A study by Salamy (1971) provides a good example of how experimentally enhanced REM motivation can increase behavioral evidence of the capacity of the individual to perceive and process information. Salamy assigned four male subjects to each of eight conditions in a $2 \times 2 \times 2$ factorial design. Half the subjects were REM deprived during the first part of the night while the other half were not awakened ("not REM deprived"). Half the subjects were given instructions to press a switch (attached to the preferred hand) three times at the onset of a tone of 35 db re-waking threshold. The other half of the subjects were given the same instructions, and in addition, were awakened abruptly if the response was not successfully executed. A successful response was defined as three presses or two series of two presses with no alpha between stimulus presentation and response. The latter group was defined as the "avoidant" group, the former as "instruction only" group. Half of the subjects were tested during REM sleep while the other half were tested during stage 2-NREM sleep. All testing was done during the last 2.5 hours of sleep when no REM deprivation was employed.

The results suggested that experimental conditions had relatively little differential effect on stage 2 responding; average successful responding ranged from 22 to 43%. The lower figure was attained by subjects in the REM deprivation-instruction only condition, and probably reflected the effect of sleep loss and the absence of a motive to respond. The effect of conditions on responding during REM sleep was dramatic. In the non-deprived condition, "punishment" elicited more response success (38%) than no punishment instructions only (14%). However, prior REM deprivation (high REM motive) elicited the greatest response success (85%) while instruction only elicited the least response success (1%). This study demonstrates the motivation to remain undisturbed in REM sleep and the capacity of individuals to process information during REM about the immediate external environment. It illustrates the problem of designing experimental conditions that can reveal the capacity to adjust while asleep, a capacity which is not always evident from mere observation of a sleeping organism.[3]

Now consider the remarkable study by Evans, Gustafson, O'Connell, Orne, and Shor (1970) which further demonstrates this capacity. Over a two night sequence, subjects were given four suggestions by an experimenter *while they were in* stage 1 (REM). For example, "Whenever I say the word 'itch', your nose will feel itchy until you scratch it." Suggestions regarding moving the pillow, the cover, and a leg, each to appropriate cue words, were also given at different times. After two suggestions were administered, only cue words (e.g.,

---

[3] There is also evidence of behavioral and electrophysiological responsiveness to external information during NREM sleep. For example, Oswald, Taylor, and Treisman (1960) demonstrated that subjects could discriminate personally significant from nonsignificant names presented auditorily during stage 2. During the presentation of the former, subjects often produced K-complexes suggestive of electrophysiological "recognition". Gastaut and Broughton (1965) reported a dialogue between an experimenter and a sleeping (stages 2 and 3) child. Despite brief EEG signs of alpha during sleep speech, the record remained basically a sleep record while the child "interacted with the experimenter". The child responded to the questions "Do you hear me?" and "Are you asleep?" by saying "Yes". Thus evaluating what the sleeping individual can do requires that we distinguish between the capacity for and presence of significant information processing vs. the relative inability to retrieve that information upon awakening.

"itch") were used on both nights. Testing occurred during the same REM period, across the REM periods of the night, and during REM periods across the two nights. No more than two suggestions were employed on a single night. In brief, the following results were obtained. First, recognizable reactions were obtained in 16 of 19 subjects (89 correct responses for 416 cue administrations of which an unknown number may not have registered or may have elicited dreaming rather than overt behavioral reactions). Occasionally a behavioral sequence was associated with alpha activity. However, the latter was lower in frequency than the waking alpha. There was no relationship between degree of eye movement activity and presence of a correct response. Postsleep recall of suggestions or responses was largely fragmentary. Despite this, correct responses to cue words were obtained at about the same frequency across REM periods of a single night and during REM periods on the second night ("carry over condition").

There were marked individual differences in the capacity to respond accurately to the cue words. Four of the "responders" who were brought back to the laboratory five months later responded to the cue work presented during REM even though they showed no evidence that they were aware of the procedure during wakefulness. Incorrect responses had a shorter latency than correct responses suggesting that "correct processing of information during sleep is slow". A total of 86 cues were inadvertently given to 11 subjects during NREM (stage 2). Only 8 responses were elicited, and these came from two of the "responder" subjects. Considering the evidence that awakening thresholds of REM and stage 2 are not significantly different, it is likely that this failure of carryover of REM-acquired responsiveness to NREM represents a state-dependent learning effect rather than differential receptivity to information. However, the latter cannot be ruled out since the information was originally learned within the context of REM states which in turn may affect the receptivity of the information.

The extraordinary capacity of some individuals to acquire chained instrumental responses during REM is illustrated by the following. "After one S had been presented with the cue work 'itch', he scratched his nose for several seconds, adjusted his pillow by pushing it into a new shape with both hands, pulled his blanket above his head, and kicked with his left leg, pausing between each successive movement. There was no EEG evidence of arousal. He had been given these four suggestions, in this sequence, during the two nights. Repetition of any of the four cue words failed to elicit further response. When the next stage 1 (REM) period occurred, presentation of a cue word again elicited the same sequence of responses, but no more responses could be elicited with another cue word. In the final stage 1 period, the same sequence occurred again. This time the S repeatedly thrashed his left leg with considerable violence. By responding in sequence to all suggestions, then failing to 'acknowledge' further stimulation, he attained a deceptively low response rate. This kind of 'response chaining' was observed with at least two other Ss" (Evans et al., 1970, p. 183).

These remarkable findings have a number of implications about the nature of REM sleep. First, they indicate that "simple" kinds of new learning can take place during sleep. However, they do not recommend sleep learning as efficient. Clearly the important thing about REM sleep is in the inventive processing of information that is already in the system (e.g., reprogramming) rather than acquiring new information or responding to old information. Second, they demonstrate that information processed during REM is relatively confined to that period, i.e., it is state-dependent. This kind of finding illustrates why much of the experience of REM sleep is lost upon awakening. It suggests that there are individual differences in "state boundaries" which in turn may determine the importance of REM sleep and the probability of REM dream recall. The potential influence of ongoing information processing and dream consciousness during testing must be considered in the full explanation of the results. Finally, individual differences in motivation to respond, detection threshold, and "preference" for behavioral vs. cognitive response surely must influence the data.

In Berger's important study (1963) of the effects of stimuli presented during REM sleep, the focus is on dream "re-cognition". Implicit in the formulation of the study was the assumption that cortical analysis of the environment continues during REM sleep. Further it is assumed that significant (meaningful) stimuli become part of the ongoing dream rather than eliciting wakefulness, especially if those stimuli do not contain information suggesting that wakefulness is required (see the earlier study of Dement and Wolpert, 1958). On the basis of GSR reactions during wakefulness, Berger selected two important names (of friends) and two neutral names which were used as nocturnal stimuli. These were presented on tape, 5-10 minutes after the onset of each REM period during 4-6 nonconsecutive nights. The name was repeated a number of times until some signs of arousal (EEG flattening) but not wakefulness (alpha) were observed, 20 seconds after which the subject was awakened and inquiry about mentation was made. The order of name presentation was random.

Because of the clinical richness of the material, the reader is urged to consult the original paper. Basically, Berger found much evidence of direct and symbolic transformation of the name stimuli. For example, after the presentation of the name Jenny (the subject's girlfriend), a dream about opening a safe with a jemmy was elicited. This example may represent incorporation by assonance, though a psychoanalytic interpretation may be more satisfying to some. Other examples include a dream response to the name Gillian which was about a woman from Chile (a Chilean, get it?). In response to "Naomi" a subject dreamed of traveling with "an aim to ski". And I'm going up with a friend who says, "Oh!" Despite the fact that some of Berger's interpretations strain credulity even in the most receptive of readers, he was able to demonstrate that both subjects and judges could match stimuli with dreams well beyond chance. There were no differences in the apparent concordance of emotional vs. neutral stimulus names and dream content.

General remarks

Thus, we have a number of studies which clearly document the degree to which the subject during REM sleep is capable of vigilance regarding the external environment. The data include responsiveness in terms of electrophysiological, behavioral, and phenomenological changes. There are other more anecdotal sources of evidence on this point.[4] We typically do not fall out of bed despite the well documented fact that there is a tremendous amount of gross bodily movement throughout the night. In addition, we are often able to awaken just prior to the onset of the alarm. Also, dreams are more conservative (less erotic, aggressive), and sleep talking less pronounced when we sleep in the laboratory than when we sleep at home. It is as though the continued analysis of an unusual external

---

[4] Recently during one of our sleep recording sessions an experimenter brought some rather pungent tacos to the laboratory. Shortly afterward, at about 3 a.m. a subject was awakened to obtain REM dream content. The subject reported that she was eating tacos! Since this was the first taco dream we have ever attained in our lab, it is probably not a fortuitous coincidence but rather a true example of olfactory incorporation.

situation tends to inhibit psychological processes. This psychological conservatism can be observed even for subjects who so wish to please the experimenter with interesting dreams that they label as "weird" rather ordinary and pedestrian dream events. Table 3-2 summarizes some of the major factors that influence external manifestations of information processing during sleep.

Assessment of the biological significance of REM vigilance must take into consideration the capacity to discriminate both the important from the unimportant, and that which urges awakening from that which does not. In addition, individual differences in detection and processing capacity (a kind of sleep intelligence) must also be involved. Dreaming is an intimate part of the vigilance process; it is a kind of re-cognition (or re-creation in both the intellectual and playful sense) which mediates overt response or the lack of it.

Popular opinion is divided with respect to the capacity of the sleeping individual. One view is that sleeping individuals can do a great deal: solve problems, learn Russian. Another view is that sleep is a waste of time during which nothing much is going on. Both are extremes that miss the mark. The truth lies somewhere inbetween and requires experimental methods of ingenious design. I am reminded of the classical experiment on latent learning done by Blodgett (1929). Rats not rewarded with food in the goal box at the end of a maze performed "poorly" compared to rats rewarded with food. The nonrein-forced rats made many "errors" while nosing their way through the maze. Of course, the stupidity was not in the rats but in the assumption that a performance curve can, under all conditions, permit direct inferences about what has been learned (what is known). For when food was suddenly made available, those "stupid" rats made no more errors on the next trial than did the rats who had been reinforced all along. What looks like an "error" under some conditions may, under other conditions, reveal something of great biological significance (exploring the environment in more detail). What seems rather limited, perhaps "stupid", about sleep may, under the proper experimental manipulations, prove to be of great psychobiological significance.

Yet in saying all this, I do not mean to romanticize the phenomenon or the phenomenology of sleep. "Experiments in nature" (Hartmann, 1973) clearly indicate that, in theory, humans might be able to get along without sleep. That is, while the instinct to sleep is typically powerful, and the functions of sleep (and dreaming) are significant, this is true because of the nature and organization of brain activity. Alter the latter and what is carried out largely in sleep could, in theory, be carried out during relaxed wakefulness. There are individuals who hardly sleep at all, and are apparently no better or worse than the rest of us. Genetic diversity includes the possibility of virtually zero sleep instinct (Meddis, 1975). There is no a priori reason to reject the hypothesis that those factors which induced the evolution of the sleep instinct, somewhat rearranged, could promote longer and longer periods of wakefulness (though a recent unpublished breeding study on mice revealed a relatively greater difficulty in the genetic selection of short sleep than of long sleep). These remarks are offered merely to put the problem in better perspective, to suggest that despite individual differences that may include a few "nonsleepers", we need to know more about the nature and function of sleep and dreaming which engages much of the time of most human beings.

I have reviewed evidence, largely from the phenomenology of the REM period, that dreaming sleep is primarily concerned with the processing (transformation, recombination, metaprogramming) of stored information more than with reception and storage of informa-tion that impinges upon the organism during sleep. Berger's (1963) study is a good example of this kind of thing. John's approach to the neurophysiology of information processing (John, 1976), typically applied to waking subjects, might be profitably exploited in the area of sleep. He has studied the EEG consequences of information input, learning, discrimination, and extinction. For example, as learning progresses, certain EEG patterns and average evoked potential characteristics emerge over different brain sites. These changes suggest temporal and formal properties of a neurological model of the external world. In addition, they indicate a certain degree of neurological "independence" or abstraction which has an effect on subsequent input (what Piaget would call "assimilation"). Under these conditions, the induced pattern is different from that imposed by the same information input to a naive organism.

Under certain conditions, an EEG pattern which typically follows as a direct consequence of a given stimulus is observed during the interstimulus interval. In fact, such a pattern may be observed when the organism is placed in the testing situation, but before the stimulus is presented, and therefore prior to, and independent of, any skeletal or autonomic responses. John interprets such a pattern as a representation of rehearsal (what, in Piagetian terms, might be called accommodation, but accommodation that is relatively stimulus free). In fact, this phenomenon can be observed on the trained side of a split-brain cat. By using the "rehearsal" or recognition pattern the p hypothesis could be used to test the acquisition of "knowledge" independent of performance. Take, for example, the classical conditioning paradigm. Let us assume that a stimulus (S) is associated with a "detection" pattern in the EEG. A UCS (e.g., shock) could be employed that is associated with an "arousal" EEG pattern. After pairing S and UCS, the S would elicit a "recognition" EEG pattern (i.e., the S would become a CS). The effect of REM deprivation on postsleep recognition could be assessed, i.e., it would be a test of memory independent of performance.

The implications for the investigation of information processing during sleep seems obvious. The ability of organisms to detect and process both novel and previously experienced information could be assessed by a combination of computer analysis of EEG characteristics and a comparison of these and dream phenomena retrieved through REM awakenings. Differences between sleep and wakefulness in reliable patterns might reveal at a neurological level the difference between the two states in information processing. Such an approach might go a long way to provide both a neurological model of "primary" vs. "secondary" processing, and a bridge between the phenomenology and neurophysiology of the dreaming process. In addition, such an approach might provide a more useful means of operationally defining the difference between states, and thus more satisfactory answers to the question of the degree to which state-dependent learning is a factor in dream recall.

Up to now I have been discussing REM sleep as responsive to the environment, how its behavioral and cognitive structure can accommodate to the structure of the stimulus situation. But we can ask a different and more interesting question. Does the information processing of REM sleep contribute to postsleep adaptation? This question will be discussed in great detail in the last chapter from the perspective of dream content. At this point, I would like to pose the following empirical question: under what conditions does REM responsiveness to presleep events mediate a more adaptive accommodation to those events? In the next section of this chapter I will describe research that has approached this question somewhat indirectly by assessing the effect of REM deprivation on postsleep behavior. REM deprivation methodology is analogous to lesion work which seeks a better understanding of what a neurological structure mediates by removing it or making it nonfunctional. Most of this work has been done on animals, and most is concerned with the sleep physiology and behavior of animals rather than on dreaming *per se*. However, implications about the nature and function of dreaming can be drawn from such studies, and there are studies of human experience that can be tapped.

2. EFFECTS OF REM DEPRIVATION ON PERFORMANCE

REM deprivation methodology

While the research on human subjects is of most direct relevance to speculations about dreaming, I will briefly discuss REM deprivation of animals which suggests a learning and memory consolidation function for REM sleep. (For more detailed reviews, see Fishbein and Gutwein, 1977, and McGrath and Cohen, 1978.) Various techniques to affect REM deprivation have been used. The most popular is that suggested by Jouvet. It takes advantage of the fact that head and neck muscles become extremely relaxed during REM sleep. Placing animals on small inverted flower pots surrounded by water allows the animal to have NREM sleep. The transition to REM sleep, with its accompanying muscular atonia, insures that the animal will either awaken spontaneously or fall into the water and awaken. Suitable controls for the stress induced by such a procedure (e.g., wetness, confinement) must be used (e.g., large flower pots). Other methods have been used, e.g., REM suppressing lesions, REM suppressing drugs, mechanical awakenings, etc. (see Vogel, 1975, and McGrath and Cohen, 1978 for discussions of the problem of control in such studies).

Regardless of the validity of the technique, we should keep in mind that deprivation of a biological event does not necessarily permit strong inferences about the role of that event. That is, "when we seriously disrupt any biochemical mechanism the resulting products may have toxic properties, but this does not prove that the adaptive value of that mechanism is the destruction of those products; under natural conditions they are innocuous chemical links in the vital process" (Snyder, 1966, pp. 124-125). One would not want to infer from the behavioral disruptions caused by choking an organism that *the* function of breathing is to prevent such behavior. Nevertheless, it would be misleading to discount the potential yield from REM deprivation methodology. We have learned a great deal about brain function from fortuitous and experimental lesions. Similarly, we can learn much about sleep function(s) by employing REM deprivation supplemented by other techniques.

There are two general paradigms which employ REM deprivation that have been used extensively in animal research. One can REM deprive, train the animal, and then either evaluate learning ability or, after a rest period, test for retention. One can train, REM deprive, and test for retention. The former, or "prior-REM deprivation" paradigm assesses the effect of REM loss on initial learning; the latter, or "subsequent-REM deprivation" paradigm is primarily concerned with the effect of REM loss on consolidation and retrieval. (Over a number of days the use of both prior and subsequent REM deprivation, or "mixed-REM deprivation" paradigm, can be employed.) Consider the following example of the REM deprivation-train-test paradigm (Hartmann and Stern, 1972). REM deprived rats spent 96 hours on inverted flower pots (6 cm). Stress control animals were immersed in cold water twice a day when they were not otherwise housed in their home cages. Non-stressed controls remained in their home cages. These procedures were followed by active avoidance task learning (to cross from a grid to a safe platform on signal to avoid shock). REM deprived animals clearly required more trials (14.3) than did either control group animals (about 9.5) to learn to avoid the shocks. AMPT (a catecholaminergic blocker) produced a performance deficit in both REM deprived and nonstress control animals while L-Dopa (a catecholaminergic facilitator) yielded performance in REM deprived animals that was midway between that of REM deprived and nonstress control performance levels. These results suggested that REM sleep is implicated in animal learning and that REM deprivation interferes with catecholaminergically mediated information processing.

A particularly elegant study strongly implicating a role for REM sleep in the consolidation of short term to long term memory was reported by Linden, Bern, and Fishbein (1975). One group of mice was given 72 hours of REM deprivation by the water pedestal technique while another constituted a REM non-deprivation control. At the end of this time, all animals were given a passive avoidance learning trial. Each animal was shocked when it entered the dark (instinctively preferred) chamber in a light-dark choice apparatus. Half of the animals was then given electroconvulsive shock (ECS) while the other half was given sham ECS. Each of these two groups was exposed to the ECS or sham ECS condition after one of eight intervals from learning: 0, 5, 15, 30, 45, 60, 180, 360 minutes. Seventy-two hours later, each of the 32 subgroups constituting the 2 (REM deprivation vs. nondeprivation control) × 2 (ECS vs. sham ECS) × 8 (learning-to-ECS, or learning-to-sham interval) design was tested for retention. Retention was operationally defined as latency to entering the dark compartment (maximum recorded time 300 seconds).

Results shown in Figure 3-2 clearly support a hypothesis regarding the function of REM in memory consolidation. First, all of the sham ECS (REM deprived or nondeprived) subgroups had long latencies (good retention) regardless of handling interval. The REM

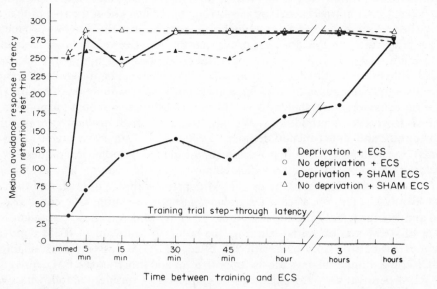

Figure 3-2 Prolonging the fixation phase of memory consolidation: Retrograde amnesic effects of ECS on paradoxical sleep (PS) deprived and control mice. Inhibitory (passive) avoidance test latencies: Mice are (1) deprived of PS for 3 days (or controls), (2) trained, (3) treated with ECS at one of several intervals after training, and (4) tested for retention 3 days (72 hours) later. Each point is based on 16 animals (from Linden *et al.*, 1975, p. 410).

nondeprived ECS subgroups also had good retention with the one exception of the subgroup given ECS immediately after the learning trial. ECS given 5 minutes or longer after initial learning had virtually no obvious effects on latency. On the other hand, the REM deprived-ECS subgroups, with the one exception of the subgroup given ECS 360 minutes after learning, had markedly short latencies (indicating poor retention). There was a clear trend for the REM deprivation-ECS subgroups to show better performance (longer latencies) as a function of the duration of the interval between learning and ECS. The marked difference in performance between two sets of REM deprivation subgroups, one getting sham ECS and showing no deficits vs. the other getting ECS and showing marked deficits, provides an elegant demonstration that REM deprivation *per se*, given prior to learning, affected consolidation rather than motivation or performance.

The method of using REM deprivation prior to learning in all animals is particularly impressive because it eliminates the problem of finding a suitable control condition to assess the effect of REM deprivation. The results of the mouse studies using this (Fishbein and Gutwein, 1977) and the more traditional train-REM deprive-test method (discussed below) suggest the following tentative conclusions. First, in its initial state, learning is in the form of a labile short term memory (STM). REM deprivation prior to learning interferes with the consolidation or strengthening of the labile STM so as to delay or prevent its transformation into long term memory (LTM). Second, REM deprivation prior to learning will therefore have minimal effect on STM, but will make it susceptible to disruptive conditions like those imposed by ECS. Third, extended REM deprivation (e.g., carried out over a number of days) may affect LTM, making it susceptible to ECS. Fourth, *brief* REM deprivation *following* learning may actually facilitate the STM-to-LTM transformation by virtue of the central arousal it promotes. That is, the disruption effect of ECS may be minimized either by REM sleep or even by brief REM deprivation (two conditions of central arousal) which follow learning and precede ECS. This is in marked contrast to the disruptive effect on learning by ECS which follows learning preceded by REM deprivation (as in the Linden *et al.*, 1975 study). These generalizations, based on mouse data, pose an interesting challenge to investigators of human learning and REM sleep.

Nevertheless, the evidence from prior REM deprivation studies is not highly consistently supportive of the hypothesis that REM sleep prepares the organism for learning. In 10 rat studies using REM deprivation prior to learning (passive or active avoidance), five supported the hypothesis, four were not supportive, and one was contradictory (see Table 3-3, p. 100, for a summary of these and other findings, and McGrath and Cohen, 1978 for details). The evidence from three human studies indicated support in two, and nonsupport in one. This is not particularly impressive considering the fact that research failing to support, or actually contradicting a hypothesis is less likely to be published. On the other hand, it is clear from the human data that the nature of the learning task is quite important in determining the effect of REM deprivation regardless of whether it comes prior to or subsequent to learning.

Now consider an example of a study using the train-REM deprivation-test paradigm. Pearlman and Greenberg (1973) gave rats training in a shuttlebox avoidance task involving signalled shock. Five groups of 10 animals each, equated for performance on the last 10 trials, were treated as follows. One group was REM deprived for two hours immediately following training (flower pot technique). The second group was given imipramine (a powerful REM suppressant). A third group was given phenobarbital. A fourth group was allowed to remain undisturbed in home cages for two hours following training and then was REM deprived. The last group was allowed normal sleep after training. Retention for the last two groups was roughly the same and significantly better than that for the first three groups. The results support the hypothesis that REM sleep mediates the consolidation of new information (learning) and the prediction that the effect of *immediate* REM deprivation (by whatever method) is to interfere with short term memory.

The subsequent REM-deprivation method has yielded relatively consistent support for the hypothesis that REM sleep participates in consolidation of new learning (see Table 3-3, and McGrath and Cohen, 1978 for details). Four of four mouse studies and three of eight rat studies were supportive (for a total of seven out of twelve animal studies), and none contradicted it. Of ten studies using humans six showed evidence in support of the hypothesis, four did not.

Thus, the training-REM deprivation-test paradigm suggests that REM sleep may be more relevant for complex, biologically "unprepared" (Seligman, 1970) tasks. For example, Pearlman and Becker (1973) compared the effects of immediate and delayed (by three hours) REM deprivation vs. control conditions on the retention of place learning ("prepared") vs. discrimination learning ("unprepared") in rats run in a Y maze. REM deprivation was carried out after each session over a number of days. By the tenth session on the discrimination task, immediate REM deprivation (affected by flower pot or drug) elicited performance that was inferior to that of subjects under control conditions (including undisturbed sleep, saline injections, delayed REM deprivation via pedestal technique, delayed REM deprivation via REM suppressing drugs). On the other hand, position learning ("prepared") was not adversely affected by REM deprivation.

The animal work on REM sleep as a state of information processing (consolidation, storage, retrieval) has raised as many questions as it has answered. It has encouraged more sophisticated questions regarding the parameters of deprivation and the nature of the task to be learned. The strength or credibility of the evidence for the information processing hypothesis of REM sleep depends on the paradigm that has been employed.

Demonstrating that REM deprivation affects behavior does not necessarily constitute evidence that the normal function of REM contributes in an important way to that behavior. Nevertheless, a combination of paradigms (e.g., augmentation of the REM of undisturbed sleep plus adverse effects of REM deprivation) would, in principle, provide a much stronger basis to argue in favor of the hypothesis. Let us consider a hypothetical example of how the problem could be approached. Suppose that we want to test a variant of the *p* hypothesis which says that REM sleep is important to processing information that is *currently* important to an organism. First, we have to select a "problem" that is graded to the organism which we will use in the experiment. We can assume that difficulty and emotional importance are two task factors that need to be defined. A task that is too easy or too difficult will probably gain little from REM sleep since no learning is involved. Clearly what is important to a rat is not, in a concrete sense, comparable to what is important to a college student. Let us use the rat because it is easier to define operationally the parameters of importance in rat-relevant tasks. Importance would be defined with respect to (a) current needs (motives or drives) and to (b) time. For example, shock-avoidance learning would be more important during the acquisition phase. That is, once the animal "knows" what to do, once the animal has "closure", the adjustment required is no longer a "current problem". It is no longer an emotional or intellective issue. We will assume that REM sleep is important only for new learning that still requires accommodation or consolidation. We will not assume that REM is necessary for this, only that REM supplements or extends the accommodation process. It therefore follows that REM sleep will be particularly important to a current concern which has not yet been completely learned at the onset of sleep. Hypothetically, the more trials the animal gets, the closer the animal will be to a state of accommodation or closure. The number of trials required will depend on the difficulty of the task, the biological preparedness of the organism for learning that task (with difficulty and preparedness being correlated), the emotionality associated with the learning, and between-trial opportunities to consolidate "off-line". At some point, a certain amount of wakefulness will suffice to complete the consolidation. Prior to this point, which we will assume has been determined beforehand, a test of the p hypothesis for REM sleep can be made. It would be predicted that the importance of REM sleep will inversely be related to the amount of wake time remaining after the last trial and prior to sleep onset: the more wake time available to consolidate, the less important the REM period to that particular learning situation.

We can set up three groups of rats, each group composed of animals who are given a sufficient number of trials to reach the point at which reliable performance requires merely additional time off line to consolidate. (Metaphorically speaking, the animal requires no further reinforcement or direct experience, but merely time to "think about it" in order to "get the idea".) Group I goes directly to sleep. Group II gets a short interval (say 1 hour) while Group III gets a long interval (say 2 hours) of wakefulness. The general hypothesis is that REM sleep will be more important to the final consolidation of learning the less waking time available subsequent to the last trial, i.e., REM sleep will be more important to Group I than to Group II, but more important to Group II than to Group III. This general prediction can be tested via two methods, and ideally, both should be used. Group I should show more signs of changes in REM characteristics (e.g., eye movement density, duration of REM periods, total REM time, etc.) compared to baseline measures. In addition, REM deprivation should be associated with more trials required to reach error-free performance in Group I animals than in Group II or Group III animals. If we can rule out performance or output deficits (retrieval), we are in a position to argue from the perspective of two paradigms that REM sleep is important to the learning of tasks, i.e., to the "solution" of current concerns.

This kind of strategy is being exploited more, and is yielding results that are favorable to the p hypothesis (see Leconte and Hennevin, 1973; Leconte, Hennevin, and Bloch, 1974). By describing some of the complexities of the problem at the relatively simpler animal level, it should be clear what a formidable task awaits the researcher who works at the human level. How do we select and grade problems for difficulty, interest, and concern so that they become relevant to the REM process? How do we control the temporal factors underlying degree of accommodation so that we can choose a point in the process which maximizes the relevance of the problem to REM? How do we deal with the fact that humans vary tremendously in intellectual ability and emotional involvement, and are as likely to assimilate the problem to their own needs as to accommodate themselves to the structure of the task? The complexity of human mental operations defies experimental control of the relevant variables. And how do we recognize the relevance of REM to specific problems in the cognitive productions of the individual? How do we deal with the incredible flexibility of the human nervous system which permits endogenous adjustments that counteract something like REM deprivation? If REM sleep is unavailable, is it not likely that NREM sleep can "take over"? The complexity of the brain function and mental operations at the human level simply defy experimental control. No wonder that results are hard to come by or are rather subtle.

REM sleep and information processing in humans

Consider the following experiment which tested the hypothesis that REM deprivation would interfere with an information processing function. Chernik (1972) gave 32 subjects a series of verbal learning tasks prior to (test for retention effects) and after (test for acquisition effects) either two nights of REM deprivation (16 subjects) or NREM control awakenings (16 subjects). A postexperimental performance task (crossing out the number three on lists of random numbers) to measure speed of scanning and two adjective checklists to assess mood were also administered. Both groups of subjects were matched on time in bed, time asleep, and number of awakenings. The REM deprivation group averaged about 10 minutes of REM (a little over 3% of total sleep time) for the two nights combined vs. about 68 minutes (about 21% of total sleep) for the controls. Although there were trends in the expected direction on the various learning, performance, and mood measures, none of the differences was statistically significant. Chernik concluded that "the results did not show any substantial effects of 2 days of REM sleep deprivation on learning, retention, mood or performance" (1972, p. 293).

I believe that this well-designed study did more than any other to dissuade investigators from the hypothesis that REM sleep has a singular status with respect to information processing. However, a number of arguments (and data) can be mustered in support of a more optimistic view. First, the animal literature suggests that we must pay attention to the nature of the task. It may be that biologically prepared tasks, especially if they tap what Jensen (1969) calls Type I (nonconceptual) intelligence, are inappropriate for testing the information processing hypothesis for REM sleep (Dewan, 1969). Or, the emotional significance of the task may be of major importance (R. Greenberg, in Chase, 1972, pp. 245, 250-251; Greenberg and Pearlman, 1974; also R. Greenberg, personal communication, May, 1973). Against both these criteria, the paired-associate and number cross-out tasks used by Chernik appear to be inappropriate.

Second, it may be that in humans, the effect of REM deprivation is a more subtle change in personality, a change which mood ratings simply do not tap and which the laboratory setting may inhibit. That this is not merely a perfunctory rationalization can be demonstrated by findings in the "split-brain" research area. Commissurotomy does not induce obvious changes in behavior or personality. The hypothesis of duality of consciousness (Sperry, 1968) is based on effects that are revealed only when rather sophisticated and inventive techniques are used (e.g., controlling visual scanning by use of tachistoscopic presentation of visual information input).

Third, there is always the possibility that while REM sleep has some unique function(s), the flexibility (redundancy of function) of the nervous system allows other states to take over during suppression of the REM state.

Fourth, it is possible that individual differences account for much of the statistical insignificance of the main effect. Perhaps REM deprivation affects only some individuals who are less likely to be selected for study in certain laboratories. For example, I will discuss in the next chapter the evidence that repressor types are in some ways more affected by REM deprivation than are sensitizer type subjects. Yet Chernik advertised for subjects by announcing that the experiment would involve sleeping in the laboratory. Since sensitizers are more likely to volunteer for such an experiment, Chernik has a built-in bias against finding effects (see Kruglanski, 1973 for a cogent discussion of volunteer artifacts). Let us consider some additional REM deprivation studies, keeping in mind the potential importance of the material, and the individual differences.

Empson and Clarke (1970) presented three kinds of information to 10 pairs of volunteer subjects. One set included a list of 32 nouns derived from four categories (e.g., animals, vegetable, etc.). A second set included five grammatically correct but meaningless sentences (e.g., "The academic liquid attended a deep bar"). These two sets of information were repeated five times before the third set was administered. This consisted of a 162 word prose passage which included anomalous information. For each pair of subjects, one was randomly assigned to the REM deprivation condition, the other was yoked to the first in order to control for awakenings. Results indicated that REM deprived subjects were slightly poorer in sentence recall, and especially poor in prose passage recall. A measure of restructuring of the sentences and prose passage yielded a nonsignificant trend supporting a "reprogramming" hypothesis for REM sleep. Thus, despite possible bias against the hypotheses (because of volunteer subjects), there was evidence that REM sleep plays some role in the restructuring or memory of material of a more complex and conceptual nature.

The potential role of REM sleep in emotional adaptation or psychodynamic regulation is suggested by a number of studies. Greenberg, Pearlman, Fingar, Kantrowitz, and Kawliche (1970) found little evidence of an effect of REM deprivation over three nights (compared to three nights of NREM deprivation) on various cognitive tasks (e.g., digit symbol subtest of the WAIS) in three volunteer subjects. However, they did find evidence of an effect on projective test measures, not with respect to the conventional determinants such as form, movement, color, etc., but in terms of psychodynamic changes, e.g., a change from inner-directed to outward-directed hostility. The authors concluded that "our earlier hypothesis about memory storage does not seem to hold true ... the need, like a computer, to discard extraneous information would probably not hold either ... [but rather] ... with dream deprivation [sic], feelings and wishes which have been kept out of consciousness now appear more overtly in the test protocols ..." (Greenberg et al., 1970, p. 9). These results are consistent with those of Fiss (1969), who found a similar effect for REM interruption, with those of Dement, Henry, Cohen, and Ferguson (1967) showing drive enhancement in REM deprived cats, and with evidence that schizophrenics are not particularly affected by REM deprivation. These results are partially consistent with those reported by Clemes and Dement (1967) who found little effect of REM deprivation on cognitive tasks (e.g., color word test, embedded figures test) or on mood ratings, but a significant effect on projective test (TAT, ink blot) measures (e.g., increased "need" and feelings, "pathonomonic verbalizations").

A more ambitious and sophisticated test of the hypothesis that REM sleep has a role in emotional adaptation was reported by Greenberg, Pillard, and Pearlman (1972). Twenty male and female college students provided baseline measures on a number of physiological dimensions (e.g., heart and respiration rate, skin potential) and were given the Psychiatric Outpatient Mood scale. They were then shown an interesting film about computer generated tones during which the physiological measures were again taken and after which the mood scale was given. A week later, subjects returned to the laboratory and the procedures (i.e., assess level of anxiety — show film — assess level of anxiety) were repeated except at this time a stressful film on autopsies was shown. During the night following this procedure five subjects were allowed uninterrupted sleep, nine were REM deprived, and six were awakened from NREM sleep. The next morning, the testing and stress film showing were repeated.

The results obtained in the presleep situation indicated that compared to the computer film, the autopsy film was more stressful (on mood ratings and on physiological measures). In addition, the REM deprived group showed less adaptation on the second (postsleep) viewing of the stress film than did the control group. Despite correction by analysis of covariance, the fact that the REM deprived group had greater "tension anxiety" *prior to*, as well as subsequent to, the postsleep viewing of the stress film than did the control group raises a question about the significance of the postfilm group differences. Does the finding indicate a failure of adaptation (supporting the general hypothesis) or does it contribute a potential artifact with respect to the pre-post analysis for the second viewing? In addition, there is some reason to question the relevance of a basically external stress in a test of the hypothesis that REM sleep is important in "psychodynamic regulation". That is, a distinction between the external threat and the internal stress may be important. I will discuss this distinction (which Greenberg has urged upon us [personal communication, October, 1972]) in more detail later.

Nevertheless, the investigators concluded that "when an individual meets a situation that is stressful for him the stressfulness is due to the arousal of memories of prior difficulties with similar situations. The person's initial defensive reaction is usually of an emergency or generalized type such as global denial or repression. Then, during the dreaming experience, these feelings from the past and the current stressful stimulus are integrated, and the individual's characteristic defenses for that particular set of emotions and memories are used to deal with the current threat. If the stress is re-experienced, he now has available his characteristic (for him most efficient) means of dealing with the threat. Thus, re-exposure to the stress should not produce the initial degree of anxiety" (Greenberg *et al.*, 1972, p. 260). This hypothesis, while only marginally supported by the data of this experiment, is consistent with the popular theories of the integrative nature of REM dreaming processing (e.g., Breger, 1967) and is actually more strongly supported by the results of a different study which I now describe.

Grieser, Greenberg, and Harrison (1972) selected subjects high on "ego strength" (thus possibly introducing a bias toward finding REM deprivation effects, i.e., those seen in repressors).[5] This procedure was utilized because it has been found that high ego strength subjects are more threatened by, and thus emotionally involved in, tasks that are interrupted prior to completion. A basic assumption tested by the study was that REM sleep facilitates defensive emotional adaptation to stress thereby permitting more rational and open acceptance and assessment of the stress. In the words of the investigators, "dreaming serves to integrate current stressful experiences with similar experiences from the past, thus enabling the individual to use his basic coping mechanisms (defenses) to deal with the current stressful situation [items which the subject is made to fail but which he believes are solvable] . . . initial reaction of the high ego strength *S*s is the repression of that material associated with a sense of failure. Only with dreaming are other mechanisms of defense

---

[5] The investigators report that repression-sensitization scores obtained on subjects did not account for significant amount of variance in recall data. However, due to the restrictive sampling of subjects, variation in repression sensitization may have been artifactually attenuated.

available for use, leading to a lessened need for repression" (Grieser *et al.*, 1972, p. 281). The major prediction of the study was that REM deprivation would interfere with the recall of uncompleted anagram items compared to a NREM awakening control condition.

The presleep anagrams task was given to each of 10 subjects per group. The task was promoted as an intelligence type test and 10 cents was paid for each word successfully recalled. Thus, ego involving motivation was maximized. The anagrams test was developed so that roughly half of each set of letters could not be solved in the 45 seconds allowed. After initial administration of anagrams, subjects were divided into four groups.

Group 1 had two hours of wakefulness prior to retesting for recall of failed or solved anagrams. This group provided a control for amount of time between testing and falling asleep experienced by the sleep group subjects. Group 2 had 10 hours of wakefulness between testing and retesting in order to control for the total wake plus sleep time interval of the subjects in the two sleep groups. Group 3 subjects were REM deprived, and Group 4 subjects were NREM-awakened in yoked control fashion (each NREM subject was paired with a REM deprivation subject in terms of number and time of awakenings). Dependent variables were ratios of (a) completed anagrams recalled to number of completed anagrams, (b) failed anagrams recalled to the number of failed anagrams, and (c) the difference between these ratios.

In general, NREM subjects recalled a greater proportion of *failed* anagrams than did REM deprived subjects though there was no difference between these groups in the recall of *completed* (nonstressful) anagrams. This latter finding supports the hypothesis that REM sleep is not especially significant in the recall of nonthreatening material, and lends support to the argument that REM deprivation is not necessarily more stressful than NREM awakenings. In addition, the finding of better recall for *failed* items than for completed items in the NREM group supports the hypothesis that REM sleep plays a role in the "reintegration of ego defenses". Finally it was found that the two sleep groups had better recall for both failed and (especially) for completed items than did the subjects in the two awake condition groups (both of which had similar and slightly less recall of failed than completed items). This study by Grieser *et al.* (1972) must stand as one of the most elegantly designed, well thought out, and convincing sources of support for a psychological theory of REM sleep and dreaming.

This important study deserves more than cursory description, and it raises some questions. First, the prediction that REM deprivation interferes with recall of failed items because it interferes with integrative (defensive or psychodynamic) processes is somewhat ambiguous. The ambiguity stems from two sources, one logical, the other methodological. The logical problem is that ambiguity inherent in the parent theory (psychoanalysis) would not necessarily lead one to make the same prediction. Seligman (personal communication, April, 1976) has suggested that dreaming about the failed items might allow a reduction of the Zeigarnik-like process of heightened recall for failed incompleted items, thereby reducing recall for them. REM deprivation should be expected to heighten recall. In addition, it might be said that dreaming would allow individuals normally disposed to use repression to continue to use repression against the failed items. That is, rather than interfering with recall, REM deprivation should facilitate recall by interfering with the smooth operation of the psychodynamic defense of choice. Nevertheless, the same laboratory has demonstrated in other studies (e.g., Greenberg *et al.*, 1972) that REM deprivation appears to interfere with emotional adaptation (suppression or repression of affects and fantasies). Presumably, the motive to repress would be maintained in REM deprived subjects. Had Grieser *et al.* been able to show that REM deprivation induced repression in repressors rather than in sensitizers, their conclusions would be even more convincing.

A methodological problem is noted in a recent review of the Grieser *et al.* (1972) study. Fishbein and Antrobus (1974) make the following observation. The subjects who were to be REM deprived initially failed significantly more anagrams (7.9) than did the NREM subjects who constituted the control group (4.7). Since, in the morning, the REM deprived group recalled 29% of 7.9 items for a total of 2.3 vs. 54% of 4.7 items or a total of 2.5 items for the NREM group, it is not entirely clear that REM deprivation had the predicted effect. The reviewers admit that the *post hoc* statistical controls did appear to handle the problem though they remain "uncomfortable" about the initial difference between the treatment groups, for "the major conclusion of the paper hangs on this one statistical manipulation" (p. 316). Nevertheless, it should be pointed out that the reviewers express admiration for the study.

A second point regards the implicit assumption that dreaming and REM sleep are synonymous. If the authors mean that REM sleep is the major physiological context within which the really important dreaming processes occur (which I believe is the interpretation intended), then there is no problem. However, it should be pointed out that a kind of dreaming, often indistinguishable from REM sleep mentation, occurs throughout the night in NREM sleep (Foulkes, 1966). REM deprivation can only restrict REM dreaming.

Lewin and Glaubman (1975) tested the effect of REM deprivation on different types of tasks for 12 subjects who served as their own NREM awakening controls. Two "production" tasks and two memory tasks (parallel sets of each to be used on REM deprivation and control nights) were used. The memory tasks included a serial memory list of 21 nonsense syllables and a free recall list of meaningful words belonging to eight categories and arranged in random order. The production tasks included a word fluency test and the Guilford Utility test. The effect of REM deprivation vs. NREM control awakening conditions on morning performance depended on the nature of the material. Specifically, REM deprivation was associated with poorer performance on various measures of "divergent thinking" such as uses fluency and originality. However, REM deprivation did not adversely affect performance on the memory tasks compared to the NREM control condition; and one measure, percentage of syllables remembered in the same serial position as presented, showed a significant REM deprivation advantage! The investigators tentatively conclude that REM sleep involves divergent (creative?) information processing. This conclusion fits nicely with anecdotally and clinically based theories about the creative function of dreaming (e.g., Krippner and Hughes, 1970 about which I will have more to say later). However, there is some ambiguity in the findings. Since there was no training prior to the differential sleep conditions, all that can be said about the REM deprivation used in this study is that it affected the *performance* (not the mediation of learning/consolidation) of certain kinds of material. That is, REM deprivation may, in some individuals, heighten unknown processes that interfere with performance immediately subsequent to sleep disturbed by REM deprivation.

Considering the importance of information processing in theories about the role of REM sleep it is remarkable how few data there are on the effect of REM deprivation on dreaming. Pivik and Foulkes (1966) reported an intensification of REM dream fantasy in repressors after REM deprivation. Also, there is enhanced eye movement activity during the REM periods of repressors subjected to presleep or REM deprivation stress (Cohen, 1975; Pivik and Foulkes, 1966). These findings are commensurate with the hypothesis that repressors under stress experience a heightened intensity of dreaming. Rechtschaffen (1964) and Fiss (1969) reported that repeated REM interruption heightens the degree of continuity of dream themes. Fiss, Klein, and Shollar (1974) reported that the dreams of two subjects (volunteers with significant psychopathology) were more intense, vivid, more clearly narrated (but not more bizarre) after a regime of REM interruption than after a regime of REM awakenings made at the end of each REM period. In addition, the interruption condition elicited more eye movement density but fewer signs of sleep disturbance (e.g., body movements, alpha, intrusion of stage 2), suggesting that interruption "purifies" while intensifying the REM process. Finally, there was evidence that REM interruption (partial REM deprivation) elicited dreams that were more clearly related to subject preoccupations established preexperimentally through clinical interviews. While these results must be considered tentative, they do seem consistent with the empirical support by the Grieser *et al.* (1972) data for the hypothesis that REM deprivation prevents defensive "relaxation". That is, the REM interruption procedure (unlike total REM deprivation) enhances the REM process, intensifies the dream experience, makes it *less* bizarre; in short, both the preoccupation and the adaptive (defensive) reaction are enhanced by conditions that "purify" the REM process. Of course this interpretation is rather speculative, but it may have some truth to it.

Consider one additional set of findings from a study reported by Cartwright and Monroe (1968). On experimental nights subjects were REM deprived during the first half of the night. When awakened, they engaged in either a fantasy or a digit span test. REM rebound was assessed during the second half of the night (the final 3.5 hours). It was defined as the difference between REM percentage for the second half of the experimental night vs. the second half of the baseline night. A negative correlation (—.45) was obtained between amount of fantasy and REM rebound. On the other hand, a positive correlation of .80 was obtained between digit span performance and REM rebound. The investigators concluded that secondary process cognitive activity necessary for good digit span performance is antithetical to the cognitive activity of the REM state, while cognitive activity during REM (reported upon awakening) that is commensurate with good REM functioning "substitutes for" lost REM functioning. These preliminary results[6] may be considered consistent with those reported by Lewin and Glaubman (1975), Fiss *et al.* (1974), Pivik and Foulkes (1966) and Cohen (1975) suggesting that REM sleep is particularly suited to divergent, emotionally significant, personally relevant information processing. However, whether these observations support a hypothesis regarding a psychological debt (e.g., need to complete a dream, need to have a certain amount of fantasy, need for a type of fantasy) independent of a physiological debt (e.g., suppressed instinct for a particular state of sleep, altered state of bioamine functioning, etc.) cannot be resolved by these data because changes in dreaming may be concomitants of physiological changes.

Table 3-3 provides a summary of the results generated to date from studies based on one or more of four paradigms used to test psychological theories of REM. The table is derived from a review of the literature reported by McGrath and Cohen (1978). An uncritical acceptance of the figures in Table 3-3 will be misleading since there are many factors which affect the results upon which they are based. For example, the type of learning/cognitive problem

---

[6] These results should be considered tentative because there are now data which are not consistent with them. I will discuss these in Chapter 4.

TABLE 3-3.　Summary of Results Generated by Research Based on Paradigms Appropriate to Testing the Hypothesis that REM Sleep Mediates Complex Adaptive Behavior

Name	General paradigm	Purpose	Subjects	Outcome[a] +	0	−
Prior-RD[b]	RD − Train	Role of REM in preparing learning	Rats	5	4	1
			Mice	2	2	0
			Humans	2	1	0
			total	9	7	1
Subsequent-RD	Train − RD − Test	Role of REM in retention/emotional adaptation	Rats	3	5	0
			Mice	4	0	0
			Humans	6	4	0
			total	13	9	0
Mixed-RD	Train − RD − Train and/or Test − RD − Train and/or Test	Related to either preparation or retention/adaptation	Rats	12	2	0
			Mice	0	1	0
			total	12	3	0
Nondeprivation	Train − Assess REM (REM%, REM density, REM latency, etc.) − Train and/or Test	Related to either preparation or retention/adaptation	Rats	5	0	0
			Mice	3	0	0
			Humans	7	11	0
			total	15	11	0

Note:　Totals refer to individual and qualitatively different conditions or studies within a report rather than reports. If the same type of REM deprivation was used to test an effect on two different kinds of task, each test is tallied. However, if REM deprivation is merely varied parametrically, those effects occurring above some predicted threshold are considered together as supporting or not supporting the hypothesis. A specifically predicted noneffect is considered support. This decision reflects the importance of the nature of task to the hypothesized relevance of REM. The failure of investigators to deal with this question produces results that may seriously bias the tallies against the hypothesis (see McGrath & Cohen, 1978, for discussion). Note also that the figures do not represent independent or equally convincing tests of hypothesis. Some of the tallies are based on more than one study or condition reported by a single laboratory.
[a]+ represents support, 0 represents nonsupport, and − represents contradictory evidence.
[b]RD refers to REM deprivation.

used in a study appears to have a significant effect on results. This and other factors are discussed in detail in the McGrath and Cohen (1978) review.

　　The research described in this and the following chapter raises at least four major methodological problems of potential theoretical significance. First, it is customary for many investigators to speak of "REM need". This term is ambiguous. With respect to the human REM deprivation studies (published between 1960 and 1975) that I am familiar with ($N=22$), the ten which deal with the "need" concept operationally define it in terms of REM *rebound*.[7] But the "need" is also manifested in changes in REM latency, and none of the studies reports data on changes during the night in REM *latency* (i.e., the latency to each REM period from prior stage 2-NREM sleep onset). Strangely, there is almost no information in the literature on the correlation between REM latency changes and REM rebound. We have found it to be quite low. Also, I suspect that some people are more sensitive to the disruption of the *timing* of REM while others are more sensitive to reduction in the *amount* of REM. The fact that latency and rebound measures of REM "need"

---

[7]　An exception is a recent study of mine which I discuss in the next chapter. I will ignore this study in the comments made here.

generally are inversely related to each other as a function of the duration of REM deprivation is no reason to ignore their functional difference.

Second, all of the 22 studies referred to above which employ a "control" condition define that condition in terms of NREM awakenings. While such a procedure controls both for a number of awakenings *per se*, and time of night of the awakenings, it does not control from number of REM *interruptions*. That is, a subject in the REM deprivation condition not only has less REM sleep, but more REM interruptions compared to a subject in the non-deprivation control group. While there is probably no satisfactory solution to this problem (REM deprivation subjects will always have more REM periods and more REM interruptions), a possible compromise might be to awaken subjects of the control condition at the estimated end of each REM period as well as during REM-NREM periods. Thus, we can at least insure that all REM periods of all subjects will be interrupted. However, even with such a procedure it is desirable to know to what extent NREM awakenings introduce sources or artifact which make difficult any comparisons between deprivation and non-deprivation groups. If a NREM awakening delays the onset of a subsequent REM period,[8] the control group might have fewer REM periods than expected. This might induce greater REM pressure than desirable. It would make it even more difficult to interpret the effect of REM deprivation vs. nondeprivation treatments on postsleep behavior. In addition, sleep onset latencies after NREM (vs. after REM) awakenings might be quite different. Many studies do not report total sleep time for the two groups. If the deprivation and nondeprivation (NREM awakening control) groups were matched on number of awakenings, it is quite possible that one group might have less total sleep time than the other because of longer sleep onset latencies per awakening. To what extent do the effects of the conditions imposed on the two groups depend on differential sleep time over and above the effects of REM restriction? Often we cannot assess this because the information is not available.

A third question is what goes on during the interval that the subject is forced to stay awake after each awakening? With few notable exceptions (Cartwright and Monroe, 1968; Koppel, Zarcone, de la Pena and Dement, 1972), none of the REM deprivation studies has utilized systematic variation in conditions imposed on the subject during these intervals. Yet the Cartwright and Monroe (1968) study, and one which we just completed, strongly imply that what the subject does (e.g., fantasy vs. intellectual effort) may have a very substantial effect on the dependent variable(s). And such differential effects may carry heuristically powerful implications of hypotheses about the functional significance of the REM process.

Finally, again with a few exceptions, the REM deprivation literature is silent with respect to individual differences. We will take up this problem in the next chapter. It is interesting to note that virtually everything that has been said about the observations and implications of REM deprivation refers to males only. Of the 22 studies on the effect of REM deprivation on REM need, postsleep performance, and characteristics of the sleep process, almost all have employed only male subjects. None has employed sufficient numbers of females to carry out comparisons across sex, and none has discussed this possibility. Of the 236 subjects run in these 22 studies, only about 7% were females. It is immediately obvious why

---

[8] Our experience suggests that NREM awakenings will have a greater effect in delaying the onset of a subsequent REM period the longer the duration of the sleep interval between the prior REM period and the subsequent NREM awakening. That is, the roughly 90-100 minute REM to REM cycle is more or less preserved if control NREM awakenings are made within 15 minutes (rather than, say 30-45 minutes) after a REM period.

it may be impractical to employ female subjects in sleep studies. However, large sex differences discussed in the next chapter strongly suggest that this individual difference variable must be addressed in the future. It should be clearly understood that virtually all of what is known about REM deprivation refers to males only, and that there is good reason to suspect that some of these comments may not apply to females.

CHAPTER 4

MOTIVATIONAL CHARACTERISTICS OF REM SLEEP

1. MOTIVATIONAL ASPECTS OF REM SLEEP

Physiological vs. psychological function(s) of REM

Does REM deprivation enhance the motive for a physiological state or a type of experience? Can we distinguish between a physiological and a psychological or phenomenological need? One way to demonstrate that a dreaming function is distinguishable from a physiological function of REM sleep is to show that REM *sleep* deprivation and REM *dream* deprivation have different effects. This was the rationale underlying a technique described by Fiss (1969). Fiss argued that the need for REM sleep is qualitatively different from the need for dreaming. Therefore while total REM sleep deprivation should be worse than partial REM sleep deprivation, total REM dreaming deprivation should not be as detrimental as partial REM dreaming deprivation (dream interruption). Fiss demonstrated that, compared to total REM deprivation, repeated REM *interruption* elicited more salient, revealing, and more dysphoric interpretations of TAT cards which were presented to the subject upon awakening. Increased anger in these stories suggested that REM interruption was more frustrating and thus more disturbing than was REM deprivation. Fiss also obtained some evidence that under repeated REM interruption across nights, subjects could avoid interruption by shortening their REM periods so that they would be in NREM sleep at the time of the scheduled awakening. These observations suggested that REM interruption is psychologically more noxious than is REM deprivation. Consider the following dream report from one of my subjects who may have been especially sensitive to the repeated REM interruptions used to obtain content reports. It comes from the sixth of seven REM awakenings:

> I was thinking about trying to suppress REM sleep so you'd leave me alone. Several times I felt myself falling into it — my heart would beat faster and I caught myself and stopped it. [The subject then describes some content fragments involving TV show characters. Again the subject explains that the thought processes included a vague awareness of physiological activation and a desire to suppress it to prevent being awakened.]

Fiss' interpretation that REM avoidance permits a functional distinction between a REM-physiological need vs. a REM-psychological (dream) need is equivocal because it is based on a questionable assumption. Fiss assumed that for a physiological process like REM sleep, the relationship between degree of deprivation and degree of disruption is *linear*, while for a psychological process like dreaming, the same relationship is *curvilinear*. Fiss' argument implies that the need for REM sleep is a motive like hunger from which it would be predicted that the more the deprivation, the more disruptive the consequences — that is, total deprivation is more detrimental than partial deprivation. However, if REM sleep is hypothesized to satisfy an instinct like elimination, then total deprivation might be better than partial deprivation. For example, interrupting the act of urination is more disturbing than (temporary) prevention! Thus, the comparative effects of interruption vs. total deprivation do not unequivocally indicate a functionally separate role for the psychological, as opposed to the physiological, aspects of REM.

Another method to separate the psychological from the physiological aspects of REM was used by Cartwright and Monroe (1968). Subjects were REM-deprived during the first half of the night only, after which they were allowed uninterrupted sleep. After each awakening, the subject was either given a digit span task or was asked to describe his dream. The investigators obtained the anticipated REM rebound during recovery sleep in the second half of the night (i.e., during the last 3.5 hours) only for subjects given the digit span task. The investigators suggested that engaging in fantasy can partially satisfy a psychological need that is normally provided by REM sleep. Therefore, REM rebound in the digit span subjects is partially the result of a blocked psychological need, and individual differences in REM rebound reflect individual differences in the need for fantasy (or the ability to obtain fantasy in states other than REM).

These data are partially congruent with some preliminary findings reported by Fiss (1969). They suggest that the ability to inhibit REM duration under conditions of continuous REM interruption depends upon the behavior that occurs immediately following awakening: when subjects are asked to engage in secondary process type behavior rather than to tell stories to TAT cards, the inhibition effect does not occur. However, the inference that primary process fantasy experienced during wakefulness is able to substitute for REM dream experience is seriously compromised by at least three considerations. First, while dreaming is certainly hallucinatory, it is not necessarily best described as primary process. Since I will deal more extensively with this issue in Chapter 6, I will not discuss it further here.

Second, Koulack (1973) recently reported a preliminary study of six subjects who were given either a dull arithmetic task or a hypnogogic reporting task for 10 minutes after each awakening during REM deprivation. The hypnogogic reporting task involved reporting whatever came to mind while the subject wore ping-pong ball halves illuminated by diffuse light accompanied by white noise. Each subject was run in each condition (half of the subjects getting the arithmetic task first, then the hypnogogic task, the other half experiencing the opposite order of conditions). As expected, REM rebound the following night was greater for five of the six subjects when given the arithmetic task than when given the hypnogogic task.

At first these results appear to confirm the Cartwright and Monroe (1968) findings and speculations. The problem is that verbal reports of the subjects under the hypnogogic condition were not especially marked by primary process or hallucinatory quality. If we wish to talk about the substitutability of certain types of experience that presumably reduce REM motivation, it will be necessary to specify more carefully what it is that is being substituted. This point is further reinforced by the evidence that REM rebound is reduced if REM deprived subjects are allowed to walk around (mild exercise) during each lost REM period (Vogel, Giesler, and Barrowclough, 1970).

Finally, the results of the Cartwright and Monroe study could not be confirmed for subjects in a recent study (which I describe in more detail below). It should be recalled that the Cartwright and Monroe study utilized a rather small sample and produced rather modest effects. Thus, the whole question of fantasy substitution for REM sleep is seriously questioned.

We can conclude two things from the results of these kinds of experimental strategies. First, there is only modest evidence that psychological events may, under certain conditions, influence the motivational characteristics of REM. Second, individual differences will have to be taken into consideration in making inferences about a psychological function for REM sleep which is separable from a physiological function. It is this assumption that provides a rationale for the following review.

What does REM deprivation do to the organism?

The "classic" REM deprivation study was reported by Dement in 1960. Using a within-subject design, Dement found that, compared to NREM awakenings, REM awakenings cause the following three phenomena: (a) increased REM pressure (attempts to get back into the REM period upon falling asleep after each awakening), (b) increased REM rebound (significantly higher proportions of postdeprivation sleep devoted to REM compared to baseline REM proportions), and (c) psychological distress. It is somewhat ironic that in his discussion of the data, Dement (like the popular press) focused on the psychological, rather than the physiological aspects as suggested by his comments about "anxiety, irritability, and difficulty concentrating"; it is just this behavioral deficit which has been least replicable in numerous subsequent REM deprivation studies (see Vogel, 1968, 1974, 1975 for the most cogent and critical reviews of REM deprivation research). For example, Dement hypothesized that "a certain amount of dreaming each night is a necessity" . . . that "pressure to dream builds up with the accruing dream deficit" . . . and that "if the dream suppression were carried on long enough, a serious disruption of the personality would result" (p. 1707). These quotes provide an illustration of how facile was the assumed synonymy of REM sleep and dreaming in the early days of modern sleep research (Cohen, 1970).

It is imperative to recognize the risk in generalizing about dreaming when these are based on REM sleep and postsleep behavior patterns that are obtained in REM deprivation studies. In fact, while the pressure and rebound effects of REM deprivation have more or less been replicated, the data do not indicate that REM sleep is necessary for biological survival or psychological well-being. Despite the motivation to return to REM sleep, organisms can survive indefinite REM deprivation (carried out by mechanical means) with little overt "symptomatology". In fact, there is now good evidence (e.g., Vogel, 1975) that individuals who appear to be at highest risk for psychological disruption (e.g., psychotic depressives and schizophrenics) are not adversely affected and, in some cases, are actually improved by REM deprivation! However, that lack of reliable evidence that REM deprivation adversely affects some humans is not evidence that REM sleep makes no contribution to behavior. On the other hand, evidence that REM deprivation does interfere with certain kinds of behavior is not unequivocal evidence that normally occurring REM sleep makes a positive contribution to that behavior.

Motivational properties of REM sleep have been inferred from the pressure and rebound induced by REM deprivation. I have discussed the hypothesis that catecholamine restoration is a principal need that REM sleep fulfills, a need that presumably builds up during REM deprivation. Stern and Morgane (1974) discuss evidence that pharmacologically-induced catecholamine facilitation during REM deprivation can reduce or eliminate REM rebound during recovery sleep. There is one additional source of evidence that catechol-amine facilitation can at least partially "substitute" for the REM process. Steiner and Ellman (1972) reported that intracranial self-stimulation (via electrodes which delivered current to reward sites, e.g., median forebrain bundle) during REM deprivation was associated with relatively little REM rebound in rats. Departing from their admittedly tentative explanation of the results, it seems reasonable to interpret the data in terms of the Stern and Morgane hypothesis (1974) that intracranial self-stimulation (ICSS) facilitates the catecholamine process thereby partially satisfying the need for REM sleep. ICSS appears to increase noradrenergic activity along a ventral tract (hypothalamus, preoptic area, stria terminalis) during ICSS (Arbuthnott, Fuxe, Ungerstedt, 1971).

An alternative explanation for these deprivation effects, diametrically opposite to the catecholaminergic restoration hypothesis discussed earlier, is that *chronic* REM deprivation permits the build-up of catecholamines (Dement *et al.*, 1967; Steiner and Ellman, 1972). I have suggested the possibility that REM deprivation might induce a gradual shift toward a catecholaminergic balance at the expense of cholinergic processes. This hypothesis could explain why chronically REM-deprived cats show heightened drive (feeding and sexual behavior, general hyperactivity) as well as the yet unexplained therapeutic advantages of REM deprivation in the psychotically depressed (Vogel, 1975). Such a hypothesis explains why electrical stimulation (either ICSS or ECS) and phar-macological agents purported to increase catecholamine activity reduce or eliminate post-deprivation REM rebound.

Selective deprivation of specific stages of sleep has been used to test the hypothesis that REM and NREM sleep serve different functions. The evidence is that while both types of sleep may satisfy a general need for rest (or the instinct for inactivity) (Johnson, 1973a), NREM sleep is more specialized for vegetative or bodily "restoration" while REM sleep is more specialized to serve a *psycho*biological function. I have already summarized some of the evidence for such a distinction (see Table 1-1). Indeed, the hypothesis that psychological processes are more important characteristics of REM than of NREM sleep is a fundamental working assumption for the organization of material of this book. However, our emphasis on REM sleep and its psychological implications should be placed in proper perspective. There is now good evidence that NREM sleep is in some ways biologically more fundamental. For example, after total sleep deprivation, NREM stages are more characteristic of recovery sleep than is REM (though it should be noted that this differential recovery is more clearly observed in humans than in animals). Stage 4 deprivation is followed by stage 4 rebound (Agnew, Webb and Williams, 1966). Total sleep loss preceding selective stage deprivation elicits significantly greater stage 4 pressure but not REM pressure (Moses, Johnson, Naitoh and Lubin, 1975b). Finally, there is greater retention of material learned presleep if the interval between training and testing is devoted primarily to NREM than to REM sleep (Barrett and Ekstrand, 1972). While both REM and NREM types of sleep have instinctive and motivational characteristics which make them important from a biological point of view, REM sleep appears to support more intense, complex, and active psychological characteristics, and thus is a more attractive object of study for psychologically oriented investigators.

2. INDIVIDUAL DIFFERENCES IN THE MOTIVE FOR REM SLEEP

REM pressure and REM rebound induced by REM deprivation suggest that REM sleep has motivational properties and, consequently, that REM sleep is psychobiologically "important". Individual differences in the deprivation-induced REM motive have not been discussed in the animal literature. Individual differences at the human level are striking and are beginning to attract empirical and theoretical attention. I will discuss the work on individual differences in the characteristics of REM sleep and dreaming which suggest that REM sleep may be more important for some individuals than for others.

Preliminary research

Cartwright, Monroe, and Palmer (1967) were the first to explore empirically the potential factors underlying individual differences in motivational aspects of REM sleep. Their preliminary work suggested that highly anxious males have greater REM *pressure* under REM deprivation while individuals who tend toward field independence (a characteristic related to concepts like good "ego boundaries", psychological compartmentalization, etc.) tend to have high REM *rebound*. In a more recent paper, Cartwright (1972) reported evidence that individuals with elevated scores on the ScK (schizophrenia) scale of the MMPI (both clinically schizophrenic or nonclinical subjects) were less likely than individuals with low ScK scores to show a differential pattern of dreamlike fantasy for REM vs. non dreamlike thought for NREM awakenings. That is, the former two groups showed a similar level of REM and NREM fantasy (measured by the Foulkes Df scale)[1] which was intermediate between the low NREM and high REM fantasy of low ScK subjects.

These findings suggested that there are individual differences in the permeability of "boundaries" between biological states. For some individuals, dreamlike fantasy is not restricted to REM sleep but rather may appear in NREM, and even in wakefulness. The careful reader will recognize, in the use of a fantasy task during REM deprivation as a substitute for REM experience, an experimental simulation of reduced boundary between states. Thus, if it is fantasy rather than a physiological REM-like process which suffices to reduce subsequent REM rebound, an argument for a general (state-independent) psychological need can be supported. As we will see, the evidence suggests rather that the degree of REM rebound seems to be a function more of the permeability of physiological state boundaries and correlated psychological characteristics (e.g., repression-sensitization, right vs. left handedness, etc.) than so-called substitutive experiences.

The boundary permeability hypothesis was consistent with some data and speculation offered by Dement and his colleagues in a number of their papers (e.g., Dement *et al.*, 1970; Dement and Mitler, 1974). They found that administration of PCPA in cats releases PGO activity (normally confined primarily to REM sleep) into NREM and wakefulness. Under PCPA conditions, there is little or no REM rebound after REM deprivation. Note too that actively ill schizophrenics (whose behavior is reminiscent of PCPA cats, e.g., frenetic, "hallucinatory") show little or no REM rebound after REM deprivation (Dement *et al.*,

---

[1] The Foulkes Df scale (Foulkes, Spear and Symonds, 1966) is a heterogeneous combination of three dimensions: recall (vs. no recall), hallucinatory (vs. thoughtlike) experience, and bizarreness (vs. conventionality).

1970; Gillin and Wyatt, 1975; Gillin, Buchsbaum, Jacobs, Fram, Williams, Vaughan, Mellon, Snyder and Wyatt, 1974). In addition, there is a preliminary report that some schizophrenics (acute onset, severe thought disorder, good prognosis) show enhanced PGO-like phasic activity during NREM (Watson, Liebmann and Watson, 1976a).

Taken together, the data suggest that the REM period is a state formed by the confluence of events (e.g., PGO, eye movement, low voltage, fast EEG, EMG suppression, hallucination) any one of which can be inhibited, separated, and/or expressed in a different state. Further, it follows that the more that these characteristics are confined exclusively to the REM period, the more they resist displacement to another state (e.g., NREM); that is, to the degree that the REM state "boundary" is relatively nonpermeable, REM deprivation will induce more intense motivation for REM restoration. Thus, individuals (e.g., acute schizophrenics) who show REM characteristics in NREM or wakefulness would not experience the same degree of "REM deprivation" as would individuals who confine all their REM characteristics to REM sleep. What about variation within the limits of normal personality? Do normal individuals vary in their need for REM sleep and dreaming as expressed by significant variation in REM intensification (increased REM pressure, increased REM rebound, increased phasic activity and dream fantasy intensity during REM)?

TABLE 4-1.   Some Characteristics Associated with Questionnaire Estimates of Emotionality Levels

Area of functioning	Repressor	Sensitizer
Physiological/medical	Organic disturbances, less medical help seeking, higher pain tolerance	Psychological problems (e.g., tension, headache); frequent medical problems
Affective-mood-temperament	Energetic, active, calm, inhibited, slow, stable, persistent, patient	Apathetic, excitable, impulsive, uninhibited, insecure, easy-going, irritable, complaining
Intellectual	Alert, ingenuous, broad and varied interests, clear thinking, original and fluent in thought, well informed, thoughtful	Coarse, constricted in thought, stereotyped in thinking, narrow, opinionated, shrewd, shallow, lacking self-direction, easily disorganized by stress
Social-work	Ambitious, enterprising, industrious, productive, strict, thorough, conscientious, responsible, practical, cooperative	Lacking self-discipline
Social-interpersonal	Competitive, helpful, honest, sincere, socially self-conscious (concerned about making a good impression), sociable, outgoing, tolerant, better adjusted	Overly judgmental, awkward, cautious, aloof, stubborn, distant, distrustful, aggressive, easily influenced, self-centered, defensive, wary

Note: This table represents a reorganization of attributes reported for the two groups by Byrne and his associates (Byrne, 1964; Byrne, Steinberg & Schwartz, 1968; Schwartz, Krupp & Byrne, 1971). It is presented to give the reader a sense of what is meant by repression and sensitization, and to make clear the fact that "repression" as used here is not a pejorative concept (quite the contrary). These characteristics are found largely for undergraduates and may not be entirely generalizable either to the same samples at a later age, to noncollege groups, or to groups with special talents. For example, sensitization plus special talents (e.g., for writing, music, physical sciences, etc.) may yield a particularly favorable mixture of traits and accomplishments. Finally, it should be noted that not all of the characteristics associated with either repressor or sensitizer groups are consistent with the general personality factor (e.g., degree of suppression of affective-intuitive experiences) which I am suggesting accounts for much of the individual differences in reaction to interference with REM sleep (discussed in this and the following chapter).

I decided to focus on one of two dimensions, i.e., extraversion and neuroticism, that appear to be fundamental in the organization of personality (Wiggins, 1968). Neuroticism (i.e., emotionality, sensitization, anxiety) emerges almost inevitably out of factor analyses of test items, has a moderate degree of heritability, and is relatively easily assessed. Table 4-1 shows some of the characteristics associated with scores at the low and high ends of emotionality scales. Since repression-sensitization, anxiety, and neuroticism scales are inter-correlated about as high (.75-.95) as their individual test reliabilities permit (Byrne, 1964; Carson, 1969; Cohen, 1970; Eysenck, 1970; Golin, Herron, Lakota and Reineck, 1967; Schwartz et al., 1971). I will sometimes refer to individuals with low scores as "repressors" and individuals with high scores as "sensitizers" regardless of which one of the scales was used to differentiate the groups. These individuals differ with regard to the degree that they experience or are willing to admit experiencing strong dysphoric emotionality. Repressors can be thought of as individuals who are either free of such feelings or "defensive" about such feelings. Individuals who score at the repression end of emotionality scales are a mix of emotional stability and defensiveness (Fisher, 1959); the latter can be thought of as a caricature of the former in that repression or defensiveness is related to measures of "ego strength" (Byrne, 1964).

Fisher (1959) has pointed out that prediction from low scores (i.e., scores in the "healthy" direction) on dimensions that measure "pathology" (e.g., anxiety, retardation) is less precise than prediction from high scores. One reason is that low scorers are more apt to be a mixture of truly healthy and health-feigning individuals. Thus, any theory that focuses on repressors rather than sensitizers may be subject to built-in "error" variance. For instance, it is not clear whether the hypothesized relevance of repression scores to predicting REM and dreaming phenomena is due to the influence of genuine ego strength or defensiveness or both. If one is more important than the other, then there will be a tendency for the *variance* in theoretically relevant measures to be greater for repressors than for sensitizers, *especially under conditions designed to increase the hypothetical REM need.*

Some examples from one of our recent studies will illustrate this point. Under conditions of REM deprivation, the variance in cumulative REM awakenings for sensitizers was 1.58 vs. 5.48 for repressors. Likewise, under REM deprivation, the variance in block design (seconds) for sensitizers was 148.77 vs. 602.19 for repressors. Finally, the variance in subjective estimation of duration of dreaming under conditions of REM deprivation was 46.22 seconds for sensitizers, 76.52 for repressors. Note that not all comparisons will generate greater variance for repressors under REM deprivation. For example, variance in mood ratings was greater for sensitizers (.78) than for repressors (.39). Repressors are simply more conservative in their ratings of mood. The point, however, is that there may be a significant degree of ambiguity in the data for the repression group.

Preliminary evidence suggested that neuroticism or repression-sensitization would be useful in accounting for much of the variation in the REM restoration motive which is elicited by REM deprivation. The basis for this assumption was as follows. First, Cartwright's speculations about the need for a quota of dreamlike fantasy (Cartwright, 1969) that nonschizoid individuals tend to confine to REM sleep (1972) suggested that repressors would have a greater REM restoration motive under REM deprivation than would sensitizers. Second, there is evidence of a modest correlation between low scores on scales tapping schizoid tendencies and low scores on scales tapping emotionality (anxiety, sensitization or neuroticism scales) (Butcher, 1969). Third, there were data showing that repressors tend to have a greater increase in certain aspects of REM intensity under conditions of REM deprivation. For example, Pivik and Foulkes (1966) showed that repressors more than sensitizers had greater dreamlike fantasy (Df scores) and more eye movement activity during a late REM period following deprivation of earlier REM periods than during a late REM period following nonrestriction of earlier REM periods. In addition, there was my (1975) study of the effect of presleep conditions on the eye movement activity of repressors and sensitizers. Stressful presleep conditions produced much more REM density, especially during the second REM period, for repressors than for sensitizers (see Figure 3-1).

A third study, that of Grieser *et al.* (1972), also suggested that REM sleep is more "important" to "high ego strength" subjects (who generally score toward the repression rather than toward the sensitization end on emotionality scales). REM deprivation induced a decrement in recall of failure — but not success — related items. Finally, a group of Japanese investigators (Nakazawa, Kotorii, Kotorii, Tachibana and Nakano, 1975a) obtained much greater REM rebound for repressors (low neuroticism) than for sensitizers during recovery sleep following a night of REM deprivation. In fact the biserial correlation between repression and REM rebound was .74. Subsequently, Nakazawa and his colleagues (Nakazawa, Kotorii, Arikawa, Horikawa and Hasuzawa, 1975b) obtained further evidence for the repression-rebound correlation.

Figure 4-1 represents a graphic summary of the moderating effects of repression-sensitization on stress- or deprivation-induced changes in REM characteristics. These

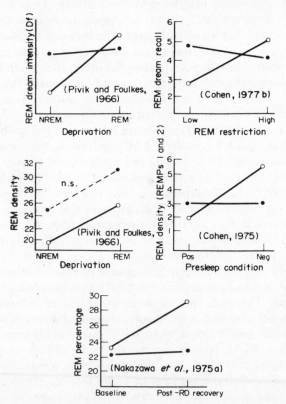

Figure 4-1   Intensification of REM sleep: repressors (open circles) and sensitizers (filled circles).

results suggest that there are individual differences in the motivational characteristics of REM: (a) changes in dreams (estimated directly via dream content analysis or indirectly via dream recall), (b) changes in phasic activity (e.g., REM density), and (c) changes in tonic motivation (REM rebound). Repressor data are represented by open circles, sensitizer data by filled-in circles. Notice that there is a tendency for repressors to respond to presleep stress or to REM deprivation with greater changes in the REM process suggesting that at least under such conditions, repressors have a greater need for REM sleep.

Further evidence

Guided by these kinds of results, I conducted a preliminary experiment (Cohen, 1977b) in which degree of REM deprivation was manipulated. The major objective was to assess the effect of neuroticism on REM pressure. At the time this exploratory study was begun, I was not sufficiently impressed by the importance of distinguishing between REM pressure *during* REM deprivation vs. REM rebound (and other effects) *after* REM deprivation. Therefore, despite evidence of a positive relationship between neuroticism and REM pressure (Cartwright *et al.*, 1967) I expected to find a negative relationship. I also expected that the performance on a complex task (Block Design) would be more adversely affected by REM restriction of repressors than of sensitizers. These expectations were based on the kinds of findings shown in Figure 4-1.

College males were randomly assigned to one of two levels of REM restriction. In the "Late" condition, the subject was awakened at the estimated end of each REM period (little restriction). In the "Early" condition, the subject was awakened as soon as each REM period began (high restriction). After each awakening, the subject was asked to report any dream experience; if there was none, he was asked to make up a dream. This was done in order to control for fantasy experience during the intervals that the subject was forced to remain awake. On the basis of Maudsley Personality Inventory neuroticism scores, the highest (Neuroticism or $N > 30$) and lowest ($N < 20$) third of the sample were selected.

The assumption that repression and sensitization are valid trait measures (rather than indicators of temporary and situationally specific deviations) was supported by follow-up data on 25 of the original 39 subjects whom we were able to contact roughly nine months later. Test-retest reliability was .79. All four of the original sensitizers remained in that category (retest $N > 30$) and eight of the original 10 repressors remained in the category (retest $N < 20$). The fact that only four of the original "neutrals" remained in that category (three changing to sensitization, four to repression) supports the rationale for eliminating subjects who score in the neutral range when conducting studies to assess the importance of a trait measure.

If we define REM pressure as the number of attempts to have REM sleep despite restrictive awakenings, then the results shown in Figure 4-2 appear to be consistent with prediction. There is a marginally significant interaction effect of degree of REM restriction and personality ($F = 4.116$, $p < .10$). However, an analysis of how these results were achieved raises two interesting questions regarding (a) the definition of REM pressure, and (b) its theoretical relationship to REM rebound. Let us address the first question.

What determines the frequency of awakenings during REM deprivation? The number of awakenings is a direct function of two latencies: (a) the latency to stage 2-NREM sleep onset from lights out, and (b) the latency to REM from stage 2-NREM onset. (Naturally, if a

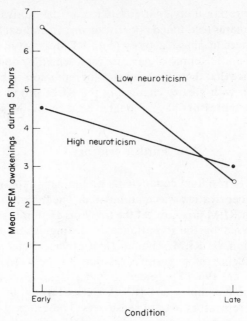

Figure 4-2   Number of REM awakenings required under two conditions of REM interruption (early or late in the REM period) for high vs. low neuroticism subjects.

subject goes directly from wakefulness to REM, the distinction between sleep and REM onset is academic.) If it makes no difference how the subject gets back into REM after an awakening, then number of REM awakenings can be used to define REM pressure. However, if REM pressure is defined as the motive to get back to the REM state *once sleep onset has occurred*, then it is necessary to distinguish between latency from lights out to sleep onset from the latency from sleep onset to REM onset.

Figure 4-3 shows both sleep onset and REM onset latencies for high and for low neuroticism subjects across the first four REM periods of each group. Now it is obvious that the more frequent awakenings for the repressor group is associated with a linear reduction across the night in REM onset latency, but not with a change in sleep onset latency. While REM onset latencies of the high neuroticism subjects are short, they do not show the nice linear decrease, unconfounded by changes in sleep onset latency, shown by the low neuroticism subjects. Thus, the overall differences in number of REM awakenings observed between the two groups in the REM deprivation condition (Figure 4-2) can largely be described as a function of short sleep onset latency plus diminishing REM onset latencies in the low neuroticism group vs. diminishing sleep onset latencies plus relatively short and unchanging REM onset latencies in the high neuroticism group. This difference makes the findings for the latter group more ambiguous from the perspective of REM motivation theory. It would appear that, although the high neuroticism group achieved about the same amount of total sleep time by the end of the night, the pattern of REM latency could be as much a function of some kind of sleep disruption as REM need. The fact that high neuroticism subjects took 43 minutes to fall asleep at the beginning of the night, as compared to the low neuroticism subjects ($X = 18, p < .005$), makes the REM onset data of the former group even more ambiguous.

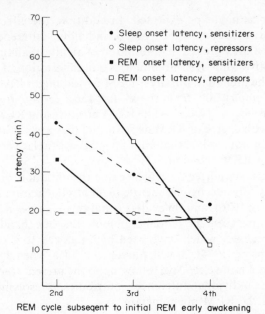

Figure 4-3   Sleep and REM onset latencies across three REM periods for high and low neuroticism subjects run under REM deprivation conditions.

We are therefore left with a number of possibilities. One is that the difference between the groups cannot be adequately assessed because the short REM onset latencies of the high neuroticism group may be an artifact of sleep disruption rather than of REM need *per se*. A second possibility is that neuroticism is not important to predicting REM pressure. However, on the basis of results of our current work (described below) it appears that males do show a negative relationship between neuroticism and REM pressure, even when sleep disturbances can be ruled out. Another possibility is that REM pressure is actually somewhat greater for high neuroticism subjects. This would be commensurate with the preliminary report by Cartwright *et al.* (1967) of a strong *positive* correlation between questionnaire-assessed anxiety level and number of REM awakenings for 10 male subjects over three nights. Our current study suggests that this may be true for *females*, but only under certain conditions.

To summarize the major problems raised by these preliminary findings: (a) Group differences in REM characteristics may be complicated by correlated differences in sleep quality induced by methodology. (b) Group differences in REM characteristics may depend on how REM deprivation is carried out and how its effects are assessed. (c) Gender, personality, and interaction effects have yet to be tested in a systematic way. (d) All of these problems are interrelated, and none has been resolved. Yet they are of sufficient importance to require further discussion. The reader should understand, however, that empirical work on individual differences in REM motivation is sparse and of a decidedly preliminary nature.

The possibility that personality and sex factors are differentially associated with different REM characteristics raises a potentially important point regarding REM pressure. When REM deprivation is carried out for a short time, the relationship between REM pressure and other motivational characteristics of REM sleep (REM quality and REM rebound) is not positive and linear as might be expected. In addition, the effect of such brief REM deprivation on pressure or rebound will depend on individual differences. We are faced with the possibility that REM pressure is a manifestation of an ultradian timing mechanism that is subject to a reset motive while REM rebound is a manifestation of a REM debt. What I am suggesting is that the motive to *initiate* a REM period might have to be distinguished, both theoretically and empirically, from the motive for a certain *duration* of REM sleep once the REM period is begun. That is, while REM pressure and REM rebound (as well as REM density) covary with degree of REM deprivation, they are not highly positively inter-correlated. Thus, one cannot assume that an individual with relatively high REM pressure will have relatively high REM rebound.

This line of reasoning is supported by evidence that the initiation, *but not the duration*, of REM sleep is markedly affected by cholinergic facilitation (Sitaram *et al.*, 1976; Sitaram, personal communication, 1976), and by evidence that there is a *negative* feedback relation-ship between REM onset centers (cholinergic) on the one hand, and other centers (adrenergic and serotonergic) which have been hypothesized to account for REM need (Hartmann, 1973; Hobson, 1974). I will pursue this idea when I describe my current research which is in part a more extensive follow-up to the present study. Suffice it to say at this point that a focus on individual differences contributes to resolving questions about the different parameters of the REM phenomenon.

Before continuing with the description of results, I would like to make a methodological point. If REM deprivation is used to test the hypothesis that REM pressure is different from REM rebound, the deprivation should be carried out for one or perhaps two **nights only.** Longer periods of REM deprivation might be associated with unknown compensatory processes to restore lost functioning. Thus, differences in the motive to reset the timing or to increase the duration of REM might be confounded with differences in ability to compensate through intensification of the REM process (e.g., more eye movement, more intense dreams, etc.) or through "leakage" of REM-related processes into NREM or wake-fulness. This difference between short term effects and more compensatory long term effects should be studied, but they do introduce complications of an unknown magnitude. The data to be described below suggest that there may be individual differences in preference for compensatory adjustments in REM timing (latency), REM quality (e.g., density), and REM duration (rebound) characteristics; these might "wash out" if only summary effects obtained after many days of REM deprivation are reported.

Studies reviewed above clearly suggest that REM deprivation has a more striking impact on certain kinds of individuals. Evidence, to be discussed in more detail later, suggests that performance on certain kinds of tasks will, especially for certain individuals (e.g., repressors, convergent thinkers, field independents), be more adversely affected by REM deprivation. In general, such tasks will be relatively more complex, and probably involve information processing that has a substantial right hemisphere component. The study just described included a postsleep block design task on which subjects were timed on the last four items. This task, requiring an arrangement of nine cubes to form a given pattern, involves a significant spatial component (Waber, 1976). In addition, there is a good deal of evidence from clinical neuropsychological assessment of performance deficits associated with disruption of the right hemisphere to indicate that Block Design performance is mediated largely by the right hemisphere (Reitan and Davison, 1974). Finally, a split brain patient has great difficulty doing block designs with his right hand (left hemisphere) which he can easily do with his left hand (right hemisphere). If the individual differences approach

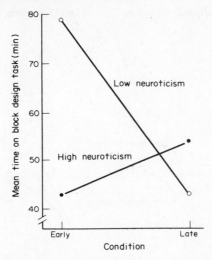

Figure 4-4   Block design performances of high and low neuroticism subjects under high and low REM restriction.

developed here is valid, and if information processing of the right hemisphere is especially prominent during REM sleep,[2] then we should expect that the adverse effects of REM deprivation on performance should be greater in repressors than in sensitizers.

Figure 4-4 shows the differential results of REM deprivation vs. control on the two groups of subjects that are in line with expectation. There was a significant interaction ($F = 7.582$, $p < .025$) determined by significant difference in repressor performance and a nonsignificant difference in sensitizer performance defined in terms of speed of design solutions. It should be noted that this effect is not due to total sleep time differences since the groups in the Early condition did not differ in total sleep time. Nor can the differences be attributed to differential number of awakenings since the correlation between number of awakenings and performance time (ignoring subject classification) was —.06. In fact, there was a tendency for performance time within each group to be *negatively* correlated with number of awakenings; more awakenings were associated with *better* (faster) performance. The differential performance patterns cannot be attributed to postsleep mood (a composite rating of energy, affect, and self-confidence) since there were no differences between the two groups in either the early or the late condition. Finally, these differential results cannot easily be attributed to differential levels of initial performance since there were no group differences in either condition on the first set of (five) block design items given subjects prior to sleep.

Figure 4-5 shows the performance, in terms of time required on each of the block designs, for the two groups in the two conditions. What is particularly interesting is that all four sub-groups have roughly the same performance on the initial item. If fatigue or some other motivational factor were operating, then there might be differences on this item. What seems to be happening is that the repressors (low neuroticism subjects) appear to

[2] There is evidence that immediate postsleep performance on the Rod and Frame test is superior when the subject is awakened toward the end rather than near the beginning of a REM period (DeKoninck, Koulack and Oczkowski, 1973). In addition, Berger and Scott (1971) reported that binocular (but not monocular) depth perception was superior after awakenings at the end, compared to awakenings at the beginning, of REM periods.

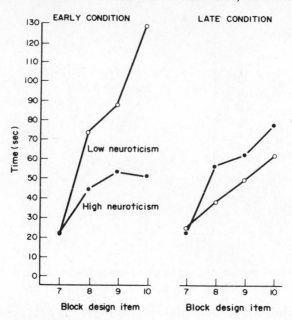

Figure 4-5   Performances on four difficult items of Block Design by high and low neuroticism subjects under conditions of high or low REM restriction.

have trouble *improving* on subsequent items on the basis of experience with prior items. It is notable that they do especially poorly on the last item, one which involves a 45 degree rotation of the design to be simulated by the arrangement of the blocks. It is noteworthy that four out of the eight repressors (but none of the sensitizers) failed to solve the last item even though they were allowed three (rather than the standard two) minutes. In addition, five out of the eight repressors and none of the six sensitizers failed at least one of the four items ($p < .05$). In fact, three of the repressors of the early condition failed two of the four items; none of the subjects in the other three cells performed so poorly.

If the general hypothesis of a differential reaction to REM deprivation is valid, then it would be predicted that repressors will respond to such a manipulation by relatively greater intensification of the REM process that occurs just prior to awakenings. One of the factors influencing amount of dream recall is the salience of the dream process. I will take up this question in Part B of the book. Suffice it to say here that any intensification of the REM process will be correlated with an intensification of the dreaming process and thus be associated with an increase in the amount of recalled dream material. If repressors are differentially responsive to REM deprivation compared to sensitizers, we should expect to see a relatively greater amount of dream recall under conditions of REM deprivation than under nondeprivation conditions in repressors compared to sensitizers. This expectation was confirmed in the REM dream recall results of the study under consideration. Initial REM period dream recall for repressors and sensitizers in the early and late conditions was quite similar. On a scale from zero to 6 that indicated amount and vividness of dream recall, there was virtually no difference among the four subgroups. However, when dream recall for the last REM period was assessed, there were noticeable differences in the expected direction (interaction $F = 5.538$, $p < .05$). Figure 4-6 shows that while there was virtually

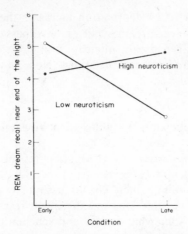

Figure 4-6   REM dream recall near the end of the night for high and low neuroticism subjects under high or low REM restriction.

no difference in sensitizer recall scores between the two conditions, the REM-early condition is associated with an apparent enhancement of dream recall by repressors in the Early compared to the Late condition ($t = 6.752$, $p < .001$). These results are all the more notable given the evidence that awakenings early in the REM period are typically associated with less dream recall and less intense dreaming than are awakenings late in the REM period (Kramer, Roth and Czaya, 1975). Parenthetically, it might be noted that the copious dream recall shown by the repressors in the REM-early condition is not due to the fact that these subjects had more awakenings than the subjects of the other conditions; the correlation between number of awakenings and amount of dream recall for this group was —.10. The results shown in Figure 4-6 strongly suggest that there are compensatory mechanisms by which the effects of REM deprivation can be reduced or eliminated. If such mechanisms are more likely to operate in individuals for whom REM sleep is hypothesized to be more important, they will tend to work against finding evidence for that hypothesis from measures such as REM rebound.

If it is especially true for repressors that REM sleep is associated with compensatory processes of the right hemisphere, there should be a correlation between intensification of REM and postsleep performance on Block Design. Specifically, repressors who show signs of increased intensification of dream processes under REM deprivation should perform better on morning Block Design than repressors who do not appear to compensate.

If dream recall can be used as an indirect estimate of the intensity of the dream process, then the obtained correlations lend further support to the hypothesis. In the REM deprivation condition, both groups showed a trivial correlation between total REM time and Block Design time (—.09 and .18 respectively). The correlation between REM period dream recall and Block Design performance of the sensitizers was also trivial (—.08). However, it was —.51 for repressors. While not statistically significant, this latter correlation is consistent with the idea that a compensatory intensification of REM can modify the postsleep performance of repressors.

To summarize, the following evidence supports the hypothesis that repressors have a greater need for REM sleep than do sensitizers: (a) REM deprivation more clearly adversely affects postsleep performance on certain tasks that are known to involve right hemisphere

S.D.— 1

mediation (Waber, 1976). (b) REM deprivation increases the intensity of the dreaming process as estimated from enhanced dream recall and vividness or clarity of recall. (c) There is a positive correlation between dream intensity and postsleep performance (negative correlation between intensity and performance time). None of these relationships is clearly evident in the data of the sensitizers.

Implications for subsequent research

Research on motivational properties of REM sleep reveals the enormously complex problem of the REM phenomenon, especially from the individual differences perspective that I have been developing in this chapter. The discussion has at least clarified some of the distinctions that will need to be addressed in subsequent research. Therefore, I will now summarize these and then, in somewhat limited and schematic form, describe research in progress which I hope will contribute to a resolution of these questions.

First, with respect to the way REM deprivation is carried out, it seems worthwhile to control and vary the kind of events and experiences that occur during the interval during which a REM deprived subject is forced to remain awake. Whether the subject engages in some sort of REM-like activity (e.g., fantasy communication) or some sort of REM-dissonant activity (e.g., solving simple arithmetic problems) may have an effect on REM parameters (latency, rebound) and postsleep functions. The differential effect of such activity may have important theoretical implications.

Second, it now appears desirable to consider the separate effects of REM deprivation on REM latency, REM intensity, and REM rebound. Another related issue is that individuals may differ with respect to their ability to compensate under REM deprivation via adjustments in any one of these three characteristics. Therefore, one subject may have less rebound because he has been able to intensify the REM process during the short interval between REM onset and awakening. I believe that this is an extremely important point. The need for REM may not be readily assessed if the degrees of freedom represented by flexibility in the REM state are not taken into consideration.

Third, and related to the second point, is the problem of individual differences in response to REM deprivation. It seems reasonable, given the evidence discussed in this chapter, that individuals differ in the motive and ability to adjust various aspects of the REM state, including those that could be thought of as indicating a need for REM. I have been emphasizing the dimension of repression-sensitization (neuroticism) as an organizing factor that helps to resolve as well as raise important questions about REM dynamics. However, two points need to be made. One is that neuroticism may not adequately represent the most relevant individual difference variable; the latter might best be operationally defined through some other, or some more direct, estimate. The meaning of neuroticism as related to REM sleep will be taken up later. The second point is that there may be other, more powerful dimensions of personality such as extraversion that not only predict REM phenomena better, but that provide theoretically powerful alternative explanations of individual differences in REM need. For example, I have suggested that individual differences in the permeability of biological states and (probably correlated) individual differences in psychological compartmentalization are related to the need for REM. I take up this hypothesis again in Chapter 5.

Suffice it to say here that other relatively easily measurable psychological characteristics may prove to be better predictors of REM need (e.g., as manifested in rebound) because they are more intimately associated with boundary permeability and compartmentalization. For example, a form of compartmentalization is lateralization of cortical function, i.e., the left hemisphere specialized for digital/verbal processes vs. the right hemisphere specialized for analogical/spatial processes. In Chapter 5, I will present some new data that show greater REM rebound for strongly right-handed (highly lateralized) than for weakly right-handed (less lateralized) individuals. In sum, while REM need appears to be positively related to estimates of biological compartmentalization of function, it is not yet clear what are the best psychological measures which are related to REM need. My guess is that such measures will be estimates of psychological characteristics whose physiological basis will prove to be associated with neurophysiological compartmentalization/boundary permeability.

Fourth, and related to the question of individual differences, is the whole question of sex differences and their possible interaction with personality factors. We know virtually nothing about the effect of REM deprivation on the REM phenomena and postsleep behavior of females. This question will be taken up shortly, but I think it important to raise it here to emphasize that virtually everything that has been said about REM from the data base of REM deprivation research refers only to males. While this selectivity derives in part from some obvious practical difficulties, and while it is not a particular failing of sleep research alone, it now seems to me to be a major shortcoming.

Now that I have made these summary comments, I want to provide a brief outline of our latest study (Cohen, McGrath, Bell, Hanlon, and Simon, 1978) which we hope will contribute to the clarification of some of these interrelated problems.

The study includes two parts that occur in sequence during a single night. During the first phase, the first 6 hours from initial lights out, subjects are either REM deprived (RD condition) or not deprived (NRD condition). During the second phase, the last 100 minutes of bed time, the subject is allowed to sleep undisturbed. Thus, the first phase provides information about latency (REM pressure) while the second phase permits assessment of both REM intensity and REM duration.

During the first phase, REM deprivation is carried out in one of two ways. During each five minute interval of enforced wakefulness the subject is asked either (a) to communicate recalled dream material or to make up a "dream" (in the event of recall failure) or (b) to repeat sets of digits forward or backward, and to engage in other simple arithmetic operations. Thus, we have an RD-digit or an RD-fantasy treatment. Two types of NRD subjects are also given either digit or fantasy when awakened. One type, the NRD-subject, is either given digit or fantasy *at the end of each REM period*. The second type, the NRD-*control* subject, is likewise treated but in addition, undergoes additional (NREM) sleep awakenings. These latter awakenings supplement the REM awakenings, and together they provide a control for the total number of awakenings achieved by the RD subjects. Thus, NRD subjects provide a baseline against which RD effects on REM *pressure* can be evaluated. On the other hand, NRD-*control* subjects provide a baseline against which RD effects on REM *rebound* can be evaluated.

One additional control group is used. The subjects of this group are permitted six minutes of REM per REM period before being awakened and given the digit task. This "RD-digit-delay" (RD-d-d) group provides a modified control for the RD-fantasy group whose

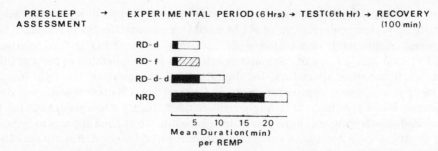

Figure 4-7   Schematic outline of sequential phases of the experiment. RD-d provides a control for REM deprivation, while RD-d-d provides a control for fantasy, against which the effects of RD-f can be assessed. The black part
of the bar refers to REM dreaming while the hatched part of the RD-f bar refers to fantasy.

subjects get about one minute of REM dreaming plus five minutes of waking fantasy. Thus,
if waking fantasy substitutes for lost REM dreaming, the REM pressure for the RD-fantasy
should be roughly equivalent to that of the RD-digit-delay (RD-d-d) control group.

Prior to the first (experimental) phase, all subjects perform two related tasks. At the end
of the first phase (six hours later) they are tested for performance on these two tasks. Thus
we can assess the effect of RD on two kinds of information processing. One task involves the
serial paired-associate learning of the meaning(s) of each of 10 "hieroglyphic" symbols. This
initial task represents a rather simple, convergent type problem, the kind not predicted to be
adversely affected by RD. The second task requires the subject to translate a "poem" made
up of five of the ten symbols. (Each symbol may be repeated one or more times throughout
the four line "poem".) This task allows for more complex, inventive, perhaps divergent
information processing, though the subject may opt for a more literal translation.

After the experimental period, recall of the meanings of the symbols (serially presented)
and a second translation of a parallel-form "poem" (made up of the five symbols not used in
the first poem) are obtained. The effect of RD on poem translation is predicted to be greater
than the effect on recall of the elements. One problem of having subjects engage in this
behavior for about 10 minutes prior to recovery sleep during the second (100 minute) phase
is that it may serve to dissipate some of the RD effects accumulated during the first six
hours. Notice that the NRD-fantasy subjects (both NRD and NRD-control) provide dream
data which permit the assessment of the relationship between dream content and poetry
performance.

A schematic outline of the experiment is shown in Figure 4-7. The effect of fantasy during
awakenings done to accomplish REM deprivation can be assessed by comparing REM
motivation in the RD-digit (RD-d) and RD-fantasy (RD-f) groups. Of special significance
is the use of delayed REM deprivation (RD-d-d) to compare the effects of waking fantasy
(RD-f) against a group that receives the same duration of dream (REM) fantasy (RD-d-d).

One further aspect of the study needs description here. Half of our subjects are male, the
other half are female. In addition, all subjects take the Maudsley Personality Inventory by
which we can estimate two important personality dispositions, neuroticism and
extraversion. Both of these dimensions have been implicated in motivational properties of
REM sleep. The possibility that there might be significant interactions of sex and
personality that differentially affect REM parameters made the question of individual
differences even more intriguing.

To summarize the organization of the study: First, we select both male and female subjects. Second, we assess personality factors, learning, and performance prior to sleep. Third, subjects are either REM deprived or experience control treatments during the six hour experimental phase which is designed to assess the REM pressure component of REM motivation and how it may be modified by awakening activity (digit vs. fantasy). Fourth, at the end of the experimental phase (after six hours) memory and performance are tested in order to assess the effects of REM deprivation as modified by type of subject and type of cognitive activity during awakening. Fifth, the subject is allowed 100 minutes during which sleep is uninterrupted. Recovery sleep is used to assess the effects of prior conditions on the duration (rebound) and intensity (eye movement activity) components of REM motivation. What follows is a presentation of results which we have obtained to date.

At the outset, it is important to note that there were no statistically significant differences within each sex (and, for the most part, between sexes) on any pre-experimental measure. Presleep measures included mood, neuroticism, and sex role orientation (masculinity/femininity). Sleep measures included initial sleep and initial REM onset latencies. Thus, at the outset of the experiment and prior to experimental manipulations, the various groups are statistically, and thus presumably psychologically, homogeneous.

Table 4-2 summarizes the major results. The N column shows the sample sizes of each group. The next column provides information on the amount of REM per REM period allowed during the experimental phase of the study. These figures constitute a strict operational definition of degree of REM deprivation as determined by experimental design (see Figure 4-7). The next column shows the total number of awakenings achieved by each group. These include both REM awakenings (determined by REM pressure) and other awakenings (both inadvertent and, in the case of NRD-control, NREM supplemental). Notice that for males there is virtually no difference across RD-d, RD-f, and NRD-control groups. (The NRD group is used only to assess REM pressure and therefore is given no

TABLE 4-2.   Comparison of Groups on Experimental and Dependent Variables (from Cohen *et al.*, 1978)

Groups	N	REM/REMP[a]	Tot. awakenings[b]	REM attempts (pressure)	REM%[c] (rebound)
Males					
RD-d	21	1.1(0.5)	6.1(1.9)	5.4(2.0)	60.6(17.2)
RD-f	22	1.5(0.8)	5.8(2.0)	5.3(1.9)	67.0(18.5)
RD-d-d	10	6.0(0.9)	5.3(2.1)	4.7(2.2)	47.6(21.5)[e]
NRD-c	20	19.1(5.3)	5.6(1.9)	3.1(0.9)[d]	46.9(12.6)
NRD	8	18.1(5.1)	4.0(0.5)	3.5(0.5)	45.8(12.2)[e]
Females					
RD-d	22	1.1(0.5)	9.5(2.4)	9.0(2.4)	61.7(13.7)
RD-f	21	1.1(0.5)	7.1(3.4)	6.5(3.3)	55.9(21.0)
RD-d-d	10	5.7(0.6)	4.7(1.5)	4.2(1.3)	51.9(15.5)[e]
NRD-c (dig)	11	20.0(5.4)	9.0(2.2)	2.8(0.8)[d]	42.9(17.7)
NRD-c (fant)	10	20.7(5.7)	7.1(3.5)	2.8(0.6)[d]	47.3(21.1)
NRD	10	18.4(3.8)	4.3(0.8)	3.5(0.7)	45.9(16.6)[e]

[a]Mean REM time (minutes) per REM period allowed during the first six hours.
[b]Includes all experimental awakenings from REM or NREM made during or at the end of the 6-hour experimental period. Brief spontaneous awakenings are not included. Numbers in parentheses are standard deviations.
[c]Percentage of recovery sleep (during the final 100 minutes) devoted to REM.
[d]These figures are probably attenuated to some degree by the influence of NREM awakenings on the duration of intervals between REM periods.
[e]These figures are not appropriate for testing the substitution hypothesis since there is no control for total number of awakenings.

supplemental [NREM] awakenings.) Also, because there was no difference in the REM pressure of males between RD-d and RD-f groups, the digit and fantasy NRD-control subgroups could be combined to provide a more reliable baseline. This lack of difference in REM pressure between RD-d and RD-f male groups is shown in the next column along with the results from the other male groups.

In contrast, it is clear that there is a marked difference in REM pressure between female RD-d and RD-f groups. This necessitated a separation of the respective digit and fantasy NRD control groups as shown in the table. However, note that each control group is comparable to its respective RD group in total number of awakenings.

Factorial analysis of variance of the REM attempt data shown in Table 4-2 yielded the following results. First, for each sex, RD was associated with greater REM pressure than NRD (noncontrol). Second, female RD-d subjects have significantly more REM pressure than either female RD-f or male RD groups. All comparisons were significant beyond the .01 level. On the other hand, the difference between female RD-f and male RD groups did not reach statistical significance. This pattern of results is confirmed by that pattern resulting from defining REM pressure in terms of changes in REM onset latency. One further observation regarding REM pressure should be considered.

During the course of the experiment a female was run who had an extraordinary amount of REM pressure. On the first night (RD-d condition) she logged 23 REM attempts. After learning that she was taking mestinon (an anticholinesterase) to control the symptoms of myasthenia gravis (a disease of the neuromuscular junction, see Wintrobe, Thorn, Adams, Bennett, Braumwald, Isselbacher and Petersdorf, 1970, ch. 377), we asked her to return for three additional nonconsecutive nights. On the second (RD-d) she had 18 REM attempts,

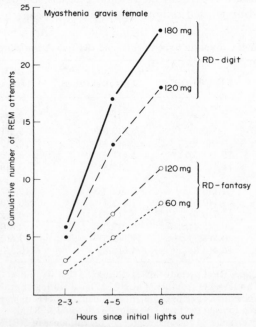

Figure 4-8 Cumulative number of REM attempts during a six hour period as affected by total daytime dosage of mestinon and by type of cognitive activity during awakenings (digit vs. fantasy). Each curve represents a single night of four nonconsecutive nights that the myasthenia gravis female spent in the laboratory.

on the third (RD-f), 8, and on the fourth (RD-f), 11. We subsequently discovered that she was varying the dosage of mestinon. The results of this combination of type of RD vs. dosage level are shown in Figure 4-8. I will discuss shortly the implications of these results. Suffice it to say here that despite high REM pressure in general, the digit vs. fantasy effect observed in the female subjects still obtained in the data of the myasthenia gravis female.

The rightmost column of Table 4-2 shows the differences among groups in percentage of recovery sleep devoted to REM. While there was a statistically greater amount of REM% for RD compared to NRD-control for both males ($p < .001$) and for females ($p < .02$), there were no within-sex differences between RD-d and RD-f groups.

Taken together, the pressure and rebound data of the males provide no support for a fantasy substitution hypothesis. That is, there is no evidence that awakenings followed by fantasy are associated with reduced REM pressure during the experimental period, or with reduced REM rebound during the recovery sleep period.

At first glance, the female data appear to provide some support for the hypothesis. Nevertheless, for the following reasons, I am at this point unconvinced. First, if we use the male RD data to provide expected values for REM pressure, the female RD-f subjects are roughly comparable. Thus, it could be argued that it is the enhanced effect of RD-d rather than the attenuation of effect of RD-f which requires explanation. A stronger argument, however, can be made on the basis of the comparison between female RD-f and RD-d-d groups. That is, an average of six minutes of predominately REM fantasy (dreaming) per REM period (RD-d-d) is associated with significantly less REM pressure than an average of six minutes of predominately waking fantasy per REM period (RD-f) (4.2 vs. 6.5 REM attempts respectively, $p < .05$). In fact, the RD-d-d results are comparable to, and not significantly different from, those of the NRD (noncontrol) group. In contrast, the results of the RD-f group are significantly greater than those of the NRD (noncontrol) group ($p < .02$). Nevertheless, until we obtain results from RD conditions that include a variety of different awakening tasks, a decision regarding the credibility of the fantasy substitution hypothesis will not be firm. In other words it is still possible that the RD-f female results constitute a weak substitution effect. Reliable sex differences in such an effect would, of course, be of theoretical interest.

Contrary to expectation, the neuroticism variable did not prove to be a strong predictor of REM motivation in the males. While there was a modest (but not significant) negative correlation between neuroticism and REM pressure for both RD-d and RD-f male groups (—.20 and —.36 respectively), no relationship obtained between neuroticism and REM rebound. REM deprivation may have been too brief, or the intervening events during the testing phase at the end of the six hour experimental period may have dissipated the effects, or the recovery phase may have been too brief. A more convincing argument can be made for the possibility that the neuroticism variable is a weak predictor because it is only an indirect estimate of individual differences in those processes which are relevant to the need for REM sleep. For example, I will suggest in Chapter 5 that individual differences in suppression of right hemisphere functions during wakefulness may be related to individual differences in REM need. While the construct of repression may indeed be of central importance to this hypothesis (Galin, 1974), questionnaire-defined differences may yield poor estimates of individual differences in this hypothetical variable.

The sex difference in REM pressure induced by REM deprivation appears to be reliable, and the difference appears to be related to the arousal at the onset of REM of left hemisphere dominant cognitive processes. This is supported by preliminary follow-up work utilizing a similar RD paradigm with a change of tasks. We have substituted a sentence memory task for the digit task and a nonverbal haptic matching-to-sample task for the fantasy task. This new set of tasks was chosen to investigate the hypothesis that the arousal of left hemisphere, REM-antithetical cognitive processes underlay the "digit effect". A more purely verbal task was developed to maximize differentially prominent left hemisphere activity and, through the use of abstract sentences, to minimize imagery and fantasy. The nonverbal task was designed to do just the opposite, The subject explores a sample configuration of cubes with the left hand, touches three other configurations while keeping the sample configuration in mind (maximizing spatial thinking), and then points to the configuration that best matches the sample. All this is done in the absence of visual cues. Verbal interaction is kept to a minimum or is entirely absent. The sentence memory and haptic tasks are carried out during each of the five minute intervals of wakefulness following REM onset awakenings during the first six hours of REM deprivation. A subject is assigned to either the RD-verbal or RD-nonverbal condition.

Our initial results based on a small sample of females are entirely consistent with the pattern obtained in the RD-digit vs. RD-fantasy conditions. The RD-verbal condition is associated with an elevation in the number of REM attempts (about 8.0) while the RD-nonverbal condition is associated with relatively fewer REM attempts (about 6.5). But further, these and the previous results are consistent in a way that requires a brief description of a different kind of analysis. It turns out that the latency to a REM period is, under conditions of REM deprivation, a function of sleep onset latency. The REM latency data of the sixth experimental hour can be divided into two categories depending on the latency to sleep following an awakening. Let us define a sleep onset latency of five minutes or less as "short", and greater than five minutes as "long". Regardless of condition, short sleep onset latencies were associated with short REM onset latencies. This was true of the females in the RD-digit and RD-fantasy groups, and it is turning out to be true for the RD-verbal vs. RD-nonverbal groups of the follow-up study. However, if the sleep onset latency is long, then the condition makes a very big difference. Specifically, for long sleep onset latencies, females in the RD-fantasy condition have long REM onset latencies while females in the RD-digit condition have short REM onset latencies. This large difference between conditions is replicating in the follow-up data. That is, under long sleep onset latencies, females in the RD-nonverbal condition have very long REM onset latencies while females in the RD-verbal condition have short REM onset latencies.

It is thus apparent that cognitive activity designed to maximize differentially prominent left hemisphere cognition at the onset of a REM period has either of two effects: (1) a tendency to reduce sleep onset latency (and thus REM onset latency), and (2) a tendency to reduce REM onset latency regardless of sleep onset latency. In other words, the reduction of REM onset latencies (i.e., increased REM pressure) in a REM deprived female appears to be relatively independent of sleep onset latency. More speculatively, it appears that the nature of cognitive activity may, under certain conditions, influence the mechanisms which are believed responsible for the timing of REM periods. The observation that REM-antithetical cognitive activity appears to accelerate REM onset under conditions of REM deprivation is at least consistent with the view that REM sleep may involve a compensatory activation of right hemisphere activity. This hypothesis is developed in the next chapter. Needless to say the status of these speculations is preliminary, but they are of sufficient interest and potential import to justify further exploration.

Further empirical work will require that attention be paid to individual differences and to

TABLE 4-3.   Factors that May Influence REM Motivation

---

1. *Individual Differences:*
   (a) gender
   (b) cognitive (field dependence, cortical lateralization)
   (c) temperament (neuroticism, extraversion)
   (d) sleep state "boundary permeability"
   (e) habitual sleep time
   (f) interactions

2. *Situational:*
   (a) quality of sleep
   (b) presleep events (controlled or uncontrolled)
   (c) interactions

3. *Methodological:*
   (a) operational definition of REM motivation (i.e., changes in
       latency, duration, intensity)
   (b) duration of REM deprivation
   (c) activity during awakenings
   (d) duration of awakenings
   (e) interactions

4. *Higher Order Interactions*

---

cognitive events associated with REM deprivation. At this point, it will suffice to point out the many factors that can, in principle, affect our inferences about the psychological significance of variation in the motivation for REM sleep. Some of the more obvious ones suggested by our recent research are summarized in Table 4-3. Clearly the complexity of the problem and the scarcity of research published to date contribute, in a negative way, to the ambiguous and unsatisfactory status of REM theory, especially from the perspective of motivational factors. Nevertheless, in the next chapter, I will attempt a modest integration of data from different research domains that I have discussed in Part A of the book. Hopefully, this integration will provide a fair summary of central ideas relevant to REM theory and will provide a biological perspective for discussions of research and theory on dreaming which constitute Part B of the book.

CHAPTER 5

THEORETICAL IMPLICATIONS

I. NREM VS. REM FUNCTION(S)

I have discussed a kaleidoscopic variety of data and hypotheses that defies integration. If one takes a nondoctrinaire position, then clearly no one theory of REM sleep appears to be completely satisfactory. However, numerous contributions from various areas of research do appear to converge on the notion that REM sleep has something to do with important processes of the central nervous system. To the degree that REM sleep function(s) can be thought of as distinct from NREM function(s), it seems reasonable to retain the popular assumption that REM sleep has more to do with brain processes while NREM has more to do with vegetative (somatic) conservation/restoration (Hartmann, 1973).

By way of summary, Table 5-1 displays some of the observations that are consistent with the hypothesis that NREM (especially delta) sleep is a somatic-vegetative process.

TABLE 5-1.   Some of the Major Evidence of the Role of NREM (Especially Delta) Sleep in Somatic-vegetative Maintenance

1. Short-term starvation is associated with increased delta sleep.
2. High presleep thyroxin level (indicating high metabolic rate) is associated with higher levels of delta sleep. Growth hormone (anabolism?) peaks during delta sleep.
3. Amount of delta sleep depends on number of prior hours awake despite possible displacement of sleep during the circadian cycle.
4. Short sleepers have equal or higher delta sleep percentages compared to longer sleepers. Extremely short (<4 hr.) sleepers have extremely high delta percentages.
5. Gradual or abrupt sleep restriction is associated with increase in delta sleep.
6. Sleep deprivation (especially if preceded by delta deprivation) is followed by high levels of delta sleep during recovery sleep. This event has temporal priority over, and is more reliable than, REM rebound.
7. Brain function appears to be reduced during delta sleep: there is slightly reduced brain oxygen consumption and increased synchrony of neural firing, and psychological events (content, consciousness) are sparse, fragmented, disorganized.

Because delta sleep is absent in neonates and in the aged, a contrast between REM and NREM function should not imply a functional independence of the two kinds of sleep. In fact, REM (in infants) and stage 2 (in the aged) may play a *relatively* greater role in vegetative maintenance than it does in normal adults. There is a tendency in theorizing about different kinds of sleep to forget that they are all variants of a phylogenetically ancient instinct which evolved different kinds of surface structure. The importance of differences in the way that inactivity is articulated electrophysiologically may be minor compared to the importance of inactivity *per se*.

A quick perusal of Table 5-2 (pp. 128-129) reveals that there is a high degree of similarity across specific hypotheses regarding the role of REM sleep in brain function and cognitive activity. That is, whatever the origin of REM sleep during evolution, it appears that REM sleep plays a role in reorganization and restoration of brain processes that mediate the flow and structure of information. This overriding idea has gained support from studies at various levels: neurophysiological, electrophysiological, behavioral, and phenomenological. The relative importance of REM sleep has been assessed by experimentally manipulating the REM period itself, by altering environmental conditions, and by taking individual differences into account. Thus, progress toward an integrated theory of REM sleep has been advanced through a convergence of contributions from neurological theory, personality theory, and behavioral experimental techniques.

A schematic representation of major theoretical ideas discussed in the REM sleep and dream literature is presented in quasineurophysiological form in Figure 5-1. The curled arrows (1) represent the idea that "restorative" processes (protein synthesis, neural reorganization, etc.) occur largely in the neocortex but also in the paleocortex and limbic system.

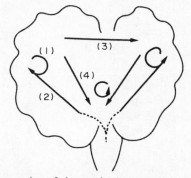

Figure 5-1   Schematic representation of changes in the central nervous system during REM sleep.

The arrows pointing toward the cortex (2) represent the idea that, periodically, the cortex receives stimulation from subcortical areas, stimulation which may mediate the "restoration" represented by (1). The horizontal arrow (3) represents the idea that there may be a significant shift from diurnal dominance by the left hemisphere to nocturnal (specifically, REM) dominance by the right hemisphere. Finally, the arrows pointing from the neocortex toward paleocortical and diencephalic areas (4) represent the idea that REM sleep is a "regressive" phenomenon, a reactivation of information processing that is more pertinent to our ontogenetic and phylogenetic origins.

These are four variants of a general theory about brain function during REM sleep. The theory can be discussed within the framework of an information processing model like the one shown in Figure 5-2. Each box represents a set of organized events. During wakefulness, information enters the system in the form of sensory information store (SIS) where it is held for a fraction of a second to permit additional attentional processes (detection, recognition) to extract a subset. If the information constitutes a "match" with knowledge/expectation/need (which is determined by some combination of prewired instinct and experience), it is either disregarded or acted upon. This effortless and relatively unconscious attentional process, guided by "old knowledge", is represented on the right side of the figure by the feedback loop SIS-Old Knowledge-A (action).

However, if the information in SIS is recognized to be complex, uncertain, affectively

TABLE 5-2. Hypotheses Regarding the Function of REM Sleep

Source	General hypothesis	Specific variants	Representative findings
Electrophysiology	Reafferentation of telencephalon (Ephron & Carrington)	BRAC represents oscillation of right and left hemisphere activation (Broughton)	High rate of cortical neuronal firing during REM sleep
Ontogeny	Endogenous stimulation of occulomotor areas promotes fetal/neonatal maturation	REM provides "cofactor" to prime NREM which is the more important stage of sleep (Feinberg)	High REM% during infancy when sleep predominates over wakefulness
Comparative (Phylogenetic)	REM supports viviparity (Allison et al.)	REM facilitates gestation (Allison et al.)	REM brief or absent in oviparous organisms; immaturity at birth correlates with REM time across species
	REM facilitates vigilance during sleep (Snyder)		Responsiveness to "meaningful" stimuli
	Endogenous stimulation of oculomotor areas (Berger)	Reorganization/stimulation of depth perception (Berger)	Better depth perception after awakening from REM than from NREM
Neurophysiology & Psychophysiology	Telencephalic reorganization and information processing	Neuronal "repair" via enhanced protein synthesis (Oswald)	Differential REM rebound after drug vs. mechanically induced REM deprivation
		Catecholamine system restoration/reorganization (Hartmann; Stern & Morgane)	REM deprivation reduces sensitivity to stimulants; stimulants reduce the adverse effect of REM deprivation on learning
		Compensatory activation of the right hemisphere (Bakan) especially during early REM periods of the night (Cohen), and especially for individuals who suppress right hemisphere during wakefulness (Cartwright; Cohen)	Damage to right hemisphere diminishes dream recall
			Individual differences in confinement of dreamlike fantasy to REM sleep
		Provide compensatory flow of information relative to waking rates (de la Peña)	Inverse correlation of waking eye movement and REM eye movement

REM Deprivation Research	Psychological adaptation (Dewan; Breger; Greenberg)	Defensive "working through" (Greenberg)
		Divergent information processing (Lewin & Glaubman)
		REM deprivation interferes more with divergent than with convergent performance
		Memory consolidation for emotionally or intellectually challenging information (Greenberg & Pearlman)
		Effect of type of material or task on post-deprivation performance
		Expression of fantasy "quota" (Cartwright)
		Partial "substitutability" of fantasy for REM experience
Clinical Psychology	Psychological adaptation/ problem solving	Infantile wish fulfillment (Freud)
		Dream interpretation
		Regression in the service of the ego; creative thinking (Krippner & Hughes)
		Anecdotes about dream solutions
		Compensatory processing of personally important experiences repressed during the day (Jung), or peripheral impressions given insufficient attention during the day (Poetzl)
		Reciprocal emphasis during dreams on unattended experiences
		Opportunity for the reintegration of cognitive and kinesthetic components of the personality (Lerner)
		REM deprivation is associated with body dissolution fantasy; exercise deprivation increases REM density and high activity dreams

Poor recall of failed items after REM deprivation

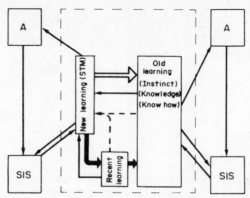

Figure 5-2   Information processing model. Information about the world which requires little new adaptation is processed automatically and with little consciousness (right side of the model). Some information about world and action will require "new learning". It will require more time, effort, and consciousness (i.e., concentration). This process is constrained by reality and influenced by old learning (knowledge that is given through instinct and experience). A subset of new learning that is especially relevant to the organism attains status (dark arrow) as "recent learning" and is held in a state of readiness to regain attention and concentration at a later time. During REM sleep the organism is, for physiological reasons, "cut off" from information about the external world as well as from relevant feedback. This is represented in the model by a dashed line which surrounds the "cognitive boxes". At this time, recent learning is integrated with old learning (represented by dashed arrows) in the form of new learning experienced during REM as dreaming. After sufficient concentration, this new learning attains the status of old learning (represented by the white arrow).

significant, etc., it will be "held" in a short term memory system for additional processing or "concentration". It will be consolidated by repetition or sustained attention (depending on whether the information is sequential or spatial). This kind of consolidation process is a relatively primitive way to "reinforce" (to make more permanent) the information, i.e., to confer LTM (long term memory) "status". Depending upon the ontogenetic and phylogenetic sophistication of the organism, the material can also undergo reorganization or coding for relationship, category, transformation, i.e., what Bartlett (1932) called "effort after meaning". This process is likely to be associated with consciousness and volition. It is represented in the figure by the feedback loop SIS-New Learning-A. But note that the process is influenced at all stages by old learning.

The result of this on-line *programming* is (a) mediation of action, and (b) relatively permanent storage of *coded* information. Presumably, the more complex, uncertain, unexpected, affectively significant, i.e., the more challenging the information, the more effort and time will be required for sufficient processing. Under such conditions, there is a greater chance for increased interference with both new information entering SIS and with the smooth organization and facilitation of action (i.e., the information "leaving" the system). It would seem advantageous to be able to apply preliminary "reinforcement" and coding sufficient to make the information relatively permanent so that, *at some later time* (i.e., off-line), under conditions of lowered demand for attention to exogenous information, the information could be reviewed. Off-line review would presumably accomplish two things. It would add "perspective" through additional categorization, interrelation, transformation, i.e., *metaprogramming*. And as a consequence, the information would be more retrievable because it would be more meaningful. The ability to transfer coded information from immediate memory (the "new learning" process) to a "recent learning" store, i.e., to store it "in the back of the mind" as it were, carries the additional advantage of

reducing proactive, simultaneous, and retroactive interference with the minimal information processing required to adjust to the immediate situation.

A consequence of this process is that learning *about* what has been learned (i.e., rule learning, metaprogramming) tends to occur off-line during "reflection". Of course, what one
learns *about* will depend on the nature of both the original programming and its subsequent
reprogramming. This will in turn be affected by the sophistication of the organism, i.e., its
ontogenetic and phylogenetic development and experience, the biological state (e.g., REM
vs. Wakefulness and the consequential shift toward relatively greater dominance by the
right hemisphere), and the nature of the raw data.

Under normal circumstances, individuals have many opportunities during wakefulness
to return to the suppressed or to the insufficiently attended. This information may have
undergone further changes while it remained unconscious (or preconscious) though these
changes are likely to be constrained by reality (represented by SIS) and "reality"
(represented by LTM or "old learning") when reflected upon during the waking state.
Reality constraints that are represented by SIS are reduced to a minimum during REM
sleep. However a relevant stimulus may alert the system with the effect either of altering the
flow of information processing, i.e., stimulus incorporation, or changing the state of the
system into one of wakefulness. This state of reduced SIS influence permits, other things
being equal, a *tendency* toward nonveridical (subjective, autistic) transformations which
are treated by the system as though they were coming from SIS. The process is therefore
experienced as real (loss of reality testing).

Under normal conditions, retrieval of information from the recent information store can
occur both voluntarily (e.g., during wakefulness) and involuntarily (e.g., during REM
sleep). Under abnormal conditions (e.g., obsessional disorders, highly threatening
situations) individuals may not be able to inhibit this information. The result is an impinge-
ment upon new learning (STM) of intense (i.e., emotional and highly conscious),
repetitious, and stereotypical information. Sleep onset insomnias may, in part, be explained
by reference to competition from such a process with normal sleep mechanisms.
Paradoxically, the use of additional, *exogenous* stimulation might be useful to induce sleep
onset. If the exogenous stimulation were informationally poor (e.g., metronome, white
noise) it would tend to distract attention from disturbing endogenous information to
monotonous, sleep-inducing stimulation.

One assumption consistent with variants of the information processing hypothesis for
REM sleep is that recent learning is integrated with (or assimilated to) old learning to yield
new structures. These, like the SIS-derived structures of wakefulness, are treated like new
learning and experienced consciously (dreamed about) during REM sleep. Thus, REM
sleep can be thought of as a REMembering process. Again, the resulting structures or
experiences may be more or less veridical as judged against some external criterion; it will
depend on the initial coding, the subjective influences during off-line coding (which could be
prelogical as well as logical), selective retrieval, etc. And all these can be affected by the
biological state of the organism, i.e., the information processing of transitional states
(ascending stage 1-NREM), stage 2, REM. The point is that these new experiences may
themselves attain sufficient "reinforcement" through attention and coding to attain LTM
status and therefore become part of what the organism knows. Kosslyn and Pomerantz
(1977) have made a similar point with respect to waking imagery. "If images are sensory
patterns that have been partially processed and stored, the question of how knowledge can
be derived from images is quite similar to the question of how knowledge can be derived

from ongoing sensory activity. Knowledge obviously is derived from perceptual representations, and there seems to be no reason why it should not also be gleaned in similar ways from mental images" (p. 60).

In other words, unless one dismisses completely the possibility that the immediate experiences of dreaming (sleep "new learning") can become permanent (though perhaps not easily retrieved, see Chapter 6), learning does take place during REM. But this learning is largely assimilative, and its effects on subsequent waking behavior will be indirect and subtle. This statement requires some additional qualification.

First, to say that dreaming is an assimilative process is *not* to say that it is necessarily autistic or unrealistic. Despite the fact that dreaming is largely reconstructive rather than reproductive, it can sometimes be quite veridical (e.g., sensible, realistic, conventional). This follows from the fact that the structures of "old learning" to which recent learning is assimilated are to some extent, at least in the normal adult, constrained by reality through evolution, maturation, and experience. Thus, the periodic weakening of the influence of SIS is not necessarily associated with the dissolution of veridical coding.

Second, that new learning will affect subsequent waking behavior will depend upon two things: (a) the amount of prior experience stored in long term memory, i.e., the "size" of old learning store, and (b) the validity of the assumption that dreaming is in fact new learning. Let us look briefly at each of these. The model assumes that the less experienced the organism, the greater will be the impact of new learning. This is a statistical assumption. That is, the smaller the n of the sample yielding results ("old knowledge") the greater the impact of a new datum (new learning) on the central tendency and organization of the sample results. Thus, a dream experience of childhood should have a greater impact on old learning than the dream experience of adulthood. In addition, the model assumes that the dreaming is analogous to the processing of SIS information during wakefulness, that it represents new learning which attains LTM status, i.e., modifies the structure of LTM or old learning. It is of course possible that this assumption is incorrect, that the dream experience is merely an epiphenomenological correlate of the playback or review of completed information processing. If dream experiences are merely examples of heightened attention to flow and perambulations of recent and old learning, a "courtesy call' paid to consciousness by unconscious processes which are more or less complete, then they would be of less psychobiological significance. However, even if we deny to dreaming the status of "programmer of a new information" (if dreaming is a reviewer rather than a director and producer), we still need to pay attention to it if we are ever to understand fully constructs like unconscious thinking, incubation, and intuition.

It would do well at this point to make explicit some additional assumptions of the proposed model. Note that the "LTM" box in Figure 5-2 is referred to as "old learning". The word "old" refers to the following: (a) Structural/functional characteristics that are "built in" or "wired in" through evolution, which mature during ontogeny, and which modify information processing during wakefulness and sleep. Thus, "old" refers to both the processes (e.g., primary processes, autonomous ego functions, etc.) and the resulting products, the latter of which are "learned" (assimilated) more through instinct than instruction. (b) Learning, influenced by instinct and instruction, that is laid down early in development and thus is temporally remote from recent events. (c) Relatively recently acquired information that is a permanent part of the LTM system (available and perhaps more readily accessible than the other above-mentioned products), information that requires relatively little additional processing.

The nature of the instinct component of "old learning" requires some additional explanation. First, we need to distinguish between (a) the instinctive *processes* that can influence anew the organization of information, and (b) the *products* of those processes which, themselves, become part of the structure of LTM or "old learning". An example of the latter would be an unresolved infantile complex (e.g., prelogical fantasies, needs in conflict, heightened emotion) which continues from time to time to influence adult interpretation of reality. Instinct as process refers to the operation of various parts of the central nervous system. For example, pontine, limbic and cortical functions peculiar to REM sleep will influence the nature of the dreaming process whatever the dream is about. I have already quoted Jouvet on the potential importance of PGO. Roffwarg *et al.* (1966) "wonder whether the eventual development of dream imagery may involve a process by which the cortex 'fits' sensory images to discharge patterns of brainstem origin established before the accumulation of sensory experience. The cortex may develop some modulating influence over these pontine discharges, but the basic discharge rhythm probably has a brainstem genesis. In this sense, the dream would truly appear to be born in the brainstem but clothed in the cortex" (p. 13). If brainstem-derived activity provides a biological substrate for instinctive tendencies in dream function during REM, the same may be said for limbic and cortical functions which are determined more by species "wiring" than by experience and instruction. For example, the activity of the limbic system could be thought of as the biological substrate of instinctive "needs" described by Freud as "id". Likewise, cortical functions peculiar to REM might be thought of as the biological substrate of Jung's concept of instinctive (i.e., species or collective) "knowledge", expressed as a tendency toward archetypical expressions.

Therefore, dreams about immediate exogenous and endogenous stimuli and recent learning will, in addition, be influenced by instinctive tendencies determined by wired in functions, and by the ontogenetically earlier products of those functions. To speak of instinctive influences on dreaming is not to degrade human information processing, but rather to give credit to its evolutionary continuity and the *natural* sources of its adaptive flexibility and creativity. It has been proposed that a function of consciousness is new learning (Kosslyn and Pomerantz, 1977). During wakefulness, external information is present in consciousness, held for a short period of time (STM) sensory, or sensory-dominated, form. Internal information (LTM or knowledge) can be extracted and *re-presented*, though these symbols of knowledge are less intensely sensory. However, in both cases, we are dealing with a neocortical process by which information can be modeled in consciousness (thought about). Thus, it is possible that new learning based on old learning is facilitated by a simulation of perception through a re-presentation of information in sensory-like form. Thus, the capacity for new learning is extended infinitely beyond the possibilities presented (in consciousness) by the sensorium. Does the consciousness of REM sleep function in a similar manner, permitting the re-presentation of recent and old knowledge in symbolic form, not merely for review but also for new learning? My guess is that this is the case.

Clearly there is a difference in the consciousness of REM sleep, and this difference is related to the relative predominance of the right hemisphere, especially during the earlier parts of the night (as described in Chapter 7, section 2). Thus, analogue coding tends to predominate over digital, the symbolic re-presentation of these in dream consciousness tends toward the spatial and imagistic rather than the verbal and numerical, and the process tends to be passively experienced rather than actively controlled in consciousness. In addition, self consciousness is largely absent in dreaming. However, lucid dreaming (i.e., including a realization of dreaming and some control over events) tends to occur later in the night, and this is in accord with evidence that (a) self-consciousness and controlled imagery is more the product of the left hemisphere, and (b) there is a tendency for relatively greater influence of the left hemisphere later, as compared to earlier, in the night.

Thus, for individuals who are representative of modern technological cultures, the *new learning* of wakefulness will tend to be dominated by (a) the left hemisphere, (b) external reality, (c) active consciousness (or the ability to retrieve and manipulate in consciousness verbal, imagistic, and numerical symbols). This is not to say that there is little or no influence on the new learning of wakefulness by right hemisphere, "internal reality", and passive consciousness (e.g., the spontaneous symbolism of daydreaming). It is to say that there is a *relative* predominance of influences during wakefulness which *tends to be reversed* during sleep (especially in the early part of the night). What I am suggesting is that new learning (not merely the activation of old information with or without consciousness) will depend on the style of cognition which in turn is constrained by the biological state of the brain. If this line of reasoning has merit, then cognitive growth is an organismic characteristic of sleep as well as wakefulness.

The model which I have just reviewed rather schematically is derived from three general sources: cognitive psychology, REM theory, and Freudian dream theory. It is offered as a heuristic device for thinking about REM research. I believe that it reflects the underlying rationale and implications of much of that research.

2. REM THEORY AND INDIVIDUAL DIFFERENCES

The remainder of this chapter will be devoted to a discussion of three potentially interrelated hypotheses about REM function that I believe have special relevance to the individual differences approach which I have been emphasizing. The first hypothesis, that of catecholamine system restoration, has been discussed at different points throughout the book. The second hypothesis says that REM sleep provides an opportunity for periodic stimulation, arousal, "reafferentation" of cortex. Thus, it concerns itself with the vertical organization of the brain (subcortical to cortical). The third hypothesis has received little theoretical and empirical attention in the sleep-dream literature. It states that REM sleep provides an opportunity for compensatory emphasis of right hemisphere information processing. Thus, it concerns itself with the horizontal or lateral organization of the brain (specifically, the neocortex).

These three hypotheses may be thought of as referring to the metabolic, the energic, and the structural/organizational aspects of brain function. However, they are not mutually exclusive. For example, metabolic activity may enhance protein building under the influence of subcortically induced activation during REM, and these events may in turn be the basis of neocortical reorganization. I have decided to focus on these three aspects of REM sleep because they are relevant to individual differences which deserve more attention. Conversely, paying attention to individual differences may provide data for the validation of these three (and possibly other) hypotheses about REM function. For example, if it is true that REM sleep provides an important source of periodic rearousal of the cortex, then individual differences in the need for periodic arousal, or individual differences in the motive to avoid extended periods of low arousal, should be correlated with a motive to restore REM sleep under conditions of REM deprivation. A formal statement regarding this individual difference approach to general hypotheses is given by Underwood (1975).

The three hypotheses proposed here constitute a subset of possible hypotheses regarding function of REM sleep in adult humans. I believe that each of them has heuristic value for theoretical advancement and empirical exploration. By focusing on these hypotheses I do not wish to imply that other REM functions of special phylogenetic or ontogenetic significance are less significant. Nor am I unmindful of the degrees of freedom permitted to theorizing given the yet unexplained complexities of the nervous system and their ambiguous relationships to poorly defined psychological phenomena. This dubious luxury is a two edged sword. We must live with speculations that prove to be wrong. But, as Claridge has pointed out, "the functional connections between various parts of the nervous system offer so many possibilities that, whatever theoretical model he erects, the behavioral scientist can scarcely be entirely wrong! This is not meant to imply that such models are valueless, but only to suggest that their main purpose is to provide a working framework for guiding further experimental research! (1967, pp. 185-186).

The biochemical restoration hypothesis

What are some of the implications for understanding individual differences in REM sleep which are provided by the catecholaminergic restoration hypothesis (Hartmann, 1973; Stern and Morgane, 1974)? Hartmann (1973) speculates that catecholamine systems mediate psychological processes loosely describable as "secondary process": critical judgement, concentration, task orientation, reality testing (i.e., being critical about unusual or bizarre circumstances), positive mood, sense of identity and free will, achievement orientation, and defensiveness. (Stern and Morgane, 1974, also speak of the importance of the catecholamine systems in mediating defensive behavior.) What is interesting to me is the general similarity of these characteristics to those attributed to repressor subjects (Byrne, 1964). Perhaps it is not too unreasonable to speculate that repressors, because of their greater commitment to "secondary process", are more likely to "wear out" their catecholaminergic systems and therefore to express a greater motive to restore REM (through increased REM duration or intensity). In fact, another variant of such a speculation has been made by Nakazawa et al. (1975b) based on their findings of an association between repression (or ego strength) and degree of REM rebound, and on the basis of earlier work (Nakazawa et al., 1973) indicating that catecholaminergic precursor (L-Dopa) reduces REM rebound. They suggest that "if, for instance, an extravert should be defined as having more intense brain function than another person who is introvertive, this would not be a hasty conclusion, we believe" (Nakazawa et al., 1975b, p. 108). Of course, in the absence of an appropriate operational definition for "intense brain function", such a statement is only suggestive.

If this idea of differences in brain processes has any validity to it, a number of predictions ought to be experimentally demonstrable. First, repressors or extraverts should be less adversely affected than sensitizers or introverts by catecholaminergically facilitating drugs (e.g., amphetamine, caffeine), especially at the end of the day, and especially after a number of days of REM deprivation. That is, these individuals should be less susceptible to behavioral disorganization due to exogenously induced catecholaminergic activation. Second, the difference in REM motivation between repressors and sensitizers should be reduced when repressors are administered such drugs presleep. This latter prediction is based on the distinction between REM function and REM process at the biochemical level (Stern and Morgane, 1974). That is, if REM sleep is a catecholaminergic restorational process, exogenous facilitation of depleted catecholamines should preempt the REM process to a significant degree (i.e., reduce the duration of REM sleep).

A further example of the heuristic value of the catecholamine restoration hypothesis is its potential for integrating ideas about REM sleep, the physiological basis of depression, and psychobiological factors underlying individual differences in personality. Seligman (1975) has recently reviewed evidence that some depressions are "helplessness" phenomena. Passivity, defeatist attitudes, physiological inertia can be simulated in animal and human subjects who do poorly in masterable testing situations after pretraining in an "inescapable condition". The latter, unlike the "escapable condition" and no treatment condition, provides experience with a (usually noxious) consequence that has only a random relationship to behaviors. After such treatment, the subject manifests behaviors which are remarkably similar to those manifested by depressed individuals in normal (escapable or no treatment) conditions.

There are two interesting things about the differential patterns of behavior that are generated in this three-condition experimental paradigm. First, there are individual differences in susceptibility to helplessness learning in the inescapable condition (Levis, 1976). Second, during the acquisition phase, "noradrenergic depletion" may play a role. Evidence for the latter comes from animal research which utilizes brain noradrenalin assays and neurohumoral manipulations. For example, in one study (cited in Seligman, 1975, p. 70) noradrenergic depletion normally induced by an inescapable condition was prevented by introducing an anticholinergic agent (atropine) which blocks septal inhibition of the median forebrain bundle. Animals treated in this way did not show the helplessness behavior which is normally observed in the inescapable condition.

If the catecholaminergic restoration hypothesis for REM sleep is valid, if repressors have a greater need for REM sleep because they more readily "wear out" their catecholaminergic systems, and if catecholamine depletion in certain brain areas (e.g., median forebrain bundle) has something to do with learned helplessness, then repressors should show a marked intensification of REM following inescapable conditions. Additional questions come to mind. Under normal conditions, are repressors less susceptible to learned helplessness than are sensitizers? What would be the effect of REM deprivation vs. NREM (control) deprivation on repressors? Would REM deprived repressors show greater helplessness in the morning relative to repressors given NREM (control) deprivation compared to sensitizers under similar conditions? That is, would the differential effect of the sleep manipulation be greater for those individuals who appear to have a greater "need" for REM (i.e., repressors) than for those individuals who appear to be less dependent on REM sleep? Or would REM deprivation interfere with the consolidation of helplessness learning in repressors, and thus be associated with *less* helplessness in the morning? We are currently running a study of learned helplessness and REM deprivation in an attempt to get answers to some of these questions.

How would the findings jibe with preliminary evidence that REM deprivation has a greater therapeutic effect on endogenous than on exogenous depressives (Vogel, 1968, 1975)? It makes little sense within the context of a catecholaminergic hypothesis for REM unless (a) the catecholaminergic restoration hypothesis for REM is not true, (b) catecholamine depletion theory of psychotic depression is not true, or (c) there is some as yet unknown "rebound" in catecholamine deprivation. Perhaps mechanically- or drug-induced chronic REM deprivation initiates a compensatory shift away from cholinergic and toward catecholaminergic functioning. REM deprivation-induced · hyperactivity observed in animals (e.g., heightened appetitive behavior, sexuality, activity) suggests that the latter possibility may be true. The fact that REM deprivation (for roughly two weeks) tends to have a therapeutic effect on those individuals (psychotic depressive) for whom catechol-amine depletion is thought to be a significant problem constitutes *the* major embarrassment for Hartmann's catecholamine restoration hypothesis for REM sleep, unless we make some assumptions.

Let us take another look at the problem. First, we know that REM deprivation is therapeutic for endogenous depressives, and in direct proportion to recovery rebound (Vogel, McAbee, Barker, and Thurmond, 1977). That REM rebound is in part a process that "restores" a catecholamine deficit is strongly implied by a number of findings, e.g., L-Dopa eliminates post deprivation rebound (Nakazawa *et al.*, 1973). Recall that there is good reason to suspect that the usual procedures do not necessarily eliminate all aspects of the REM state. It is possible that while the drive for REM builds up there is *partial* "recovery" of catecholamine systems, and that the greater the pressure, the greater the recovery. These assumptions would fit both the findings of a therapeutic effect (partial recovery) for individuals with a presumed catecholamine system deficit and the continuing need (rebound).

These assumptions are consistent with other observations regarding endogenous depression. With respect to REM sleep, there is now good evidence that the mechanism of REM initiation is cholinergic. This evidence comes from (a) Hobson's work on FTG cells of the brain stem, (b) latencies by cholinergic facilitation, plus (c) earlier research done by Jouvet and Hernandez-Peon which strongly implicated cholinergic processes underlying REM sleep (see Chapter 1). It is becoming increasingly apparent that a distinction must be made between those mechanisms that account for the initiation of REM (REM latency) vs. those which account for the duration of REM once it has been initiated. Second, with respect to endogenous depression, there is some reason to believe that an imbalance between cholinergic and adrenergic processes favoring cholinergic dominance operates in a number of endogenous depressives (Davis, 1975), especially in the retarded (bipolar) types (Baldessarini, 1975; Davis and Janowsky, 1975; Maas, 1975). This imbalance would fit nicely with Kupfer's (1976) review of evidence that there is a short initial REM onset latency in endogenous ("primary") depressions, but not when they are in remission. Is it possible then that REM deprivation, like tricyclic antidepressive medication (e.g., imipramine, desipramine), which is known to be anticholinergic (Silverstone and Turner, 1974), initiates a gradual shift from a cholinergic to an adrenergic emphasis in the central nervous system? Such a shift could explain the antidepressive effects.

What is the significance and relevance for REM theory of the observation of individual differences in personality between endogenous depressives (i.e., bipolar depressives and lithium-responding unipolar depressives) vs. other depressives (specifically, tricyclic responders)? The former do not seem to show much evidence of neurotic and immature behavior either premorbidly or during the psychotic phase while the latter do (Donnelly, Murphy and Scott, 1975; Kupfer, Pickar, Himmelhoch and Detre, 1975). Is there a tendency for the former group to be "repressor" persons who come from repressor-type families while the latter are exaggerations of the sensitizer personality? Such a distinction would help to explain why the relatives of neurotics (presumably including depressives) are not elevated on neuroticism scales (Slater and Cowie, 1971). Perhaps we are dealing with problems of classification. Some depressions are associated with low neuroticism (repression) and some with high neuroticism (sensitization). One problem with applying results from REM research on personality to questions about clinical disorders is that the two may be psychologically and physiologically discontinuous. Perhaps an endogenous psychosis includes a breakdown in the functional effectiveness of what is normally an effective REM process.

This is, in principle, a testable speculation. It generates the prediction that individuals who have high REM rebound after REM deprivation are more apt to report a higher incidence of *endogenous* depression in their relatives. My guess is that those individuals who show minimal REM deprivation effects (e.g., sensitizers, introverts) are likely to report a relatively higher incidence of "nervous breakdown" and schizophrenia in their relatives. Conversely, if you selected subjects who have a first degree relative diagnosed as depressive with neurotic personality (hysteroid, immature, anxious, demanding) or subjects who have a first degree relative equally depressed but without those neurotic features, the latter group of subjects would tend to show more REM intensification under conditions of REM deprivation than would the former group.

While catecholamine restoration is a heuristically powerful hypothesis, it does not readily explain a number of hypotheses about REM sleep (see Chapter 1). Consider the following. (1) There is some reasonably consistent evidence (largely from work on animals) that relatively high noradrenergic levels are associated with increased activity and improved performance on simple, speed-related tasks, e.g., digit symbol; conversely, there is similar evidence that high levels of acetylcholine are associated with lower activity levels and improved performance on more complex tasks that require delay, reversal of habit, restructuring, e.g., block design (Broverman *et al.*, 1968). (2) There is some evidence that relatively high levels of catecholamines are associated with shorter durations of REM sleep while relatively high levels of acetylcholine are associated with shorter latencies to REM sleep (Hartmann, 1973; Sitaram *et al.*, 1976). Thus, the catecholamine restoration hypothesis predicts a tendency for *short term* REM deprivation to be associated with relatively low levels of catecholamine and relatively high levels of acetylcholine. If this is true, then we would expect REM deprivation to have an adverse effect especially on tasks requiring speed rather than complex restructuring, and to lead to lower rather than higher activity levels (cf., Broverman *et al.*, 1968). But just the opposite tends to be true. That is, REM deprivation, when it does have a documentable effect, tends to increase activity levels, drive levels, affect (Dement *et al.*, 1970), selective (narrow) attention (Koppel *et al.*, 1972), and tends to have an adverse effect on more complex tasks of the restructuring variety (e.g., those requiring perceptual reorganization and divergent thinking). This kind of evidence, in the light of our relative ignorance of other neurotransmitters and their mutual interactions, suggests that the hypothesis may have to be revised. In any case, I believe that a simple "catecholamine restoration" hypothesis cannot, in itself, account for many observations on the effect of REM deprivation of normal or clinical samples.

I have said a great deal about the REM process as a motivational state. A separate motivational factor for REM dreaming has not been established. That is, a need for REM sleep may not represent a need for a psychological experience (fantasy) rather than for a biological event. Some have suggested ways to differentiate REM sleep from REM dreaming functions. For example, Cartwright and Monroe (1968) reported that waking fantasy could reduce REM rebound in REM deprived individuals. These preliminary findings suggested that the motive for REM is partly psychological. However, the data from our current study provide little support for this idea. Perhaps the substitution of dreamlike activity during NREM sleep under conditions of REM deprivation might also be associated with less REM pressure (Cartwright *et al.*, 1967). However, such evidence of state boundary permeability could not be taken as evidence of the substitutability of a purely psychological experience independent of more fundamental shifts in REM characteristics at the physiological level. At present, there is no unequivocal evidence that the need for REM, which we infer from signs of REM intensification, is basically a need for a certain kind of psychological experience which is more or less independent of the biological state of the organism. If there is any validity for the fantasy substitution hypothesis, it will require the induction of fantasy which is most similar to REM fantasy. But that would require a biological substrate that is similar to REM sleep, and substituting such a state would effectively cancel out the REM deprivation! At best, one could argue that REM sleep/dreaming displaced in time would reduce the need for REM sleep dreaming which occurs normally at other times. While the evidence is sparse, I do not believe that waking fantasy (daydreaming) or transitional state (stage 1-NREM) "dreaming" is a particularly effective substitute for REM sleep/dreaming. In fact, demonstrating that stage 1-NREM cannot substitute for lost REM would constitute strong evidence for the unique function(s) of REM sleep and REM dreaming despite the superficial similarities.

However, saying this, I do not mean to suggest that the nature of dream content is of little interest in the experimental exploration of the REM motive. Quite the contrary, if we accept the belief that there is a psychophysiological bridge carrying information and influence both ways (Akiskal and McKinney, 1975), then information about the biological characteristics of REM sleep should have implications about dreaming, and information about dreaming should have implications about the biological substrates of REM sleep (Bertini, 1973; Hartmann, 1973). Despite this, we have next to nothing to go on with respect to the changes in the dreaming process (other than characteristics like intensification of dreamlike fantasy) associated with a heightening of the REM sleep motive under conditions of REM deprivation. Perhaps this reflects the rather primitive state of dream analysis. I will have some comments later about the nature of dream content in repressors and sensitizers under different kinds of presleep conditions. However, this information will not be sufficient to advance significantly our knowledge of the role of dreaming *per se* in the expression or mediation of the hypothesized REM motive.

Restoration of optimal levels of cortical arousal

This hypothesis stems from the discussion of REM-NREM dynamics provided by Ephron and Carrington (1966). They have characterized REM sleep as a mechanism of endogenous restimulation of the cerebral cortex which occurs after a period of NREM sleep. They speak of the reafferentation properties of REM sleep, and consider them to be of great importance to the maturation of brain function in the developing neonate (Roffwarg *et al.*, 1966). The implication of such a view of REM sleep for an individual differences approach may prove quite useful.

Before discussing the relevance of this approach to questions of individual differences, a brief comment on the potential importance of the function of periodic cortical arousal is in order. First, we have already seen that learning during sleep generally requires a certain degree of cortical arousal (usually inferred from EEG characteristics of low voltage and fast activity). Cortical arousal can be elicited by subcortical (reticular) stimulation. Such artificial experimental stimulation can (a) enhance learning when it occurs during post-trial consolidation, and (b) eliminate the performance decrement of amnesiac agents when the stimulation precedes the administration of the agent (Bloch and Fishbein, 1975). In addition, there is growing evidence that during the activated state of REM, information already in the system is consolidated (allowing recall and adequate postsleep performance) and to some extent is reorganized (allowing more creative adaptation). During REM sleep, "cortical centers may process the information *as though it were from some external source*" (Bloch and Fishbein, 1975, p. 161, italics added).

What all this suggests is that a kind of learning during REM may take place which simulates learning during wakefulness, and this learning, though lost to recall through its state-dependency (Cohen, in press; Evans *et al.*, 1970), may have as much or more influence on the development of the organism as learning during wakefulness. The vividness of experience, heightened as it is by inhibition of sensory input and motor output (i.e., organismic isolation), and the lack of reality testing (i.e., naive acceptance of the experience *as though real*), provides the potential opportunity for a kind of complex learning (metaprogramming) in which both the "environment" and the "reactions" are orchestrated (assimilated) by the subject. Though the average human adult may spend as much as two hours in REM sleep, those two hours may in a sense be functionally comparable to two hours of intense wakefulness during which assimilation rather than accommodation is the rule (Piaget, 1962).[1] This may be especially true for infants and children and for preliterate peoples for whom distinctions between fantasy (dreaming) and reality (wakefulness) are least developed. After all, if early childhood learning continues to have important and lasting effects on adult behaviors (temperament, career choices, marital decisions, etc.) then much of this "learning" may be the metaprogramming of REM sleep. For example, sometimes sudden onset of fears or interests that are incomprehensible on the basis of knowledge about a child's waking experiences may be explainable, in principle, on the basis of endogenous and perhaps fortuitous events that arise during REM (or sleep onset) dreaming. (I am grateful to Martin Seligman for reminding me of this potentially important aspect of dream psychology.)

Rosenbaum (1972) has spoken most eloquently about the role of early fantasy as a source of learning. "Because neonates are unsophisticated judges of fantasy and 'reality', their assimilations of fantastic and 'realistic' percepts are indiscriminate. Consequently, their cognitive frameworks tend to internalize both kinds of percepts equally; cognitive structures which embody fantastic information are formed as readily as structures which embody realistic information. Later, when the distinction between fantasy and reality is learned, fantasy structures are modified and are subordinated to reality structures. Those fantasy structures which are displaced or absorbed become cognitive residues that are rectified in fantasy" (1972, p. 480). The point is that these "residues" are in one form or another permanent and at least indirectly influential.

Piaget's discussion of "unconscious symbolism" (personal, subjective, dreamlike) is consistent with the hypothesis of endogenous REM learning. He speaks of affective

---

[1] REM would then be a unique condition for which the concepts of independent and dependent variables are relatively meaningless. The philosophical implications of such a view of REM sleep are profound. Despite its "regressive" features, REM sleep becomes a model of the highest level of independence from the immediate environment permissible without rejecting psychological determinism. The REM state provides one of the best examples of the fallacy of conceptualizing cognitive and instrumental behavior as merely "dependent variables".

schemas which dominate ludic (play-related) and dream symbols, "a summary blending of the various feelings aroused by them and it is these schemas which determine the main secondary symbols [affective language], as they often determine later on certain attractions or antipathies for which it is difficult to find an explanation except in unconscious assimilation with earlier modes of behavior" (Piaget, 1962, p. 176).

Learning without awareness need no longer be thought of as a paradox of knowing and not knowing. Research on commissurotomized patients suggests that the right hemisphere can know without awareness. Modern information processing models include perceptual awareness, both sensory and cognitive in nature, which may not attain permanence in long term store. The interference hypothesis for memory is consistent with the view that much of what is momentarily perceived consciously (and which *could be* coded and rehearsed so as to be retrievable) may attain long term store without being easily retrievable. Yet there is good reason to believe that such information can influence behavior.

For example, Nisbett and Wilson (1977) describe a study by W. Wilson in which subjects showed no consciousness that certain tone sequences had been presented in the unattended channel of a dichotic listening task. They were unable to discriminate beyond chance those sequences from a set of new ones in a subsequent test. However, when asked to rate the sequences, they indicated greater preference for those presented during the dichotic listening task, that is, those that were familiar though unconscious. Rather than interpreting this effect as reflecting the failure of material to attain long term store, it can be thought of as an example of the effect of available but inaccessible information. This idea is certainly not new to dynamic psychology. It merely reinforces, through empirical demonstration, the possibility that nonrecalled dream experiences may, especially in childhood, have two kinds of influence. First, they may effectively alter long term storage, thereby constituting a *direct* influence on what the individual knows. Second, they may influence the individual's attitudes and feelings about aspects of the environment (e.g., aversions, incentives), thereby constituting an *indirect* influence on what the individual will learn during wakefulness.

How could we test the hypothesis that nonrecallable experiences during REM sleep influence waking thought and action, i.e., effectively change the individual adaptively or maladaptively. Recall the work on REM learning and state-dependent recall by Evans *et al.* (1970). It might be possible to use personally more meaningful stimulus sentences during REM. These could be tailored both to the affective life of the individual and to the testing conditions of the experiment. Would the subject, like the hypnotized individual made amnesic for instructions, demonstrate changes in appetite or aversion after REM inductions? Would such evidence support inferences about "learning" on the basis of naturally (endogenously) arranged experiences during REM?

Having reiterated the potential importance to the individual of REM sleep let us consider the question of whether there are individual differences in the "need" for such a central state of arousal.

Let us assume for the moment that for optimal functioning, a cortex requires a certain amount of arousing information flow from subcortical centers (especially reticular and limbic). It is reasonable to assume that there are individual differences in the complexity of the cortex (and therefore individual differences in need for arousal) as well as individual differences in chronic levels of arousal. To the degree that there is a mismatch between the need for, and characteristic availability of, such arousal, one might expect that there would be individual differences in the tendency to restore an organismically determined balance. For example, individuals who tend toward excessive sensation-seeking may be individuals whose characteristic level of subcortical activation is insufficient relative to cortical requirements. Therefore, just as the REM period is thought to restore cortical reafferentation after a period of NREM low arousal, during wakefulness individuals may engage in instrumental activities that, through the activity itself or through the increased information input insured by that activity, provide the necessary arousal.

If this line of reasoning has merit, there should be evidence that (a) arousal-promoting activity can at least partially "substitute" for REM sleep, i.e., be related to less REM rebound after REM deprivation, and (b) individual differences in traits related to periodic sensation-seeking should be relatively highly correlated with REM rebound after REM deprivation which presumably reduces an important source of endogenous stimulation. There is preliminary work suggesting that there is a reciprocal relationship between intracranial self-stimulation (ICSS) and REM rebound; ICSS reduces REM rebound while REM deprivation increases ICSS activity (Cohen, Edelman, Bowen and Dement, 1972; Steiner and Ellman, 1972). Another study reported that light exercise (having subjects stroll around the lab) during the estimated duration of each REM period was associated with 5.8% less REM sleep on the initial recovery night than was the no exercise control awakening condition (Vogel et al., 1970). Finally, there are data suggesting that evening exercise is associated with less REM sleep than nonexercise control conditions (Desjardins, Healey and Broughton, 1974). These data are consistent with the idea that, in part, REM sleep serves as a source of arousal.

With regard to individual differences, it can be predicted that individuals whose characteristic level of arousal is low (e.g., relatively slow EEG) and who tend to restore periodically the required arousal (e.g., through excessive bouts of motor activity or sensation-seeking) will be especially likely to show REM rebound after REM deprivation. An obvious prediction would be that the subset of "hyperactive" children who show slow EEG patterns should show more REM rebound after REM deprivation, and less after treatment with stimulants. Another prediction is that physically active, sensation-seeking individuals should show a greater REM motive. I know of only one set of published findings that are in accord with this prediction, those of Nakazawa et al. (1975a, 1975b), who found greater REM rebound in extraverts than introverts. According to Eysenck's conceptualization, extraverts are cortically less active, tending to get bored more easily in dull situations (Eysenck, 1967). The fact that there is a correlation between extraversion and sensation-seeking scales (Farley and Farley, 1967) reinforces the idea that individual differences in need for REM may be related to need for periodic arousal after periods of low arousal.[2]

Compensatory right hemisphere information processing

Let us now consider the hypothesis that REM sleep is particularly specialized for right hemisphere information processing. The heuristic value of hemisphere-specialization theory goes without question. If anything, it may seem to explain too much, and like other

[2] Farley and Farley (1967) reported evidence that male extraverts are apt to subscribe to the following kinds of items from the sensation-seeking scale developed by Zuckerman, Kolin, Price, and Zoob (1964): (1) I would like to try some new drugs that produce hallucinations. (2) I sometimes would like to do things that are a little frightening. (3) I would like to have the experience of being hypnotized. (4) I would like to try parachute jumping. (5) I prefer friends who are excitingly unpredictable. (6) I often find beauty in the "clashing" colors and irregular forms of modern paintings. (7) When I feel discouraged I recover by going out and doing something new and exciting.

"breakthroughs" in psychiatric research, may prove to be more fashionable than substantive with regard to explaining sleep phenomena. Nevertheless, let us briefly explore some of the implications of the hypothesis that REM sleep functions are related to lateral (horizontal) organization of the cerebral cortex. Simply stated, the hypothesis proposes the following: (a) A major characteristic of REM sleep is heightened activity of right hemisphere processing. (b) This heightening of activity can be thought of as compensatory for the predominant left hemisphere-mediation of information processing during wakefulness. (c) Conditions (situations, traits) associated with relatively heightened left hemisphere orientation during wakefulness will, other things being equal, tend to be associated with especially heightened right hemisphere activity during REM. (d) Such conditions will be associated with greater need for REM, e.g., REM deprivation under such conditions will be associated with higher REM rebound or relatively greater postsleep performance deficits, especially on tasks that require substantial right hemisphere mediation.

The heart of the general proposal suggested here is the notion of a compensatory shift of mode of information processing during REM sleep. If the terminology of the following statement is translated into that of hemisphere lateralization terminology, it can stand as a good representation of the proposed hypothesis. "For a day experience to be elaborated within memory it might be necessary that material learned along the lines of secondary process thinking be transformed so that it will tie in with the highest possible number of related experiences. This requires a shift in the functional organization of the psychic apparatus which allows for a regression to the most primitive way of functioning without disorganizing itself, and without losing the adaptive control of reality. REM sleep, with its intense activation and modulation of the most primitive brain centers, seems to meet the requirements for this shift in a typical although not exclusive manner" (Bertini, 1973, p. 62).

While I favor the idea that this compensatory process represents a shift toward paleocortical (e.g., limbic) influence on cerebral function, I am suggesting that there is also a shift toward right hemisphere influence of information processing. The notion of shift in mode of processing is analogous to suggestions in the clinical literature on dreaming that there is a kind of restorative process that corrects "imbalances" in waking emphasis. Jung's (1933) theorizing about the role of dreaming to restore the integrity of personality comes closest to this kind of thinking. (Evidence of the suppression of right hemisphere is reviewed by Searleman, 1977, pp. 521–522.)

The clinical literature is not the sole source of speculation about the compensatory aspects of cognitive functioning. For example, Rosenbaum (1972) has offered a theory regarding the importance of fantasy as a reflection of the motive to reify or actualize cognitive structures that have been displaced by those which guide adult behavior. He argues that during development, those structures (primary process?) which are displaced, suppressed, or subjugated by reality considerations take on the status of "residues". He proposes that residues always tend to seek reification in consciousness and behavior. "But residues become residues because they are not reified. They are displaced or absorbed by new structures which *are* reified and which, consequently, can become predominant in the cognitive framework. As long as these new constructs remain predominant, it can be presumed that they find continual reification in the environment and that residues do not. This means that if residues are to be reified, they must be reified in some environmentally anomalous way. Furthermore, their reification should not be reprehensible to predominant structures but should at least be granted a special context to prevent contradiction of new structures" (1972, p. 475). Dreaming provides such a context. And if the right hemisphere plays a special role both in the mediation of repressed/suppressed residues (Galin, 1974) and in the mediation of dream imagery, it can be argued that it may do so through a compensatory exaggeration of function during REM sleep.

Regardless of whether one takes a physiological or a phenomenological perspective with regard to the hypothesized compensatory function of REM dreaming, the approach suggests that the process will be of special importance to those individuals whose waking cognitive and personality styles constitute a suppression of those characteristics that have been attributed to the REM process. Both the general hypothesis regarding compensation and its derivative application to individual differences will be taken up shortly.

Before discussing the evidence for right hemisphere compensation during REM sleep it would be useful to discuss a potential moderator variable that may affect results from which need for REM is inferred. This variable may be called psychophysiological compartmentalization. Compartmentalization refers to the degree that psychological and physiological events have what Mandler (1975) calls "tightness and invariance of structure", the degree to which they have exclusive function. This idea is based on evidence of individual differences in the degree to which REM phenomena (e.g., PIPs, eye movement, intense dream activity) are confined to REM sleep (Cartwright, 1972; Dement *et al.*, 1970). The more that REM sleep is compartmentalized, other things being equal, the more REM deprivation should intensify the REM process and disrupt waking processes that are mediated by REM.[3]

The relationship between physiological operational definitions of REM compartmentalization and REM rebound has not been adequately established. There is indirect evidence from the work of Dement and his colleagues that under conditions of reduced REM compartmentalization (conditions which induce "leakage" of REM processes into other states) there is reduced REM rebound after REM deprivation. Watson, Liebmann, and Watson (1976b) have recently reported a nonsignificant positive correlation (.31) between the frequency of PGO-like phasic events during NREM sleep and a Rorschach measure of psychopathological thinking. They also found a highly significant positive correlation (.70) between the frequency of these phenomena and human movement responses (reflective of inner fantasy). These data, obtained from a group of 23 hospitalized schizophrenics, are consistent with hypotheses regarding psychophysiological compartmentalization. In addition, there is evidence that acute schizophrenics have less psychophysiological compartmentalization and little or no REM rebound. Also, if it is reasonable to expect a relationship between psychological and physiological compartmentalization, then the findings of high REM rebound in field independent individuals is consistent with the general idea that deprivation-induced REM need will tend to be higher for individuals whose REM periods have a more exclusive function. And this will be the case regardless of whatever specific function one hypothesizes for the REM period (e.g., catecholamine restoration, reafferentation, right hemisphere compensation).

If this line of reasoning has merit, then it should be expected that additional evidence for relatively high REM rebound will be obtained for individuals who are highly specialized or

---

[3] This hypothesis is consistent with data that suggest that arousal and the motive to resume functioning is determined by interruption of any well organized, familiar sequence of behaviors, and by the discrepancy between the interrupted and interrupting phenomena (Mandler, 1975, pp. 162-163).

compartmentalized, e.g., field independents, individuals whose REM periods are much more dreamlike than their NREM periods (Cartwright, 1972), individuals who are genetically unrelated to schizophrenics, and who are not subject to high anxiety of other kinds of disorganizing emotionality. In addition, unless REM function is entirely different in children, one should expect a tendency for infants and children to show less REM rebound. There is one unpublished study of the human newborn, and one published study of neonatal vs. juvenile rhesus monkeys (Berger and Meier, 1966) whose results are roughly consistent with this expectation.

With this potential modifying variable in mind, we can now focus attention on those individual differences and conditions that are relevant to the hypothesis that REM sleep provides the opportunity for compensatory right hemisphere information processing. If this hypothesis is valid, then REM sleep should be especially important for individuals who, during wakefulness, are especially likely to (a) emphasize left hemisphere functioning at the expense of right hemisphere functioning, and/or (b) tend to suppress right hemisphere functioning, and individuals (c) whose left and right hemisphere functions are highly compartmentalized (i.e., who show a high degree of lateralization of cortical function). The expression vs. suppression of affective, intuitive, subjective, sensual behavior has been recently attributed to left vs. right hemisphere dynamics (Bakan, 1971; Galin, 1974; Schwartz, Davidson and Maer, 1975).

Descriptions of certain personality variables strongly suggest the tendency for left hemisphere emphasis and dominance over the right hemisphere during wakefulness (Dimond, Farrington and Johnson, 1976; Galin, 1974; Geschwind, 1975; Searleman, 1977). Two personality variables appear to be especially relevant: repression as estimated by repression-sensitization or neuroticism type questionnaires, and field independence estimated by behavioral tasks such as the Rod and Frame, Embedded Figures, and Block Design tests. For example, field independent or cognitively differentiated individuals show a high degree of articulation of experience of the world, self, and body. Characteristics of field independent individuals include (a) a high degree of *analytic* ability, that is, capacity to separate the relevant from the irrelevant (vs. a more diffuse and global style); (b) active and objective approach (vs. a passive, intuitive, and subjective approach); (c) relatively greater *control of impulses* and moods via defense mechanisms of intellectualization and isolation (vs. greater impulsivity and a tendency to use massive repression or denial), (d) more stable GSR and less manifest anxiety or aversions, (e) a more well defined sense of identity, as well as more self-confidence. Witkin, Dyk, Faterson, Goodenough and Karp (1962) summarized data from a number of studies by saying that "persons with a relatively global field approach [field dependents] are more apt than analytical people [field independents] to show open anxiety reflecting, presumably, less effective controls" (Witkin *et al.*, 1962, p. 169).

Note the similarity between the characteristics of field independents and those of repressors (Byrne, 1964). Also note that the concept repression used here as a description and throughout this book refers to suppression/control over affect and impulse, not necessarily of thoughts or ideas (e.g., denial, massive repression, the kind of characteristic more likely to be demonstrated by field dependent individuals). Also note that many if not all these field independent characteristics are similar to those attributed to greater left hemisphere orientation. Therefore, such individuals may represent a higher degree of left vs. right compartmentalization and possibly a tendency to suppress both right hemisphere and paleocortical/diencephalic functioning. This latter statement is supported by findings such as those reported by Bertini (1975). Under conditions designed to induce free association (instructions plus *gansfeld*) field independents' productions were *less* fluent, perceptual, bizarre, affective, vivid than were field dependents' productions.

However best estimated, the tendency toward repression may be related to REM function. First, during wakefulness, the left hemisphere tends to dominate over/inhibit the right (Dimond *et al.*, 1976; Geschwind, 1975; Searleman, 1977). Second, repression may be an exaggeration of this tendency (Galin, 1974), especially a tendency toward inhibition of affective/emotional processes which appear to be mediated by the right hemisphere (Davidson, Schwartz, Pugash and Bromfield, 1976; Dimond *et al.*, 1976; Gainotti, 1972; Tucker, Roth, Arneson and Buckingham, 1977). Third, if REM sleep provides an opportunity for compensatory expression of right-mediated processes (see below), then the REM period may be more important to repressors than to non-repressors. This is simply another way of suggesting that there are individual differences in the exclusivity of REM function.

Table 5-3 shows the three aspects of left vs. right differentiation which may have implications for REM function theory, plus some ways that they might be operationally defined for research purposes. In addition, the table includes some experimental manipulations that might be used presleep to effect a differential exercise on the right or the left hemisphere. Preliminary results relevant to left vs. right hemisphere differentiation theory of REM function suggest that REM sleep is in some sense more important for individuals who are highly compartmentalized and who tend to emphasize left and suppress right functioning during daytime. In addition, it is hypothesized that presleep manipulations which exercise the right hemisphere will tend to reduce the need for REM sleep. For example, it has been reported that meditation (TM) produces a significant reduction in REM percent (17.2%) compared to nonmeditation conditions for the same subjects (25.8%)

TABLE 5-3.   Possible Factors Relevant to a Right Hemisphere Compensation Hypothesis for REM Sleep

A. Individual Differences in Left vs. Right Differentiation:
   1. *Compartmentalization:*
      (a) Confinement of REM phenomena to REM sleep, e.g., PIPs[a], muscle atonia, fantasy, etc.)
      (b) Left vs. right EEG amplitude for REM vs. NREM sleep
      (c) Cognitive differentiation (e.g., field dependence)
      (d) Cortical maturation
      (e) Handedness (degree of lateralization of cortical functions)
   2. *Suppression of right hemisphere functioning:*
      (a) Repression
         (1) Questionnaire estimates of the trait
         (2) Discrepancy between the presence of definite physiological signs of "rest" phase of the BRAC vs. relative absence of psychological/behavioral signs (e.g., fantasy, prelogical thinking, rest)
      (b) Left vs. right hemisphere emphasis during wakefulness in cognitive style (e.g., right vs. left looking, preference for art vs. science, low vs. high imagery/daydreaming frequency/intensity, etc.)
      (c) Individual differences in metabolic activity in left vs. right hemisphere (e.g., assessed by radioactive xenon methodology)

B. Experimental Presleep Induction of Left vs. Right Hemisphere "Exercise":
   1. *Verbal-analytic vs. tactile-form recognition tasks*
   2. *Convergent vs. divergent tasks*
   3. *Exercising the left (vs. the right) hand in eye-hand coordination tasks*

[a]Phasic integrated potentials (or PGO-like phenomena) of the extraocular muscles. These are discussed in Chapter 7, section 1.

(Becker and Herter, 1973). Such manipulations are suggested in Table 5-3. The effects of such manipulations would not be large, but the hypothesis would not require large effects. In fact, in the light of our difficulties in replicating a fantasy substitution effect (see Chapter 4), it might be hypothesized that the degree to which psychological experience during wakefulness can mobilize the right hemisphere exclusively, the less pressure for REM will be shown.

It is possible that we are dealing with a number of dimensions of individual differences each of which may make a relatively small independent, and possibly additive contribution to the motivation for REM sleep. For example, repressiveness (right hemisphere suppression) and field differentiation (psychological compartmentalization plus left hemisphere emphasis) may each contribute to a need for REM. If this line of reasoning is valid, then those individuals who show the strongest REM intensification under conditions of REM interference will be field independent repressors with a strong bias toward left hemisphere-mediated behaviors.

The hypothesis that REM sleep represents a tendency toward right hemisphere compensation appears to boil down to two variants. (1) *Passive compensation*: the right hemisphere dominates because dominance by the left is diminished. Diminution of left dominance could occur in two ways. The similarity between catecholamine-mediated processes (Hartmann, 1973) and those purported to be mediated by the left hemisphere (Bakan, 1971) suggests that catecholamine depletion affects the left more than the right during the early REM periods of the night. On the other hand, diminution of left dominance may be attributed to the relatively lower levels of subcortical arousal that presumably affect the left more than the right hemisphere (as suggested by my discussion in Chapter 1, see Figure 1-5). Are catecholamine restoration and periodic subcortical arousal functionally related? Is catecholamine restoration facilitated by subcortical arousal, or are both the products of pontine-initiated events (PGO)?

If the diminution of left dominance is not a mere artifact of diminished levels of subcortical arousal rather than some intrinsic state of depletion, then the passive variant of the right hemisphere compensation hypothesis predicts that REM deprivation should more adversely affect those behaviors that are most exclusively mediated by the left hemisphere. That is, REM deprivation would interfere with the (catecholaminergic?) "restoration" of left hemisphere capacities.

(2) *Active compensation*: This variant of the hypothesis indicates that there is an active emergence of the right hemisphere. The assertion of function may take advantage of a relative diminution of left functioning, but it is significant in itself. During sleep when the normal channels of cognitive reification (to borrow Rosenbaum's terminology) are unavailable, alternative channels become predominant. The active variant of the right hemisphere compensation hypothesis suggests the prediction that REM deprivation will more adversely affect right hemisphere-mediated behaviors.

If, as it is likely, both passive and active compensation is the rule, then a certain degree of ambiguity will characterize our predictions about the kinds of behaviors that would be affected by REM deprivation. While I tend to favor the active compensation variant, it could be argued that many of the available data are consistent with either variant. For example, if repressors or field independents show a greater need for REM, it may be due either to suppression of right hemisphere functioning or left hemisphere depletion or both, i.e., the price paid for suppression of right is depletion of left.

To determine the relative importance of variants of hemispheric differentiation theory of

REM sleep, better operational definitions are needed for independent, intervening, and dependent variables. For example, independent variables could be defined in terms of right vs. left hemisphere tasks and cognitive (and personality) styles as suggested in Table 5-3.[4] Intervening variables could be measured in terms of catecholamine levels, or left vs. right EEG amplitude ratios (Galin and Ornstein, 1972) or regional cerebral blood flow (Risberg, Halsey, Wills, and Wilson, 1975) during presleep conditions. Dependent variables would include those indicating REM need, e.g., REM rebound. Table 5-4 shows examples of such findings that I believe are consistent with the right hemisphere compensation hypothesis, and which, taken together, appear more consistent with the active compensation variant. Needless to say, they do not constitute a very impressive data base. What will be required is research designed specifically to test various aspects of the hypothesis.

I have suggested that REM compensation theory might profit by considering the relationship between individual differences in personality or cognitive style and individual differences in REM rebound. There is another dimension which may be more relevant than these for testing REM compensation hypotheses. Hardyck and Petrinovich (1977) have reviewed evidence that handedness is a fairly good indirect estimate of the degree to which cortical functions are differentially associated with one or the other cerebral hemisphere. The evidence is based on diverse kinds of studies, e.g., dichotic listening tasks, loss and recovery of function subsequent to localized cerebral damage, etc. It appears that individuals with strong right-hand bias are more highly lateralized for cortical functions than are individuals with weaker right or weak left biases, especially those with familial left-handedness. In addition, there is some evidence, though not as impressive, that females tend, on the average, to be somewhat less lateralized than are males (Bakan and Putnam, 1974; Levy, 1972). The logic of the right hemisphere compensation hypothesis for REM sleep, as outlined above, suggests that the duration of REM sleep after REM deprivation should be greater for the more highly lateralized individual. That is, the strong right-hander is more compartmentalized (cortically differentiated in terms of lateralization of function), may therefore be better able to suppress or inhibit right hemispheric functions during wakefulness, and therefore should be more sensitive to manipulations which eliminate REM time. I can now report evidence which is consistent with this derivation.

Subjects were given a handedness questionnaire composed of 10 activities (e.g., writing, drawing, throwing, etc.). They rated their preference for either right (scored positive) or left (scored negative) hand from strong (2) to weak (1) or no preference (0). Averaging over the 10 items yielded a right preference score that could vary from—2 through zero to 2. Prior to analyzing the results, it was decided to categorize subjects with scores from 1.6 to 2.0 as strong right, subjects with scores from zero to 1.3 as weak right (or ambidextrous) and anyone with a negative score as left. Since there were very few left-handers, we will focus on the subjects of the other two groups, a total of 46 (26 male and 20 female undergraduates).

Each subject spent a single night in the sleep laboratory. During the first six hours after initial lights out, the subject was either REM deprived or run under control conditions. REM deprivation was carried out by awakenings made at the onset of each REM period such that only about 1.0-1.5 minutes of REM per REM period occurred. Subjects in the control condition were awakened at the estimated end of each REM period (thus allowing

[4] Of course, in the real world, situations and individual differences are *not* likely to be independent. Left hemisphere "types" are likely to be attracted by, and seek out, left hemisphere-related situations. For example, Horn, Turner and Davis (1975) reported that high school repressors are far more likely to *choose* scientific college majors than are sensitizers.

TABLE 5-4. Findings Relevant to the Hypothesis that REM Sleep Is Particularly Concerned with Right Hemisphere Information Processing

	REM sleep/dream characteristics	REM motivation	REM deprivation effects
A. General	(1) Affective, intuitive spatial quality of dreams (2) EEG evidence of a shift toward relatively greater right hemisphere activation from NREM to REM sleep (3) Adverse effect of right hemisphere lesions or commissurotomy on dream intensity and dream recall (4) Spatial (e.g., Rod and Frame Test, depth perception) ability is better at the end of REM periods than at the beginning	(1) REM rebound reduced by fantasy task during wakings, not reduced by "secondary process" task (2) REM pressure: minimized by right hemisphere type tasks, maximized by left hemisphere type tasks done during awakenings (female)	(1) Adverse effects on divergent, but not convergent, task performance
B. Individual differences	(1) High ScK individuals have less exclusive confinement of dream-like fantasy within REM sleep (and show less REM rebound) than low ScK individuals (2) REM deprivation or presleep stress has a relatively greater effect on EM activity of the REM sleep of repressors than of sensitizers (3) Dream recall frequency is higher for males and females with a "feminine" rather than a "masculine" sex role orientation (4) REM onset latency throughout a deprivation night is positively correlated with amount of dream-like fantasy (repressor subjects only)	(1) Repressor and field independent individuals have greater REM rebound than field dependent, and schizophrenic individuals (2) Relatively greater lateralization of cortical function (estimated by gender and handedness) associated with higher REM rebound	(1) Relatively more adverse effect on block design performance of repressor than sensitizer individuals (2) Some evidence that REM deprivation induces more dysphoric mood in repressors and "compensators" (3) High ego strength individuals are more likely to repress ego threatening information after REM deprivation

about 18-20 minutes of REM per REM period) plus, in some cases, during intervening stage 2-NREM. Thus, REM deprivation and nondeprivation subjects were comparable with respect to the total number of sleep interruptions during the first six hours of the night. During each awakening the subject was asked to report dream content or to make up a fantasy. This procedure lasted for five minutes. During the last 100 minutes, sleep was uninterrupted. If the logic of the REM compensation hypothesis is sound, and if lateralization of function can be inferred from handedness, then the following predictions should be supported: (a) Strong right-handers should show greater REM rebound during the last 100 minutes of sleep than should weak right-handers. (b) Males should tend to show more REM rebound than females. (c) Evidence of familial left-handedness in weak right-handers should be associated with the least REM rebound.

For the first analysis, REM rebound (REM%) was assessed as a function of strong or weak right-handedness under conditions of REM deprivation ($n = 30$) or nondeprivation ($n = 16$). Figure 5-3 shows the results. Aside from the obvious effect of REM deprivation ($p = .003$), there was a significant interaction ($p = .028$). REM deprivation appears to have virtually no effect on weak right-handers while it has a powerful effect on strong right-handers ($p < .005$).

Let us now consider the subjects run under conditions of REM deprivation. If we divide them into male and female groups who are either strongly or weakly right-handed, we find that, as expected, the males show higher REM% than do females ($p = .012$), and strong right-handers show higher REM% than do weak right-handers ($p = .016$). There is no interaction. The results are shown in Table 5-5. As predicted, REM% is highest for strong right-handed males and least for weak right-handed females.

Finally, the prediction that REM% would be lowest in weak right-handed subjects with familial left-handedness was also supported. Since there were almost no strong right-

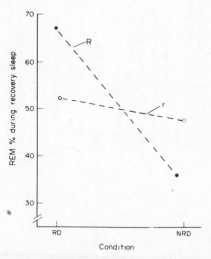

Figure 5-3   REM% during the last 100 minutes of a night after six hours of REM deprivation (RD) or REM nondeprivation (NRD) for groups with strong (R) or weak (r) commitment to the right hand.

TABLE 5-5.   REM% During Post-REM Deprivation Recovery Sleep for Male and Female Individuals with Strong (R) or Weak (r) Right-handedness

Sex	Handedness	
	R	r
Males		
$\bar{X}$	76.7	59.6
s.d.	18.9	13.5
n	7	10
Females		
$\bar{X}$	58.9	40.0
s.d.	22.5	19.5
n	8	5

handers with familial left-handedness, these (four) subjects are eliminated in the following analysis. Table 5-6 shows REM% for strong right-handed, weak right-handed, and weak right-handed plus familial left-handedness. The overall relationship is statistically significant ($p < .05$) indicating a significant difference between the right and weak right plus familial group ($p < .02$). While the difference between any two adjacent pairs of groups does not reach statistical significance, the three groups do line up as one might expect if these categories reflect degree of lateralization.

The literature suggests that individuals with strong left-handedness are probably as highly lateralized as individuals with strong right-handedness. Only 3 individuals run under the REM deprivation condition indicated left-handedness (negative score on the handedness scale). The mean handedness ratings for these three individuals was —1.6 (indicating relatively strong left-handedness), and their mean REM% was 68.3 (s.d. = 11.6), a figure that is virtually identical to that of the strong right-handers (67.2).

While handedness was associated in a theoretically meaningful way to REM rebound, there was no difference between strong or weak right-handedness groups in REM pressure (number of REM attempts during REM deprivation). This differential association of two, REM characteristics (pressure vs. rebound) and an external variable (handedness) provides further support for the argument that when we speak of the motive for REM, we need to specify which characteristic (REM pressure, REM%, REM density) we mean. While these three characteristics do covary with degree of REM deprivation, they are not highly

TABLE 5-6.   REM% During Post-REM Deprivation Recovery Sleep for Males and Females with Strong Right-handedness (R), Weak Right-handedness (r), or Weak Right-handedness plus Familial Left-handedness ($r - l$)

	Handedness		
	R	r	$r - l$
$\bar{X}$	70.8	59.1	46.6
s.d.	21.1	19.7	13.4
n	11	8	7

positively intercorrelated as one would expect on the assumption that they are merely different ways of estimating the same function.

Taken together, these results provide preliminary support for the hypothesis that individual differences in compartmentalization and perhaps suppression of right hemispheric function are associated with individual differences in a compensatory motive to restore lost REM time. In addition, they provide support for the idea that right hemispheric activity is an important feature of the REM process.

Throughout this book I have tried to develop the implications of individual differences in the data. I have discussed or will discuss individual differences in eye movement density, quality and quantity of sleep, arousal thresholds, resistance and reaction to REM deprivation, capacity to respond to signals presented during sleep, in the capacity to dream about topics suggested presleep, in the content of dreams, and in the ability to conceptualize problems during dreaming and to use the products of this intellectual work. There is no doubt in my mind that separately, additively, or interactively, these differences relate to differences at the biological level with as yet barely appreciated implication for REM theory.

In my judgement, the potential contribution of individual differences to an understanding of the nature and importance of REM sleep has not been given the attention that it deserves. We have seen that in every area of sleep research there is an enormous amount of variation in the data. This variation might profitably be explored by controlling enduring subject differences (traits) as well as by trying to control situational factors. For example, if it is true that REM sleep is particularly geared to exercising normally suppressed right hemispheric functioning, then individual differences in such suppression might explain some of the variation in REM deprivation effects. Perhaps the apparently greater importance of REM sleep to some individuals can be understood as an expression of a fundamental neuropsychological "style" that underlies personality characteristics such as conventionality, or cognitive style characteristics such as field independence. In this section of the book I have taken a psychobiological approach in order to draw implications for the dreaming process from data and theory on the physiological context of REM sleep. It seems to me that cross-fertilization between personality and REM sleep theory is not only possible but desirable. While I have attempted to apply concepts from personality to REM theory, it is becoming more and more apparent to me that REM research may provide important insights regarding the biological basis of personality differences. The two fields should profit greatly from mutual influence.

In speculating about the data on REM sleep, I and others have tried to draw out implications in the form of testable hypotheses. This is particularly important since speculation is really the easy part and often contributes to a sense of knowing more about a phenomenon than is truly the case. One of my colleagues has suggested that the value of speculation is relative to its consequences. Consequences can be either practical or theoretical. Clearly, I have tended to develop speculations that lead to testable hypotheses that are more theoretical than practical. However, if these derivations eventuate in a better understanding of the phenomenon, they may indeed have practical implications. As Rechtschaffen has said, in order to know what is good sleep or enough sleep we need to know what sleep does (Rechtschaffen, 1971). I would add that there is evidence, at least with respect to REM, that sleep may "do" different things for different people. For example, sleep characteristics (both normal and abnormal) and sleep function must be related to variation in temperament, as well as in situational factors. Selection of pharmacological and/or behavioral therapeutic approaches to insomnia will benefit from a greater understanding of the effect of personality, situation, and interaction effects on sleep. Thus, in a very real sense, practical consequences are often implied in theoretical consequences of speculation. Only in the context of further research will it be possible to evaluate the validity and usefulness of concepts like fantasy quota, psychobiological state boundary, suppression of right hemisphere functioning, catecholaminergic restoration, defensive processing, and ultimately, REM need.

This part of the book has been devoted primarily to a consideration of empirical data from which a psychobiological analysis of dreaming might be made. I have focused on REM sleep rather than NREM sleep for a number of reasons. For example, there are more data on REM sleep, and the psychological experiences during REM are generally more organized, informationally rich, and more readily subject to experimental investigation. I have tried, where possible, to draw from the biological facts of REM sleep implications about dream theory which for too long has been articulated from a nonbiological, nonempirical, purely psychological perspective. The rationale for focusing on psychobiological roots of dreaming is that there is continuity in biological functioning from wakefulness to sleep, that this continuity underlies both waking and sleeping experiences, and that dreaming reflects the *milieu intérieur* as much as the external environment. And while it is true that we are rather limited in what we can say about the symbolic *meaning* of dreams from such a perspective, there is much that can be said about biological factors that influence both *content* and *function* of dreaming. If one is interested only in dream symbolism, perhaps there is little of value that such an approach can add *at the present time*. However, no large theory of dreaming that considers dream content and dream function as well as dream meaning can be complete without considering the various sources of biological determinants of which the REM sleep data are representative.

Part B

Psychological Approaches
to Dream Content

. . . a man defines himself by his make-
believe as well as by his sincere impulses.

Albert Camus

CHAPTER 6

DETERMINANTS OF DREAM RECALL

The validity of a theory is limited by the quality of its data base. Hypotheses about the content and function of dreaming derive from dream report data. The validity of these data, their availability and accuracy with respect to the original experience, is affected by a number of factors. These include consciousness during the original experience, short and long term memory, motivation, fatigue, verbal skills, and the compatibility of waking retrieval processes with information encoded during sleep. In a sense, a dream report is twice removed from the dream; it is a report of a memory of an experience. No wonder that under normal conditions so little dream material is available to the average person.

Ideally, a dream report should constitute faithful *reproduction* of the major events and characteristics of the experienced dream. However, in practice we can only hope that the ostensibly well-recalled dream is minimally characterized by the other two aspects of recall, namely reconstruction and deduction. *Reconstruction* (transformations, elaborations, interpretations) may promote an understanding or appreciation of the individual but may create obstacles in empirical research on the nature of the dream as it was actually experienced. *Deduction* is the process by which the subject logically fills in details of what must have been, and thus may do damage to the faithful rendering of experiences which may *not* have followed rules of logical sequencing that govern similar experiences during wakefulness. I know of no study that has explored the degree to which subjects differ in their ability to employ reproduction rather than reconstruction and/or deduction in the recall of incidentally observed visual events that serve as stimuli during wakefulness. Are there individual differences, associated with reliable and objective personality/intellectual characteristics, that experimenters could be alerted to in order to select good recaller subjects? In this sense, "good recallers" would not be frequent or plentiful recallers, but *accurate* recallers.

A weak criterion for judging the validity of the dream report is the requirement that there be a general similarity between the contents of the report (e.g., its length, quality, etc.) and concomitant physiological or verbal (i.e., sleep talking) events. Against such a criterion, the dream report obtained in the laboratory after a REM sleep awakening appears to be a credible datum. However, dream theories are developed on the basis of dream report data that vary in terms of (a) quantity (e.g., how much material at what point in the night, under what conditions?), (b) quality (how well or selectively recalled?), (c) sample bias (what kinds of individuals provide the data, what kinds of influences come from the investigator?). A clinician working with patients is likely to develop hypotheses about the nature and function of dreams that differ from those of his or her academic counterpart whose dream data come from college subjects whose sleep is interrupted in the laboratory. This is not a trivial difference we shall see; hypotheses have ranged from the romantic view of dreaming as more creative and insightful than waking thought to the tough-minded though minority opinion that dreaming is the chaotic assembly of essentially random events generated by a central nervous system in the state of "idle". Clearly, we ought to pay attention to factors that affect dream recall, if only to rule out potential confounds in studies on situational and dispositional factors that affect dreams.

1. THE REPRESSION HYPOTHESIS

Basically there are three general hypotheses regarding access to the dream experience via the dream report. (1) *Repression hypothesis*. This hypothesis holds that defensiveness with respect to inner experience interacts with the content of dreams, and this may affect dream recall and/or reporting. First, defensive operations (censorship) may occur during dream-work so that an emotionally neutral or safe dream is consciously experienced. Second, a threatening dream that was consciously experienced during sleep would, upon awakening, elicit repression or simply suppression (i.e., unwillingness to report the experience). This second variant of the repression hypothesis suggests two kinds of predictions: (a) Repressor-type individuals will tend to have less dream recall than nonrepressor types. (b) Conditions which increase the likelihood of threatening dream content will, especially in repressors, reduce the probability that dreams will be recalled.

(2) *Salience hypothesis*. This hypothesis states that dream recall is positively correlated with neurophysiological arousal during REM, imagery ability, emotional impact of the experience, i.e., factors that are more likely to heighten consciousness and attract attention during the dream.

(3) *Interference hypothesis*. This hypothesis states that dream recall will be inversely correlated with events during dreaming, during awakening, and after awakening which interfere with the consolidation or retrieval of memories associated with the dreaming experience. Variables that are loosely categorizable within the framework of the interference hypothesis include, for example, state-dependency or "boundary permeability" between sleep and wakefulness, and degree of attention to the dream memories rather than to external information.

I have discussed in detail the evidence for all three hypotheses in a review paper (Cohen, 1974d). What follows will be a more selective discussion of highlights of this research and their methodological and theoretical implications.

With respect to the first variant of the repression hypothesis — that dream content may reflect defensive transformation of threatening material into disguised and neutral or safe dreams — there is virtually no good empirical evidence. Hall (1966) points to numerous examples where individuals dream about an obnoxious event openly and directly even though, at other times, these same individuals might dream about such events in more symbolic fashion. "Moreover, there is no lack of dreams in our collection in which the most distasteful and shameful things happen. Fathers and mothers are murdered by the dreamer. The dreamer has sex with members of his family. He rapes, pillages, tortures, and destroys. He performs all kinds of obscenities and perversions. He often does these things without remorse, and even with considerable glee" (Hall and Nordby, 1972, p. 14). Of course, it is just as reasonable to speculate that it is the (periodic) failure of repression which explains such reports. Since the data base for arguments regarding the disguise function of dream symbolism rests on psychodynamic theory and clinical interaction, we cannot yet evaluate these ideas from a scientific perspective.

The second variant of the repression hypothesis — that repression of obnoxious dream experiences upon awakening accounts for variation in dream recall — has generated a great deal of empirical work. This variant of the repression hypothesis is aptly described by Freud who says "that during the night the resistance loses some of its power ... [and] ... having gained its full strength at the moment of awakening, it at once proceeds to get rid of what it was obliged to permit while it was weak" (1955, p. 526). This "after expulsion" version of the repression hypothesis has been the subject of correlational and experimental research.

Since much of the evidence bearing on the repression hypothesis comes from questionnaire or diary measures, it will be useful briefly to mention that such measures demonstrate acceptable levels of reliability. A number of years ago I obtained estimates of dream recall frequency from three different measures that were provided by a group of college students. The first measure was a variant of an eight-step dream recall frequency questionnaire (Q-DRF). The second was a check-list on which subjects recorded the presence or absence of dream recall (no details were asked for) over a 30 day period. The first 25 days of recorded information were used, each day scored zero or 1 with total range of 0-25. Later, the subjects were asked to fill out a dream diary sheet on each of three consecutive days describing any dream content they could remember. Recall of any material was scored as "recall". Thus, the range of possible scores was 0-3.

Table 6-1 shows the intercorrelation matrix for the three measures of dream recall frequency, male correlations above and female correlations below the diagonal. Clearly, despite motivational problems that contribute to error variance, there is a reasonable degree of redundancy in these measures. Also, in terms of consistency over time, when recall for the second week was correlated with recall during the fourth week, the correlation for 125 males was .64, for 203 females .52. The predictability of performance measures of dream recall frequency from Q-DRF estimates is illustrated by results shown in Table 6-2. That is, high recallers report dream recall more frequently on both the checklist and diary tasks than do low recallers. This kind of result has been replicated a number of times for both males and females. For example, in an earlier study of females, of 34 high recallers (estimated from the

TABLE 6-1.   Intercorrelation Matrix for Dream Recall Questionnaire (Q-DRF), 25-Day Recall Checklist (25-Day) and 3-Day Dream Diary Task (3-Day)

	Q-DRF[a]	25-Day[b]	3-Day[c]
Q-DRF	–	0.54	0.56
25-Day	0.69	–	0.54
3-Day	0.37	0.47	–

Note: Male data above, female data below the diagonal. Based on samples of 133 males, 205 females. All scores based on the number of dreams recalled (vs. not recalled) estimated from each measure. All correlations are significant beyond the 0.01 level.
[a]Range of possible scores: 0-14.
[b]Range of possible scores: 0-25.
[c]Range of possible scores: 0-3.

TABLE 6-2.   Mean 25-Day Recall Checklist and 3-Day Dream Diary Performance of Highest
and Lowest Self-rated (Q-DRF) Dream Recallers

Criterion	High recallers[a]	Low recallers[b]	$p<$	r_{pb}
25-Day				
Males (N = 65)	13.9	6.1	0.0001	0.65
Females (N = 99)	16.4	5.8	0.0001	0.77
3-Day				
Males (N = 59)	2.1	0.5	0.0001	0.70
Females (N = 118)	1.8	0.9	0.0001	0.42

[a] Recall most mornings of the week or more.
[b] Recall less than once a week.

Q-DRF), 20 or 59% reported two or three dreams on a three day diary task while only two
out of 22 low recallers (9%) performed as well.

Correlational approach to individual differences

An obvious first prediction, that repressors should have less dream recall, gained attention
when Schonbar (1959) reported what turned out to be an inordinate and nonreplicable
correlation between repression-sensitization scores and dream recall (.59). Since that time
modest, barely significant correlations (at best around .25, often lower, sometimes negative)
tended to cool whatever enthusiasm existed for the hypothesis that a repressive life style
inhibits dream recall (Schonbar, 1965). For example, Cohen and Wolfe (1973) reported
evidence against the idea that infrequent dream recall is the product of the *rejection* of inner
life. This is not to say that dream recall is uncorrelated with a tendency toward the practical,
conventional, and external. In fact, there is some evidence for such a correlation, weak
though it may be. The point is that these correlational data do not demonstrate that poor
dream recall is the result of a *rejection* of inner life; rather, they may indicate a lack of skill
based on memory capacity, imagery capacity, and attitudes developed during socialization.

For example, Cory *et al.* (1975) reported that frequent dream recallers were significantly
better than infrequent recallers on tests of short-term, long-term, and incidental memory.
(In addition, they found no difference between the groups on anxiety. In fact, they found a
marginally significant *positive* association between repression and dream recall!) This study
represents a significant improvement over earlier studies that could find no relationship
between dream recall and memory (e.g., Barber, 1969; Cohen, 1971). The Cory *et al.*
findings, along with results indicating poor dream recall in subjects with short-term
memory defects (Greenberg, Pearlman, Brooks, Mayer and Hartmann, 1968; Torda, 1969),
constitute strong evidence that individual differences in memory account for some of the
individual differences in dream recall. In addition there are correlational data suggesting
that a positive attitude toward visual fantasy (daydreaming, imagery) and a divergent
cognitive style are associated with good dream recall (Austin, 1971; Hiscock and Cohen,
1973; Holt, 1972; Schechter, Schmeidler and Staal, 1965; Singer and Schonbar, 1961).
There is also an interesting study showing high dream recall in the deaf, especially the
congenitally deaf, along with evidence that their dreams are more colorful (Mendelson,
Siger and Solomon, 1960).

There is additional evidence for the idea that dream recall is affected by skills and attitudes which are developed within certain social conditions rather than a reflection of repression. Consider my study of the dream recall frequency of twins (Cohen, 1973a). Male and female identical twin pairs ($N = 54$), same-sex dizygotic twin pairs ($N = 34$), same-sex sibling pairs ($N = 32$), and same-sex friend pairs ($N = 42$) were each divided into subgroups depending on whether they were currently living together or apart. Results shown in Table 6-3 indicate that there was a significant main affect for together vs. apart ($p < .05$) and a significant difference for related (all sibs) vs. unrelated ($p < .03$). While MZ twins were more alike than were DZ twins, nontwin siblings were as alike as MZ twins. Thus, a genetic hypothesis for dream recall frequency (at least measured by questionnaire) could not be accepted. These results support the hypothesis that to some extent, similar socialization and life style factors are reflected by similarity in dream recall. Since it was choice more than circumstance which determined living conditions, we can assume that similarity in dream recall frequency reflects the operation of common rather than complementary attitudes (Seyfried and Hendrick, 1973). Having said this, it should be noted that correlations between dream recall frequency and specific personality measures have been weak, trivial, or inconsistent (Cohen, 1974d). However, these disappointing findings are more damaging to the repression hypothesis because factors that are found to be associated with dream recall (e.g., memory; field dependence) can be interpreted as psychodynamically neutral.

Sometimes a failure to find evidence for a hypothesis yields information of some methodological or theoretical interest. Such is the case with the relatively small correlations between estimates of repression and estimates of dream recall frequency. Consider two estimates of the repression disposition. One is derived largely from psychodynamic tradition which tends to view the relative absence of anxiety and other dysphoric affects as a sign of "ego strength" and the healthy or defensive "binding" of affect. Measures related to this somewhat vague concept of repression derive from emotionality questionnaires (e.g., Bryne Repression-Sensitization Scale, Eysenck Neuroticism Scale, Taylor Manifest Anxiety Scale, IPAT [Cattell] Anxiety Scale, etc.). These highly intercorrelated scales have been used to test the prediction that there is a relationship between relatively low dream recall frequency and scores at the repression end of the scale. As we have seen, such correlations have been found though they have been relatively small and not particularly reliable.

The second type of repression estimate derives from the comparative-developmental tradition which tends to view the relative absence of anxiety and other dysphoric affects as a ing increasing differentiation, specialization, and integration of function. The relative

TABLE 6-3.   Similarity in Dream Recall Frequency Expressed in Mean Intrapair Difference Scores for Same-sex Monozygotes, Dizygotes, Nontwin Siblings, and Friends Living Together or Apart

Living condition	Group			
	Monozygotic	Dizygotic	Sib	Friend
Together				
X	2.37	3.18	2.00	4.33
SD	1.82	2.04	1.55	3.41
Apart				
X	4.00	5.57	3.81	5.62
SD	3.21	3.41	3.46	3.83

absence of anxiety is roughly commensurate with good psychological "boundaries" including the separation of thought and affect. Thus, a less differentiated cognitive style would tend to be associated with two kinds oi psychological phenomena: diffuse, global, more intuitive thinking patterns and a tendency toward anxiety and impulse expression. Measures of perceptual articulation (e.g., Embedded Figures Test, Rod and Frame Test, Block Design, Tilted Room) are often used to infer a disposition to use repression. However, this concept of repression is somewhat different from that reflected in the more psychodynamic tradition. It refers to a tendency to block out chunks of cognitive information rather than to suppress affect. Thus, field dependents are described as using "massive repression" and "denial". Clearly, if one believes that failure to recall dreams is due to repression, then it would be predicted on the basis of the comparative-developmental view, that field dependents would tend to have less dream recall than field independents. In fact, some findings consistent with the prediction have been reported (e.g., Schonbar, 1965; Witkin *et al.*, 1962) though they are not always significant (Cohen and Wolfe, 1973) nor do they account for much of the variance in dream recall frequency estimates.

The interesting contradiction in these findings, regardless of the strength of the reported relationships, is that individuals who tend to score at the low end of emotionality scales ("repressors") are similar to individuals who tend to score in the field independent direction ("nonrepressors"). If one looks at the published descriptions of personality characteristics and behaviors of questionnaire-defined low emotionality "repressors" (see Chapter 4, p. 108), one finds rather similar characteristics: a tendency toward analytical thinking, conservatism, emotional stability, self-confidence, self-esteem, impulse control, etc. Of course, this makes a great deal of sense from both the psychodynamic and cognitive differentiation perspectives. The latter would hold that there should be a tendency for individuals with well differentiated or "bounded" styles to have good "ego strength", i.e., to cope more effectively in a complex world. The similarity between repressor and field independent styles also makes sense in terms of psychodynamic formulations which attribute "binding" properties to the "energy" that would otherwise be freely expressed in affect and impulse. However, the similarity between repressors and field independents is *not* reflected in predictions about dream recall frequency, since field dependence, rather than field independence, is taken as an indication of the habitual use of repression.

How can we account for reports that there is a tendency for questionnaire-defined "repressors" to have low dream recall frequency while there is a tendency for field dependents also to have low dream recall frequency? There are at least two possibilities. One is that there is so much bias in what gets published that the findings represent an artifact of editorial policy rather than a reflection of the real world. The other possibility is that the emotionality and cognitive style dimensions are less correlated than suggested by the personality descriptions in the literature. If this is the case, then it would be expected that a combination of field dependence and repression would yield very low dream recall frequency while the combination of field independence and sensitization would be associated with very high dream recall. I know of no such analysis in the literature. But if such an analysis did reveal *strong* relationships in the predicted direction, it would explain the low correlations found when the competing effects of the two separate dimensions are not taken into consideration. Thus, if field dependence and low emotionality each has a depressing effect on dream recall, but if in fact these two dimensions are uncorrelated or somewhat *negatively* correlated, the effects of each will tend to cancel out.

Situational effects

Let us now consider some of the evidence that bears upon a prediction derived from the after-expulsion variant of the repression hypothesis. This prediction states that conditions that presumably stir up threatening dreams which are "candidates for repression" (Goodenough, 1967, p. 139) will, especially in repressors, be associated with less dream recall. Since the hypothesis fares rather poorly, I will discuss here only a few examples from my own research that reasonably represent the kind of disconfirmatory evidence that is more thoroughly reviewed elsewhere (Cohen, 1974d).

In one of these studies (Cohen and Wolfe, 1973), we tried to effect a diminution of dream recall by telling subjects that dreams are important sources of information about latent or manifest psychopathology. We hoped to demonstrate at least a suppression if not a repression effect. If ever there was experimenter bias in a study, it was here. Yet despite the apparent credibility and acceptability of our cover story, the manipulation was associated with a tendency toward *more* rather than less dream recall; and this increase was accounted for largely by the *infrequent* reporter subjects (the supposed repressors)! This finding is compatible with the more parsimonious view that interest or curiosity, rather than defensiveness with regard to dreams, accounts for more of the variance in dream recall. Perhaps this is because most individuals are not threatened by dreams and, in reasonably nonthreatening conditions, are willing to communicate them. For those individuals who have an inordinate personal investment in their dream life (e.g., patients in psychoanalysis), repression may be a significant factor in dream recall. The point of this discussion is not to challenge the concept of repression, but merely to question its utility in accounting for the variance of the dream recall of relatively normal populations.

A more direct test of the repression hypothesis was carried out in two studies which I reported in 1974 (Cohen, 1974a, 1974b). Results of the first study (Cohen, 1974b) showed a positive association between dysphoric mood and dream recall, especially for subjects who tend to be poor recallers. In this study, female subjects filled out presleep mood scales and dream diary sheets (the next morning) for a period of five days. A within-subject comparison was made between dream recall after the night associated with the highest self-confidence rating vs. dream recall after the night associated with the lowest self-confidence rating. Results are shown in Table 6-4. The relatively larger percentage of contentless than dreamless reports in the positive mood condition is particularly interesting in the light of the hypothesis that contentless experiences are phenomenological representations of the

TABLE 6-4. Mean Percentage of Three Types of Dream
Diary Report Associated with High- and Low-self-confidence
Ratings of Forty Subjects with Significant Mood Fluctuation

Type of report	Self-confidence rating	
	High	Low
Content	34*	63*
Contentless	36**	18**
Dreamless	29	19

$*p < 0.01.$
$**p < 0.06.$

process of repression (Witkin, 1969, p. 32). Evidence which I will discuss later suggests rather that such reports are caused by psychodynamically neutral distractions and state-related interference rather than cognitive escape from internal threat (repression).

In the follow-up study (Cohen, 1974a), 81 college females filled out presleep mood and morning dream diary sheets. The association between dysphoric affect and heightened dream recall was again observed but the relationship was weaker. Again, the effect was observed for the infrequent recallers (62% recall vs. 39% recall for worse vs. best mood nights respectively) but not for the frequent recallers (40% vs. 42%).

Now consider the data from the Cohen and Cox (1975) study that bear on the hypothesis that individuals subjected to ego threat, especially repressors, are less likely to recall dreams. Table 6-5 shows that for neither REM nor NREM awakenings was there a significant conditions (stress vs. positive) $\times$ personality (repressor vs. sensitizer) interaction effect on any measure of dream recall which was elicited by the experimenter. On the other hand, the recall data derived from diary reports filled out by the subjects after alarm clock awakenings did reveal a pattern similar to that found in the home dream reports of the female subjects in the two previous studies (Cohen, 1974a, 1974b). The proportion of subjects with diary recall

TABLE 6-5.   Variables Associated with Dream Material

| | Presleep condition | | | |
| | Positive | | Negative | |
Variable	$\overline{X}$	n	$\overline{X}$	n
Experimental awakenings[a]				
Sensitizers	3.80	10	3.00	12
Repressors	3.33	9	3.00	9
REM reports per subject[b]				
Sensitizers	1.60	10	1.42	12
Repressors	1.67	9	1.22	9
NREM reports per subject[b]				
Sensitizers	0.60	10	0.75	12
Repressors	0.56	9	0.67	9
REM units per report[c]				
Sensitizers	2.61	9	2.50	11
Repressors	2.30	9	2.71	7
NREM units per report[c]				
Sensitizers	1.83	6	1.86	7
Repressors	1.60	5	1.60	5
Time per REM report[d]				
Sensitizers	4:41	9	4:25	11
Repressors	4:39	9	4:34	7
Time per NREM report[d]				
Sensitizers	4:22	6	5:10	7
Repressors	3:35	5	4:12	5

[a] Refers to awakenings for all subjects to obtain reports or (occasionally) to adjust electrodes. ns refer to subjects who recalled at least one REM or NREM dream.
[b] ns refer to subjects who recalled at least one REM or NREM dream.
[c] ns refer to subjects who recalled the indicated type of dream material. The values represent amount of dream material per report based on scale from 1 (fragmentary) to 4 (rich, detailed, developed) used by independent judges demonstrating good interrater reliability (rs 0.90).
[d] Time based on within-subject averaging across indicated type of awakenings which yielded dream recall, and then averaged over subjects.

(of a dream experience occurring just prior to awakening) in the positive condition was .38 (.50 for REM, and .27 for NREM awakenings); in the negative condition the respective figures were .61 (.89 and .43). When the data from the 12 most frequent recallers (estimated by pre-experimental questionnaire) were removed, the relationship was even stronger: .33 for the positive condition and .71 for the negative condition ($p < .03$). While confirming previous results, the difference between experimental vs. diary findings suggest that, whatever the effect of conditions and personality, it can largely be eliminated by a task-oriented condition which focuses the subjects' attention on the dream and elicits sufficient motivation to report despite fatigue and external distraction. As we will see, both the salience and interference hypotheses can account for these and other results better than can a repression hypothesis.

Another set of results from the Cohen and Cox (1975) study is worthy of mention because it directly contradicts a different prediction generated by the repression hypothesis. Data from eye movement measures taken on these subjects were reported in a separate paper (Cohen, 1975). I have already described the results (see Figure 3-1). The interesting thing about them is that they could be interpreted as supporting a repression hypothesis. Recall that in the negative condition, the repressors had greater REM density than did the sensitizers, while in the positive condition, the repressors had less REM density than did the sensitizers. A variant of the repression hypothesis makes the following argument. First, attempts to suppress fantasy during wakefulness is associated with increased eye movement activity (Antrobus, Antrobus and Singer, 1964). Second, poor dream recallers are repressing (e.g., not focusing on dream material long enough to consolidate memory traces that would be strong enough to survive awakening). Therefore poor recallers should have more eye movement activity during REM than good recallers. Antrobus, Dement, and Fisher (1964) did find such a relationship.

However, Cohen and Cox (1975) found no relationship between habitual dream recall frequency and eye movement density, no relationship between dream recall frequency and repression vs. sensitization, and no relationship between REM dream recall and REM density (see also Molinari and Foulkes, 1969). Another problem is that the Antrobus *et al.* study may have confounded fantasy inhibition and mental effort. There is ample evidence that both eye movement activity (see Chapter 7, Section 1) and pupil dilation (Craik and Blankstein, 1975) are increased under conditions that call for cognitive effort (e.g., Klinger, Gregoire and Barta, 1973). Suppressing fantasy may simply be more difficult than producing fantasy, or it may require thoughtlike cognition which appears to be associated with relatively high amounts of eye movement activity.

The oculomotor avoidance hypothesis is important, not because it is supported, but because it is derived from a methodologically sophisticated approach to the problem of objectifying a rather elusive, "on-line" phenomenological event. The approach attempts to establish a psychophysiological correlation that exists outside of sleep, i.e., cognitive avoidance and eye movement density. It is assumed that eye movement density during REM represents similar cognitive activity during sleep. A similar approach has been reported by Bell and Stroebel (1973). Preliminary evidence (Bell, Stroebel and Prior, 1971) suggested a relationship between physiological recordings of scrotal muscle activation and anxiety content in the interview material. Again, on the assumption of a continuity of this kind of correlation during REM sleep, Bell and Stroebel predicted that REM content, elicited at the moment that such physiological patterns were observed, would be more dysphoric. Such a relationship was found. The interesting thing is that there was no evidence that these physiological patterns were associated with a failure to recall content. Similarly, Goodenough *et al.* (1974) found no evidence that REM periods characterized by relatively high amounts of physiological turmoil (pre-established as characteristic of the subjects in their stress film condition) were associated with relatively less recall; in fact, just the opposite tended to be the case. Unless the assumption of continuity of psychophysiological correlation is rejected, these findings constitute fairly strong evidence against the repression hypothesis.

The results shown in Table 6-5 suggest that REM and NREM dream recall elicited in the laboratory is not markedly affected by presleep conditions and level of repression. One objection to the assumption that repressors should show a marked diminution of dream recall under stressful conditions is that dreamwork could neutralize potentially threatening latent content by creating safe experiences that are more acceptable to waking recall. If that were the case, it would be expected that the dreams of repressors who are subject to stressful presleep conditions should be more mundane, pedestrian, conventional. The evidence is mixed. While the dreams did tend to be affectively bland, they were not inherently less interesting or exciting (at least to judges asked to rate the dreams blindly). A major problem with data that are consistent with a repression hypothesis is that they usually are consistent with other, empirically more substantiated and theoretically more parsimonious, hypotheses (see Goodenough *et al.*, 1974).

In sum, the available data suggest that repression probably contributes little to the variation in dream recall for most individuals.

2. ALTERNATIVE HYPOTHESES: SALIENCE AND INTERFERENCE

Salience of dream experience and dream recall

For the two alternative hypotheses — salience and interference — there is relatively more consistent empirical support. In addition, those findings which are consistent with a repression hypothesis are fully explainable within the context of either one or both of these alternative hypotheses (Cohen, 1974d; Goodenough *et al.*, 1974). Let us start with evidence for the salience hypothesis which states that recall is facilitated by the subjective impact (e.g., emotionality, vividness, intrinsic interest) of the dream experience. The most obvious evidence comes from differences in dream recall from REM vs. NREM awakenings. Psychophysiological parallelism is evident in the association between the "brain storming" (Jouvet, 1974) and vegetative turmoil of the REM period and the salient quality and ready recallability of REM experience. Since there is no reliable way to assess the nature of the dream independently of the process of recall, it is possible that better memory rather than better dreams is associated with REM sleep. However, the sleeptalking data do suggest that the REM experience itself is more affective and coherent.

During the night REM periods become physiologically more irregular in activity and (up to about the third REM period) longer. If this evidence of greater activation is correlated with more salient dream imagery, then we should expect a corresponding increase in dream recall quality (amount and clarity). Figure 6-1 shows recall data for REM dreams elicited at three points in the night, and for presleep waking behavior during the ten minutes prior to arriving at the laboratory. The latter estimates were elicited from subjects when they first

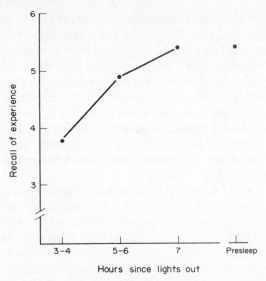

Figure 6-1   Dream recall across REM periods of a night compared to recall of 5-10 minutes of waking activity upon arrival at the lab.

arrived at the laboratory. Recall quality is based on a seven point scale which taps the amount and clarity of the experience. Notice that for the ten subjects who provided data at each of the four occasions, there is a gradual increase in recall quality from earliest to last REM periods, the recall of the last REM period being commensurate with recall of events during 5-10 minutes of prior wakefulness. Since dream recall is at least in part a function of verbal processes, it is possible to interpret the increase in recall as an indication of a gradual increase in the influence of the left hemisphere across REM periods of a night. This hypothesis is discussed at length in the second section of Chapter 7.

In addition, there is evidence that dream recall is better for long than for short sleepers (Cohen, 1972a; Taub, 1970a, 1970b). Presumably long sleepers are more likely to awaken from a more activated REM period. (It is also possible that their awakening thresholds are lower, awakenings more abrupt, and therefore the material is more easily retained in memory — see Shapiro, Goodenough, Lewis and Sleser, 1965.)

Compared to the REM vs. NREM data and the REM-to-REM data, the within-REM data are not clearly supportive of a salience hypothesis. That is, there does not seem to be a reliable difference in REM dream recall after awakenings from phasically active vs. phasically quiescent REM periods. For example, there is no reliable difference in recall for REM awakenings during eye movement bursting or lack of eye movement activity. However, there are at least three reasons not to interpret these findings as contradicting the salience hypothesis. First, there is little evidence of a *marked* and reliable correspondence between salience of the dream experience and phasic activity of the REM period (Firth and Oswald, 1975). Second, laboratory conditions tend to maximize REM retrieval and thus to minimize the effect of differences in dream salience.

Third, there may be as yet unknown interactions between the salience of the dream and interference factors which, under laboratory conditions, tend to favor interference factors. Under ideal conditions for REM dream retrieval, differences in dream salience may not be as important in determining recall as differences in interference factors. If this latter qualification is true, then manipulations designed to affect dream salience should be more readily observable under less ideal conditions for obtaining dream reports (e.g., home dream recall, NREM dream recall, using infrequent dream recallers).

Consider the following prediction from the salience hypothesis: factors that intensify the dream experience will have a relatively greater impact on the dream recall of infrequent than of frequent recallers. Evidence for such a prediction comes in two forms: (1) infrequent recallers tend to have less salient dream experiences, and (2) variation in presleep stress, presumed to be correlated with dream salience, is associated with greater variation in the dream recall of infrequent recallers than of frequent recallers. For example, Hiscock and Cohen (1973) reported evidence of a positive association between waking imagery ability and habitual dream recall.[1]

The rationale for this study was that frequent recallers differ from infrequent recallers in terms of an ability to form salient images both during wakefulness and during dreaming. From a pool of about 648 undergraduates who completed a questionnaire, 286 became eligible for participation by indicating frequent (at least every other morning) or infrequent (not more than once a week) dream recall during the prior two week period. The final sample included 15 male and 19 female frequent recallers and 26 male and 11 female infrequent recallers. Each subject learned each of two paired-associate lists of 10 concrete nouns each of which was paired with a number from one to ten. The two lists were matched for number of syllables, frequency, rate of presentation, and imagery value (I), concreteness (c), and associative meaning (m) as defined in Paivio, Yuille, and Madigan (1968). After learning the first list, each subject was tested for recall by randomly presenting each of the 10 numbers and requesting the appropriate noun. The recall measure constituted performance on trial 1.

Prior to trial 2, each frequent or infrequent recaller subject was assigned to an imagery or association condition. In the imagery condition, the subject learned rhyme words, one for each number (one-bun, two-shoe, etc.) and was then asked to combine the rhyme word and the list word into a complex image (e.g., a pencil in a hot dog bun) in order to facilitate recall. In the association condition, the subject was asked to combine the rhyme word and the list 2 word associatively (i.e., to say mentally "one-bun-pencil") in order to facilitate recall. Recall of list 2 words constituted performance on trial 2.

Figure 6-2 shows the results for the two frequent and two infrequent recaller subgroups on the two trials. There were no significant differences among the subgroups on trial 1 (paired-associate recall in the absence of specific instructions). On trial 2, better recall was associated with frequent recall ($p < .03$) and imagery instructions ($p < .01$). The expected interaction between the two main effects did not reach statistical significance. That is, recall in the imagery condition relative to the association condition for frequent recallers was no greater than that for the infrequent recallers. However, the imagery condition did produce better recall (trial 2) for frequent recallers than for infrequent recallers in the absence of such a difference on trial 1.

It is not clear why the infrequent recallers were slightly *adversely* affected by the association instructions while the frequent recallers appeared to benefit from them. The

---

[1] If intense visual imagery is mediated by brain structures that are responsible for processing visual information from the external world, and if questionnaire estimates of "good imagery ability" are valid, then intense imagery should interfere with perceiving external visual input. A recent unpublished study found evidence that good imagers failed to perceive as much input while engaged in imagery as did poor imagers. Engaging in auditory imagery does not have the same detrimental effect on processing visual input (Singer, 1975).

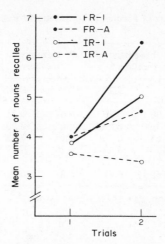

Figure 6-2   Mean number of nouns recalled by frequent dream recallers (FR) and infrequent dream recallers (IR) for baseline (trial 1) and for either imagery (I) or for association (A) instructions (on trial 2).

former effect, entirely unexpected, contributed, in a negative sense, to the failure to obtain the expected interaction. It is interesting to note that on two postexperimental measures of visual imagery (a short version of the Betts questionnaire of clarity and intensity of imagery, and the Gordon test of imagery controllability) the frequent recallers scored significantly higher in imagery capacity. No difference between the two groups obtained on a test of auditory imagery. While not unequivocal, these data are consistent with the hypothesis that individual differences in dream recall frequency are a function of differences in visual imagery.

The Cohen and MacNeilage (1974) study was a more direct test of the REM dream salience-dream recall relationship. We studied REM dream recall across three of four laboratory nights. There were 16 male subjects, eight frequent and eight infrequent recallers selected on the basis of both questionnaire and home dream diary. A total of 131 REM awakenings were made, 68 for frequent and 63 for infrequent recallers. As expected, the percentage of REM awakenings yielding at least a fragment of recall was greater for the frequent than for the infrequent recallers (96 vs. 75 respectively) averaged over the three nights (see also Lewis, Goodenough, Shapiro and Sleser, 1966, for virtually identical figures). Interestingly, when material was recalled, about the same amount was available for frequent and infrequent recallers. Thus, comparisons between content variables for available material were not confounded with quality of material.

Table 6-6 shows the difference between the two groups on four dimensions of dream salience. These differences seem to reflect a difference in the quality of dream experience rather than an artifact of recall.

An interesting finding emerged from dream diary measures that were recorded spontaneously by the subjects when they awoke by alarm (and in the absence of the experimenter). Differences between the two groups in this diary measure of recall were greater when the subjects awakened from NREM than when they awakened from REM. Of the 64 alarm awakenings (16 subjects, four nights each), 24 occurred out of REM (12 for each group) and 26 occurred out of NREM (16 for high, 10 for low recallers). REM awakenings yielded diary recall percentages of 95% and 75% for frequent and infrequent recallers

TABLE 6-6.   Comparison of Frequent and Infrequent Recallers for Dimensions of
Dream Salience

Dimension	Frequent recallers		Infrequent recallers		Comparison	
	$\bar{X}$	SD	$\bar{X}$	SD	t	r_{pb}
Vividness (V)	1.00	0.37	0.67	0.31	1.859*	0.44
Bizarreness (B)	0.36	0.17	0.25	0.23	1.213	0.31
Emotionality (E)	0.61	0.30	0.25	0.28	2.335**	0.53
Activity (A)	0.77	0.28	0.79	0.17	<1	—
Mean sum salience [(V + B + E + A)/4]	0.69	0.16	0.46	0.21	2.323**	0.53

Note: For each comparison, df = 14, N = 8 per group.
*$p < 0.10$.
**$p < 0.05$.

respectively; NREM awakenings yielded diary recall percentages of 75% and 25% for
frequent and infrequent recallers respectively. The difference in diary recall between the two
groups was significant only for the NREM awakenings. These results are consistent with the
hypothesis that under typical (home) conditions, the difference in dream recall between
frequent and infrequent recallers is greater for NREM than for REM sleep awakenings.

Now consider the following set of data which were obtained from a subgroup of subjects
from the Cohen and Cox (1975) study for whom we had dream recall frequency questionnaire ratings. Ten frequent and ten infrequent recallers were selected such that half of each
group had been run in the positive and half in the negative presleep condition. Under the
positive condition (that condition most nearly approximating the condition under which
the Cohen and MacNeilage subjects were run) there was a marked difference in mean sum
salience scores between the frequent and infrequent recallers ($p < .01$). Under the negative
condition, the difference was virtually nonexistent because the salience scores of the
infrequent recallers were relatively high and comparable with those of the frequent recallers
of both conditions. These and the prior results are therefore consistent with other findings
(e.g., B. Barber, 1969) suggesting that normally, there is a difference in dream salience,
especially NREM dream salience, favoring frequent recallers. Under emotional stress, these
differences tend to wash out because of the increase in dream salience of infrequent
recallers. A similar interaction between imagery and arousal has been observed when LSD
is used. Subjects whose imagery is estimated to be relatively weak require high doses to
produce psychedelic intensity comparable to that induced by lower doses in subjects with
good imagery ability (T. X. Barber, 1971).

Under natural conditions, differences between frequent and infrequent recallers in dream
recall are due to differences in dream salience, that is, *other things being equal*. The problem
with this assumption is the phrase "other things being equal". Let us consider one "other
thing" which may not be equal: probability of awakening from REM sleep.

If dream recall can largely be predicted by knowing what sleep stage an individual
awakens from, perhaps frequent and infrequent recallers do not have the same ratio of
REM to NREM awakenings. Consider the following argument proposed by Webb and
Kersey (1967). If dream recall is largely a function of awakening from REM sleep, then the
percentage of subjects reporting recall of a dream on any particular day should be the

multiplicative combination of (a) the probability of awakening from REM sleep and (b) the probability of dream recall from a REM awakening. Webb and Kersey found that 37.5% of a group of 762 subjects reported having had a dream that morning. The probability of awakening from REM sleep was estimated at about .45 (on the basis of data from 32 subjects run three nights in the laboratory). They estimated that the probability of dream recall from REM awakenings was .85. The combined probabilities of awakening from REM (.45) and REM recall (.85) yielded .37, a figure that is virtually identical to the questionnaire findings. Of course, this rather impressive statistical finding tends to simplify a rather complicated phenomenon. Nevertheless, it does serve to remind us of the importance of the psychobiological state of the individual upon awakening.

Let me now engage in a bit of speculation regarding the dynamic relationship between REM sleep and dream recall. Suppose that a major determinant of dream recall is the probability of awakening from REM sleep. Is it possible that infrequent recallers tend habitually to awaken from NREM sleep? On the baseline night of the Cohen and MacNeilage study (1974) during which there were no awakenings, five of seven frequent recallers awakened from REM sleep while five of seven infrequent recallers awakened from NREM sleep ($p < .13$). Is it possible that at least *some* infrequent recallers have the ability to exit from REM into NREM prior to awakening, and is the ability partly *motivated* by a need to complete a REM period?

There are two sets of data which are relevant to this question. First, regarding the ability to avoid REM awakenings by returning to NREM, recall the preliminary data reported by Fiss (1969). Fiss found that after a number of REM interruptions, subjects terminated their REM periods by changing their sleep patterns to NREM prior to the scheduled awakening. Second, recall the evidence that I presented earlier on the apparently greater need for REM sleep under certain conditions displayed by repressors: evidence that presleep stress and/or REM deprivation increases the eye movement density, dream salience, dream recall, and REM rebound of repressors more than of sensitizers. This evidence suggests the tentative hypothesis that a relatively greater need for REM sleep will be associated with a tendency to avoid REM interruption under conditions that both stimulate the need for REM and permit the avoidance of REM interruption. This will occur only for individuals with the ability to execute the avoidance behavior. Perhaps such a hypothesis can explain why there is at times an association between repression and infrequent or poor dream recall: not because repressors are "expelling" the dream but because certain individuals are more "protective" of their REM experiences. Thus, rejection of the repression hypothesis does not imply a rejection of a psychodynamic view of dreaming and dream recall. It does require that we specify more clearly what the dreaming process does, and what are the individual differences in those processes.

There is one further set of data which makes somewhat equivocal *some* of the evidence for the salience hypothesis and which illustrates the importance of experimental control over sleep variables. It is now evident that subjectively poor sleep in otherwise normal individuals is associated with (a) more frequent awakenings from REM sleep, and (b) more frequent termination of sleep out of, or in close temporal proximity to, a REM period (Baekeland, Koulack and Lasky, 1968; Tanaka, 1975). Considering the differential dream recall for REM vs. NREM sleep, it is obvious that individuals who experience presleep stress (and therefore subjectively less satisfying sleep) will, other things being equal, tend to have more dream recall simply because they are more likely to awaken from REM sleep. Thus, the results of the two home dream recall studies that I described earlier (Cohen,

1974a, 1974b) could have been due to the effect of stress on stage of final awakening rather than the effect of stress on dream salience. That the salience hypothesis cannot be entirely ruled out is suggested by other data from studies where stage of sleep and quality of report were controlled (Cohen and MacNeilage, 1974; Cohen and Cox, 1975). However, even with such controls, it is possible that under certain kinds of stress, the awakening thresholds of REM sleep are lower. Thus, better REM recall could be a function of better retrieval rather than better (more salient) encoding. Until it can be shown that enhanced dream recall occurs under stress despite insignificant differences in awakening threshold, a retrieval factor may turn out to be more important.

The data on stress and REM sleep suggest a connection between anxiety measures, sleep time, and dream recall. That is, to the extent that there is a positive interrelationship between sensitization, longer sleep time, and less satisfying sleep, there will be a tendency for dream recall (because of REM awakenings) to be somewhat enhanced (Cohen, 1972a; Hartmann, 1973; Taub, 1970a, 1970b).

In short, while I am reasonably confident that the data support the hypothesis that differences in dream salience (the encoding aspect) play a role, I am inclined to believe that factors which affect the retrieval process (e.g., arousal threshold, postsleep distraction) are more important determinants of both the probability of recall and the quality of the report (e.g., amount of material, clarity of recall).

Factors that interfere with dream recall

There is relatively little direct empirical evidence regarding the interference hypothesis. An obvious source of support is that conditions that maximize attention and motivation, namely experimenter-supervised inquiry, yield much higher percentages of recall than are usually obtained at home (or even in the laboratory on a spontaneous diary task simulating home conditions; see Cohen and Cox, 1975). A more direct test of the effect of immediate postsleep distraction on dream recall was reported by Cohen and Wolfe (1973).

The sample was composed of 86 male and female college students who were randomly assigned to an experimental or control condition. Subjects were asked to fill out a dream diary sheet the next morning upon awakening. The experimental subjects were asked to call the weather number immediately upon awakening and write down the temperature for the day prior to reporting dream material. Control subjects were asked to spend roughly the same amount of time (about 1.5 minutes) lying quietly in bed prior to filling out the diary form. Of 40 control reports, 63% had content, 18% were contentless, and 20% were dreamless. Of 46 experimental reports, 33% had content, 43% were contentless, and 24% were dreamless. The difference in patterns for the two groups was significant ($p < .01$). Note that the experimental manipulations had virtually no effect on the percentage of dreamless reports but a marked enhancement of the contentless experience. A follow-up study (Cohen and Wolfe, 1973) included a replication of the telephone distraction manipulation crossed with a condition which maximized or minimized the subject's attention or interest in the dream reporting process. Roughly half of each of the distraction and nondistraction (dream focus) subjects were told that dreams provide information on latent or manifest psychopathology. These "high salience" subjects were also informed that their dream reports would be assessed in the light of results of their personality scores which would be presented to them the next day. They were told that the personality and dream data could reveal

TABLE 6-7.   Percentage of Diaries with Dream Content

Presleep condition	Postsleep condition		
	Dream focus	Distraction	Combined
High salience	63	26	43
Low salience	45	32	39
Combined	54	29	

evidence of latent psychopathology. The rest of the subjects were told that they were participating in a normative study on dream content. Results shown in Table 6-7 indicate that the telephone manipulation (distraction) again had the effect of reducing dream content reports ($p < .02$). In addition, the effect of the "threatening" cover story was to enhance dream recall, but only in the nondistraction (dream focus) condition. These results are clearly consistent with a straightforward postsleep interference hypothesis.

Regarding the potential for the awakening process to interfere with dream recall, I have suggested (Cohen, 1976) that there may be individual differences in the psychobiological "distance" between the sleep-dream state and the waking state. That is, the absence or fading of a dream upon awakening may be a function of the state-dependency of the dream experience (Evans et al., 1970; Overton, 1973). As Broughton (1975) suggests, "Indeed, it may be that man (and certain other animals) have three somewhat separate and more or less state-dependent streams of mental activity occurring in wakefulness, NREM sleep and REM sleep, respectively, with his 'picking up where he left off' as he re-enters each state, and with relative difficulty of his consciously using material from one stream (e.g., from NREM psychic activity) in either of the other two (e.g., in REM sleep or waking psychic activity)" (p. 222).[2]

A study by Chute and Wright (1973) provides an excellent example of the kind of state-dependent phenomenon that I suggest may be operating to affect dream recall. Immediately after a one trial passive avoidance learning acquisition trial, rats were either administered sodium phenobarbital (drug) or saline (nondrug). Twenty-four hours later, half of each group was tested for retention under either drug or nondrug conditions. As expected, best performance (longest latencies to previously shocked response) was recorded for the two groups of rats for whom consolidation of learning and testing occurred under the same states (either drug-drug or nondrug-nondrug). The other two groups, for whom consolidation and testing occurred under different states (drug-nondrug, nondrug-drug), performed significantly worse. Note that there were no differences among the groups for acquisition latency. I am suggesting that retrieval of dream content will be affected by the degree that the awake individual is "in tune with" the dream experience. If a dream is to a large extent a right hemisphere-mediated process, individuals with good right hemisphere "skills" should report higher dream recall frequency.

Let us look at this question of the relationship between hemisphere laterality and recall a bit further. If we accept for the moment some preliminary generalizations about cognitive and personality styles and cerebral orientation (Bakan, 1971), certain predictions about individual differences in dream recall can be tested. Specifically, individuals with a tendency

---

[2] Our inability to recall childhood events, especially those that occurred during sensorimotor and prelogical periods, also may be state-dependency-determined. If so, these experiences are still available (stored) but normally not accessible (retrievable) except under special conditions (e.g., dreaming).

toward subjective, intuitive, affective, global, artistic, expressive life styles, compared to individuals with a tendency toward objective, analytic, pragmatic, instrumental, scientific, affectless life styles, have been hypothesized to be more right hemisphere-oriented. One operational definition of hemisphere orientation that has been suggested by a number of investigators is direction of eye movement. Despite specific conditions, a tendency to look leftward is assumed to be an overt though admittedly crude estimate of the dominance of the right hemisphere (Bakan, 1971; Gur and Gur, 1975; Schwartz et al., 1975). Let us consider two characteristics that may be related both to hemispheric dominance and to dream recall.

At the risk of appearing male chauvinistic, it is reasonable to predict that individuals with a feminine orientation (described in more detail in a later chapter), and therefore with a presumed orientation toward behaviors and experiences mediated by the right hemisphere, should be better recallers of dreams. (We have already seen that individuals with a commitment to a humanities rather than an engineering major tend to recall dreaming more frequently [Schechter et al., 1965].) The data to be presented come from a follow-up study of sex-role orientation and dream content. Unlike the earlier study (Cohen, 1973b), male and female subjects were preselected on the basis of both masculine and feminine scales (rather than on the basis of a single bipolar masculinity-femininity scale). On the basis of median splits of each of the two scales of the Personal Attributes Questionnaire (Spence, Helmreich and Stapp, 1975), 47 males and 52 females were selected from a larger group of 937 undergraduates to represent (for each sex separately) (a) androgyny (high-high), (b) masculinity (high masculine, low feminine), (c) femininity (low masculinity, high femininity), and (d) undifferentiated (low-low). Cells were filled over a two semester period and ranged from 10 to 15 subjects per cell. Dream recall frequency was defined by assigning a score of 0 (no recall), 1 (fragmentary or sparse recall), or 2 (complete or long dream) to each of 14 dream diary protocols filled out by each subject at home, adding scores and dividing by 14. Interrater reliability (based on subject totals) was .997.

Table 6-8 clearly indicates that both male and female subjects with a relatively predominant feminine orientation had significantly higher dream recall frequency. This difference replicated across the two semesters. Between-sex differences were not statistically significant. While these findings do not constitute direct evidence of a cerebral hemisphere dominance effect, they are at least consistent with the hypothesis that a tendency toward right hemisphere mediation will facilitate recall of largely right hemisphere information (dreams).

A somewhat different though related approach to the question of hemisphere "preference" and dream recall was carried out on the basis of a report by Gur, Sackeim and Gur (1976) who suggested that classroom seating might provide an unobtrusive estimate of

TABLE 6-8.   Mean Dream Recall Scores for Males and Females in Each of the Four Masculinity and Femininity Groups

	Undif.	Andro.	Masculine	Feminine	Overall
Overall group mean scores	0.644	0.765	0.500	0.802	
Females	0.637	0.694	0.405	0.830	0.642
Males	0.650	0.835	0.596	0.774	0.714
First semester	0.748	0.750	0.428	0.732	0.665
Second semester	0.539	0.780	0.572	0.872	0.691

hemisphere dominance. That is, individuals who prefer to sit on the right side (and therefore who tend to look to the left) are more right hemisphere dominant. These investigators reported that males who prefer to sit on the right reported more psychopathological symptoms than males who prefer to sit on the left. The relationship was reversed for females.

We gave out questionnaires to five groups of about 30 undergraduates each. They were asked to indicate seating preference by placing a mark on a diagram of a classroom which showed a set of left, middle, and right rows. In addition the subjects reported dream recall frequency on the standard questionnaire (scored 0-14) and filled out the Maudsley Personality Inventory. A total of 57 females and 82 males responded to all questions. For neither sex did the Maudsley neuroticism scale correlate with seating position. However, sex differences in seating preference were quite remarkable and admittedly unexpected. Males rather evenly distributed themselves across the three seating categories: preferences for left, center, and right were 28%, 37%, and 31% respectively. However, for females, the corresponding figures were 12%, 42%, and 47% respectively. The difference between sexes in left vs. right preference just misses significance at the .05 level with a conservative chi square test. Since the finding derives from multiple replications across small groups of students tested independently it appears to be reasonably reliable, though its interpretation is not immediately apparent.

With regard to dream recall, the male data are consistent with expectation. That is, males who prefer to sit on the right (left lookers) reported significantly higher dream recall frequency (8.11) than did males preferring to sit on the left (5.41) ($t[49] = 2.202, p < .05$). Results for females were in the opposite direction (right preference recall, 6.85; left preference recall, 7.43). However, the nonsignificance of this relationship and the small number of left preferences make cross-sex comparison difficult. Thus, at least for males, there is reasonably consistent though indirect evidence from the perspective of hemisphere dominance theory that habitual dream recall is related to the tendency toward right hemisphere dominance. These relationships are not particularly striking but they do suggest an alternative approach to the problem of explaining individual differences in dream recall frequency. Thus, correlations between dream recall estimates and personality qualities such as "intuitive", "artistic", "creative", or life styles and career choices that reflect such characteristics, can be reinterpreted. Rather than reflecting freedom from repression, they may indicate a neuropsychologically defined skill, e.g., predominance of right hemisphere-mediated processes, relative absence of interference by left-mediated processes. In short, good recall would be an indication of relatively less state-dependency for the dream with respect to the waking state.

If state-dependent phenomena are determined by the psychobiological "difference" or "distance" between states, then individuals with more distinct "state boundaries" (Cartwright, 1972) would presumably be more readily affected. For example, it would be interesting to test the correlation between state-dependency of memory, e.g., information learned during an alcoholic state recalled in the nonalcoholic state vs. dream recall. If those more affected by state differences were less apt to recall dreaming (especially NREM dreaming, since NREM is apparently psychobiologically more distant from wakefulness than is REM dreaming), this would support a state-dependency factor. There is some evidence to support such a notion. For example, there tends to be a correlation between auditory awakening thresholds and dream recall (Zimmerman, 1970). That is, the more difficult the transition from a sleep stage to a wake stage, the less likely that dreams will be recalled (assuming equivalence in other factors such as dream salience, postsleep distractions, etc.). Deficit in dream recall could be due to disruption of fragile short-term memory (effect on consolidation) or the failure of the decoding processes of wakefulness to match up with encoded products of sleep. After a *temporary* failure to recall a dream upon awakening, the phenomenon of suddenly recalling a dream later in the day might be a function of the basic rest activity cycle (simulating, or more closely approximating, the REM period in which the dream originally was experienced) in conjunction with external cues.

It is relatively easy to demonstrate the effects of postsleep distractions or the effect of awakening on dream recall. It is much harder to establish a role for interference *during* dreaming. In fact, at this "level" the distinction between interference and salience is academic. Interference with attention to, or consciousness of, dreaming can be thought of as a reduction of salience. Recall that Antrobus *et al.* (1964) hypothesized from data on waking behavior that eye movement density during REM indicates an attempt to avoid paying attention to dream events. Any process involving attention deflection during dreaming would presumably be associated with less dream recall if attention during sleep is required for the optimal encoding and memory storage which can withstand the transition from sleep to wakefulness.

The pioneering work of Dement and Wolpert (1958) suggests another potential source of on-line interference with dream recall. They were particularly interested in the relationship between body movement and both the nature of dream content and the length of dream narratives. With regard to the latter, they found that reports which were shorter than expected (on the basis of the duration of the REM period) were often associated with body movement that had occurred prior to awakening. In other words, the length of reports appeared to be a function of the duration of that part of the REM period which followed a spontaneous movement and prior to experimental awakening. If we can assume that the length of the narrative is roughly correlated with the amount of material remembered, then to some extent dream recall or its absence may indeed be a function of the immediacy of body movement just prior to awakenings. Thus, poor recallers might, as a group, be more likely to have a body movement just prior to awakening from REM sleep. Under typical (home) conditions that do not impose maximal attention and motivation to recall dreams, variation in intensity, duration, and timing of body movement or general neuromuscular tension might contribute substantially to variation in dream recall beyond the contribution of stage of sleep from which the individual habitually awakens.

In fact, muscle tension or overt body movement may be considered to be an example of two kinds of influence on dream recall — salience and interference — that might operate at a number of "levels" or stages (from the dream experience to postsleep recall). Muscle tension might interfere with recall by reducing the sensory salience of the experience as well as by producing competing input during attempts at recall. Differences between dream recallers and nonrecallers as well as differences between REM and NREM recall may turn out to be substantially dependent on differences in neuromuscular tension. Habitual or situational deficiencies in imagery and dream recall may be characteristic of individuals who "may be somewhat hyperkinetic types, restless, twitchy, or otherwise motorically engaged" (Bugelski, 1971).

Consider one other hypothetical source of interference during the dreaming process that might affect dream recall. We have not distinguished between the information processing and conscious experience aspects of dreaming. The former could be thought of as the deep structure, the latter, the surface structure. Presumably, the experienced dream is a product of the translation of deep structure into imagistic and verbal characteristics of consciousness. In principle, it is possible that anything that interferes with this translation (e.g., anything that blocks consciousness) would affect dream recall. (How the absence of consciousness affects the nature of the information processing is an entirely different matter.) Let us assume that the imagery quality of dreams is particularly dependent on right hemispheric functioning, while verbal aspects are more intimately tied to left hemispheric functioning (assuming the case of the typical right-handed individual). It is possible that damage to the right hemisphere might reduce dream recall, not because the information processing of dreaming is affected, but because the information processing of both hemispheres fails to get translated into conscious imagery. Thus, I am suggesting that salience and interference aspects of the dreaming process are intimately related.

Evidence which can be considered at least consistent with this speculation is discussed by Galin (1974). Patients with right posterior lesions report a diminution of dream recall as well as an inability to imagine. There is, in addition, a reduction in both imagery and dream recall, as well as a diminution of the salience of recalled dream content, in commissurotomized patients (Hoppe, 1977). There is evidence that chronic alcoholism eventuates in a relatively greater degree of deterioration of the right than of the left hemisphere (Jones and Parsons, 1975). If it could be shown that frequent dream recallers who became chronic alcoholics experience a marked diminution of dream recall, this would constitute further evidence for the speculation.

Figure 6-3 provides a summary of factors that are hypothesized to affect dream reporting.

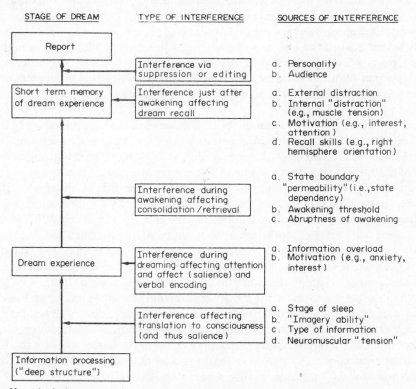

Figure 6-3   Hypothetical sources of interference with information processed during sleep and awakening.

Different stages from information processing to reporting are shown in association with potential sources of interference. Salience factors which were discussed previously can largely be derived from the relative absence of interfering factors at the information processing and dream experiencing levels. Factors or characteristics shown on the right of the figure include the physiological, the psychological (both dispositional and situational), and the environmental. Presumably, for those individuals and in those situations that are characterized by vivid consciousness during sleep, good imagery ability, verbal encoding, relatively low awakening thresholds, high recall motivation and little external distraction, dream accessibility is maximized.

Implications

The problem of dream recall implies two kinds of issues, one methodological, one theoretical. Regarding the first, it should be clear that any study which focuses on dream content analysis must control for the quantity and quality of dream report data (Hall, 1969; Van de Castle, 1969). Unless one has evidence of a predicted difference or change in some categories but not others, one must assume *a priori* that the better the dream recall (frequency, amount, and quality), the higher the probability of finding evidence for the presence of any category. As we have seen, individual differences in REM dream recall reported in the laboratory are less subject to such bias than are reports written at home. Also (in this case, fortunately) there is relatively little evidence that variation in dream recall is markedly associated with important personality differences. Thus, laboratory studies which focus on the relationship between dream content and personality factors are less likely to be markedly biased against the null hypothesis since differences between groups in the quality of dream reports will not be too severe. However, control of dream recall quality is probably a more important requisite in home dream studies where individual differences in habitual dream recall frequency and *some* personality variables (e.g., repression-sensitization) are suspected.

The major theoretical implication of the dream recall data is the limitation that it places on our knowledge about the dream experience. Despite our working assumption that a reasonably well-recalled dream has some validity, it must be granted that the dream report is a limited datum. This is especially true of NREM reports and reports obtained from early REM periods. For example, suppose that we are interested in changes in the dream experience during the night. If our subjects are not especially good dream recallers (some investigators only use good recallers but this has the effect of introducing unknown sources of bias), then it will be difficult to compare the quality of dream reports obtained early in the night with the quality of reports obtained later in the night; this is especially true of NREM reports. Therefore, if we control for recall quality, our early reports will constitute a highly biased sample since most of these dream experiences are poor in quality. If we use all reports, then the poor quality of the earlier reports will introduce unknown biases against finding evidence of certain characteristics that may in fact be experienced but may not be as readily reportable. Evidence that memory and/or motivation accounts for some of the differences in recall quality is scanty. Sometimes later in the night, subjects spontaneously clarify earlier reports of poor quality so that it is clear that the dream experience was more organized and "logical" than the earlier report suggested. Therefore, while I believe that these are real differences in the quality of experiences associated with early REM periods (see Chapter 7), memory and/or motivational factors cannot be ruled out.

Therefore, to the degree that retrieval adversely affects the dream report, our inferences about the nature and function of dreaming will be affected. It is often held that dreaming is a "primary process": "vague, irrational, absurd, nonsensical, and extravagant — a kind of temporary madness reflecting an alien, archaic world beyond the laws of time or space or logic or morality" (Snyder, 1970, p. 124), "nonsensical, feeble-minded, meaningless or strangely crazy" (Hawkins, 1969). According to Hartmann (1973, Ch. 12) those very characteristics of mature and healthy ego functioning which we take for granted during wakefulness (e.g., evaluation, discrimination, judgement, impulse delay, concentration) are markedly absent in dreaming (due to the "shunting out" of catecholaminergic systems, normally mediating such functions, which require "repair" during sleep). Such characterizing of dreaming may be consistent with hypotheses about symbolism and disguise, but it is clearly inconsistent with the hypothesis that during sleep problem-oriented thought, even problem solving, can occur. The concept of "regression in the service of the ego" requires both "regression" (flexibility, associative loosening, childlike playfulness, etc.) *and* "ego", and thus cannot be applied to dreaming unless both take place during sleep. The primary process view of dreaming tends to rule out the "ego" aspect, leaving the dream, at best, a source of raw material and inspiration. For a number of reasons, the least legitimate one being my fondness for the hypothesis that dreaming has problem-solving capability, I believe that such a view requires a great deal of qualification and revision.

First, it is clear that many REM dream experiences are rather mundane, ordinary, minimal modifications of daily events both past and present, with little or no confusion, distortion, bizarreness. I have found this to be the case, as have others (see especially Snyder, 1970). Aside from the hallucinatory intensity of the dream experience (which does *not* correlate with bizarreness or "regressiveness"), it appears that dreaming may approach the depth, flexibility, logic, and intuitive power of·wakeful thinking — *sometimes, and under some conditions*. This needs clarification. First, it may be that REM dreaming, compared to thinking is *statistically* better described as *tending* toward primary process. Second, this tendency appears to be maximized by certain personality characteristics (as dream content studies, which I will describe later, seem to show). Emotionally disturbed individuals, especially under stress, should be expected to experience more disturbed dreams. Third, laboratory conditions will tend to minimize the trend toward primary process as suggested by some (but not all) studies that compare laboratory and home dreams (Hall and Van de Castle, 1966; Weisz and Foulkes, 1970). I spoke of the capacity of the individual while in REM sleep to show evidence of vigilance which includes a kind of defensive cautiousness and conservatism in dreaming.

Fourth, our impression about the content and sequencing of dream events is affected by the quality of dream recall. In the absence of clear and objective external markers for dream events, the primary process nature of dream content may to a large extent reflect the relatively poor memory, low motivation, and fatigue factors associated with immediate post-sleep functioning rather than the nature of the dream experience itself. Such distortions are likely to be even further magnified by nonoptimal duration between waking and reporting, and by personality factors that bias dreaming toward more pathological organization. Dreams that appear to be sequentially fragmented, disjointed, mixed up may in fact be a *series* of dreams. Consider the findings of Dement and Wolpert (1958) regarding the relationship between the distribution of body movements during REM sleep and the sequencing of dream content. Of 35 REM periods punctuated by body movement, 21 (60%) were associated with fragmented dreams (containing two or more apparently unrelated themes). Of 42 REM periods without such body movement, only 10 (24%) were associated with fragmented dreams. Thus, body movement may be an external marker for the breaking up of attentional or cognitive sets, and may be thought of as inducing new dreams rather than bizarre dreams. Good recall of REM experiences, under conditions of periodic body movement, may therefore give the impression that dreaming is more disorganized than is actually the case. The frequent body mover may simply be one who has a lot of different things to dream about rather than a person whose individual dreams are disorganized.

Fifth, our impressions about the nature of dream content may be affected by the quality of dream reporting which is determined both by subjects' *and* interviewers' biases and selective emphases. A good example comes from the work of Molinari and Foulkes (1969) and Foulkes and Pope (1973). These studies demonstrated that, compared to spontaneous REM dream reports given under relatively unstructured conditions, more carefully structured reports obtained under the same REM conditions showed evidence of secondary process ("secondary cognitive elaboration") which was not evident in the spontaneous reports. It is quite possible that some of the characteristics which define "good ego functioning" are simply harder to remember or more readily taken for granted. Dement captures the problem best when he suggests that "our task in describing the dream world is roughly as difficult as if we were strolling casually without a care down the Champs-Élysées, and we were suddenly plucked into the dream world to the accompaniment of a raucous buzzer where in the dim light of a dream bedroom a shadowy figure would begin a relentless interrogation about what we had just been doing. One would surely forget a few things" (Dement, 1975, p. 291). And clearly, if the experimenter (or clinician) and the subject (or patient) conspire consciously or otherwise to focus on the unusual, the bizarre, and the affective, then generalizations (and theories) about dreaming will clearly be biased.

Figure 6-4 shows "ego functioning" ratings made by 10 subjects who reported REM dream content at three points during the night, and who produced ratings of recalled prelaboratory behavior as well. Ego strength was a composite rating of seven scales such as judgement, impulse control, social adjustment, etc. Notice that by the last hour, ego strength ratings are comparable to levels associated with presleep waking behavior. That this change is not merely an artifact of better recall later in the night is indicated by similar results for subjects who produced good quality dream reports at each point during the night. In short, our knowledge of and hypotheses about the nature of the dreaming experience will be affected by a number of factors which have not been given sufficient empirical attention: personality, presleep events, temporal factors, memory factors, communication factors (that is, both reporting and listening).

Sixth, I would like to suggest that the excessive emphasis on the primary process quality of the dream may be based on a bias for recalling *dreamlike* imagery at the onset, but even more likely, at the termination of sleep states. Foulkes and Vogel (1965) went to great lengths to document empirically the dreamlike quality of sleep onset mentation. In this excellent study they clearly demonstrate that such mentation is characterized by many of the features that mark the REM dream. However, it is my impression that they did not go far enough, that for many people, hypnogogic and hypnopompic imagery is *more* dreamlike (or should I say "dreamy"?) than is REM mentation. It is also my impression that there may be rather interesting individual differences related to being a night person or a morning per-

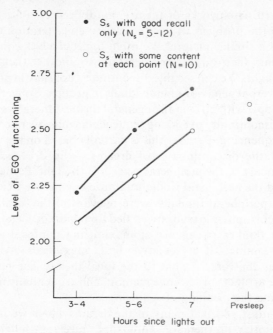

Figure 6-4   Ego function ratings for REM dreams compared to ratings of presleep behavior.

son in the degree that sleep onset or sleep termination fantasy is relatively fantastic. For example, some people drift off to sleep gradually, spend much time in stage 1-NREM sleep onset, may even be arousable momentarily during which time they utter some of the most fantastic nonsense. These same people may awaken abruptly in the morning clear headed and without dream recall. On the other hand, there are people who go rather directly into stage 2-NREM after a short sojourn through stage 1, but at the end of the night, waken gradually while grappling dreamily with transitional mentation that mediates rather irrational forms of communications. What I am suggesting is that much of this mentation is the primary process of *transitional phases* between the more familiar biological states of "real" sleep and wakefulness, that this mentation is *not* REM mentation, and that much of this mentation is presumed to be equivalent to REM mentation. All I wish to emphasize here is that transitional mentation, rather than REM mentation, may be the actual source of much of what is known clinically or informally about dreaming. It thus serves as a further source of bias against which interest in REM sleep and dreaming must contend.[3]

My seventh point regarding factors that distort our picture of dreams has to do with dream sequencing. Hypotheses about the adaptive significance of dreaming (programming information, problem-confrontation, problem-solving, insight, etc.) imply a minimum of good ego functioning which should be reflected in the organization of at least some dreams. Even REM reports sometimes give the impression that dreams are sequentially rather

---

[3] The dreaming experiences of ascending stage 1-NREM may explain why people report "dreams" when they awaken from afternoon naps which typically do not contain REM stages. Individuals who take afternoon naps for psychological reasons rather than to make up for lost sleep, that is, appetitive rather than replacement nappers, have light sleep patterns (including much stage 1-NREM) and much shifting sleep staging (Evans, Cook, Cohen, Orne and Orne, 1977). These sleep characteristics of appetitive nappers are thus especially conducive to the recall of dreamy mentation, though clearly this is not REM recall.

disorganized, haphazard patchworks of themes, hardly representative of a capability for sustained attention to the problem. However, careful consideration of the sequencing of *waking* thought yields a similar picture! We often find ourselves concentrating on something someone is saying, then shifting momentarily to another theme, then returning to the original line of thought. We can see this discontinuity not only in private thoughts but in the sequencing of the verbal behavior of individuals in groups. Conversational themes shift rapidly from topic to topic with no overall or general theme. I therefore think that we tend to underemphasize the discontinuity of waking sequencing while overemphasizing the discontinuity of dreaming sequencing. Perhaps this is partially based on the vivid pictorialization and dramatization of the discontinuities of dreams — in dreams, we may give equal "weight" to both the focal and the peripheral aspects of thought. Perhaps such a democratization of the focal and the peripheral would minimize cognitive efficiency during wakefulness. However, if the peripheral thoughts were relevant to the focal, efficiency might be *enhanced*. While the schizophrenic tends to get tied up in nonfocal associations that are not relevant, the creative thinker is capable of maximizing nonfocal associations that *are* relevant. Perhaps dreaming, at its creative best, maximizes vivid dramatization of peripheral associations that are relevant to the focal theme. The point is that apparent discontinuities may be artifacts of selective memory and sequentially nonvalid reports, and of difficulty interpreting the meaning of sequences.

Having said this, I must add that many of the dreams which we have collected do not show gross discontinuities or thematic anomalies, rarely include impossible physical transformations of objects, and never include impossible combinations of features of animate objects, e.g., rabbits with antlers. I must agree with Snyder who says that "the form and content of dreams typically reported in the laboratory are highly disappointing and 'undreamlike'. They are rarely fantastic, surrealistic, or even impressionistic, but just plain representational. The self is almost always the central figure, usually interacting with other people around very ordinary activities and preoccupations, and generally talking about them.[4] Far from being bizarre, or exotic, the general run of their plots is remarkably mundane, plausible, sedentary, and uninteresting to anyone, with the possible exception of the dreamer" (1971, p. 528).

Thus, studies of factors that affect dream recall suggest that theories based on the home dream recall of clinical samples will be quite different in emphasis from theories based on the lab (REM) dreams of normal samples. Factors such as personality, physiology, social situation, interviewing style will determine the character of dream reports and therefore what we think dreams are like and what we think they accomplish.

---

[4] The presence of secondary process in dreams has been underestimated because most data have traditionally come from disturbed subjects who selectively report nonrepresentative samples of total dream life. (A subject whose waking life is not characterized by a high degree of secondary process should not be expected to generate dreams rich in secondary process.) We now know that there is far more intelligent and intelligible verbal activity during dreaming than ever was suspected (e.g., see Chapter 7; also see Snyder, 1970).

CHAPTER 7

PHYSIOLOGICAL CONTEXT OF REM DREAMING

1. PSYCHOPHYSIOLOGICAL CORRELATES OF REM

The remarkable thing about REM sleep is the prominence of biological activity from the cellular to the behavioral (gross motor) level. It was this activity, coupled with evidence of correlated reports of rich and varied dream experiences, that led to an explosive growth of research on dreaming during the fifties and sixties. It did more than anything else to establish the face validity and scientific respectability of dream reports. The heart (and soul) of classic sleep research is the attempt to draw psychophysiological parallels: that is, to establish correlations between specific physiological events and dream characteristics. Much of the excitement in this area of inquiry has dissipated because of relatively low yield, and I think, because it is often difficult to infer causal relationships from such findings. After reviewing some of the major physiological characteristics of REM sleep, I will discuss the correlational findings that have emerged during the last few decades.

Of course, the most striking characteristic of REM sleep is the eye movement activity. Eye movements occur as sporadic isolated events and as bursts or trains of relatively long duration. In contrast to the slow, rolling eye movements of NREM sleep, the eye movements of REM are marked by conjugate celerity. In contrast to the REM sleep eye movements of neonates which tend to be vertical, those of the adult human tend to be oblique. In contrast to NREM sleep, autonomic activity (e.g., heart rate, blood pressure, respiration) in REM sleep is usually characterized by heightened *variability*. Muscle tonus, especially in the head and neck regions, is often at its lowest level during REM sleep. Yet despite this diminution of tonic levels, periodic outbursts of gross muscle movement are even more characteristic of REM sleep than of NREM sleep. These movements run the gamut from twitching to turning over, and tend to be distributed in greater frequency at the beginning or end of REM periods. It is not known whether there is a correlation between such movements and more complex, goal oriented, organized behavior such as sleep talking (in both REM and NREM) or sleep walking (NREM). Finally, REM sleep is characterized by periodic durations of penile tumescence, not only in adult males, but also in infants and the aged.[1] All of these physiological variables have been studied in relation to dream content elicited from REM periods. After discussing some methodological and theoretical issues, some of the highlights of this correlational research will be presented.

---

[1] The clinical usefulness of REM tumescence for distinguishing between psychogenic (vs. biogenic) impotence has been demonstrated in a study by Beutler, Karacan, Anch, Salis, Scott, and Williams (1975). Waking impotence, despite the capacity for full tumescence during REM, was related to the combined factors of at least one MMPI scale score over 70 and a 60 or greater elevation on the Mf scale.

Methodological problems

The first issue is the validity of the dream report. Although I discussed this problem in Chapter 6, it requires some additional attention here. Clearly, the report is an account of a memory of an event and thus is twice removed from the original experience. Needless to say, prior to the onset of REM research, there were few external validity data for dream reports. However, reports obtained from subjects awakened rather abruptly from REM (and NREM) sleep have acquired a sort of scientific, though sometimes grudging, acceptability because their characteristics can, in principle, be related to external, observable validity indicators (see Rechtschaffen, 1967). Following the suggestions of Stoyva and Kamiya (1968), consider the case of two REM dream reports: one is short, undramatic, visually sparse, involving little activity on the part of the dreamer; the other is quite the opposite. If the former report is associated with REM characteristics such as short duration, respiratory regularity, and few eye movements, while the second report is characterized by longer duration, respiratory irregularity, more eye movement, etc., then one is more confident that, in general, REM dream reports are valid. This assumption is further supported by evidence that sleep talking is highly correlated thematically with REM dream content elicited moments later (even in the absence of recall for the talking episode) (Arkin, Toth, Baker and Hastey, 1970).[2] Much of the research on psychophysiological correlates is concerned with differences in objective REM characteristics and their association with variation in REM dream reports. As such, it provides evidence for the validity of dream reports.

The original impetus for the scientific investigation of dreaming came from early work on the difference in dream reports elicited from REM vs. NREM sleep. These studies revealed that REM reports were characterized by vividness, organization, emotionality, and recall quality generally not found in NREM reports. In fact, using rather strict definitions for "dreaming", early investigators believed that REM sleep was synonymous with dreaming sleep. NREM reports were interpreted merely as artifact, at best the recall of prior REM experiences rather than true dream experiences associated with NREM sleep. This position is clearly no longer tenable because there is good evidence that mentation often indistinguishable from REM dreaming can occur during sleep onset and NREM sleep (especially during stages 1 and 2 later in the night, and particularly for light sleepers or good dream recallers) (Foulkes, 1966). However, generally speaking, the more dreamlike, better recalled, more affectively toned experiences of REM appeared to make sense in the light of "the vegetative turmoil of REM periods" (Snyder, 1971). And indeed, the focus of laboratory dream research has largely been on the phenomenology of REM sleep. In short, the validity of dream reports can be assessed from the perspective of psychophysiological correlates.

A question about the validity of dream reports obtained in the sleep laboratory is raised by comparing the quality of REM dreams to the quality of home dreams. I have discussed this issue in the previous chapter. Suffice it to say here that a number of investigators have challenged the psychological relevance of the lab dream on the basis of data suggesting that lab dreams are more mundane, conventional, impoverished. Overstating the point, Hall says: "The hope that neurophysiology would illuminate a psychological phenomenon has been dashed . . . it is true that one can collect many more dreams in the laboratory than at home over the same period of time, but this is no advantage if the laboratory dreams are of

---

[2] A critical review of methods used to validate reports about waking imagery is given by T. X. Barber (1971).

little significance." These lab dreams "lack the dynamic significance of home dreams. They are 'little' dreams." Hall concludes that "our understanding of dreams, it seems, will have to come from psychological analysis, just as Freud and Jung have said" (1967, pp. 103, 104). When applied to the understanding of dream content, especially its meaning, Hall's comments have a certain face validity though they are a bit extreme. However, as I hope to show through the literature reviewed in this book, an understanding of some aspects of dream content requires the investigation of the biological context within which the psychological events operate. That lab dreams are more mundane than are home dreams may be true but does not negate the value of lab dream data to understanding the psychobiological events of sleep. If we keep in mind distinctions between the different scientific objectives regarding the psychological aspects of sleep (the dreaming process, dream content, dream meaning), then the following statement by Hall appears to be excessive: "There may be a biology of dreaming but it is dubious whether there is a biology of dreams" (Hall, 1967, p. 103). To embrace this view with enthusiasm would, in my opinion, constitute a premature foreclosure.

A second, closely allied issue is the quality of the data that go into psychophysiological correlations. The more specific the relationship sought, the more important it is to have accurate, carefully described, detailed reports. Highly motivated, verbally proficient, good dream recallers are essential if Type II errors (rejecting as a chance finding a true relationship) are to be avoided (Gardiner, Grossman, Roffwarg and Weiner, 1975). In addition, on the physiological side, studies typically isolate one or a number of discrete variables rather than look at *patterns*. The dream is embedded in a complexity interrelated fabric of shifting physiological states which emerge from a confluence of individual physiological variables (Dement and Mitler, 1974). While it is easier to measure an isolated variable, it is likely that dream content is associated with emergent properties of physiological activity rather than isolated physiological events. Thus, focusing on isolated variables may give the false impression that there is little psychophysiological relationship during sleep. Related to this problem is the frequent failure to consider widespread individual differences (Hauri and Van de Castle, 1973a, 1973b). It is well known that an affective experience may be associated with a decrease or an increase in heart rate in different individuals, or that heart rate may be a relevant variable for one subject while respiration may be more significant for another. Hauri concludes that "because of individual response specificity, global and replicable correlations between dream content and physiological parameters are unlikely to be found" (1975, p. 278). Low intrasubject and intersubject correlations among heart rate and other autonomic characteristics (McCanne and Sandman, 1976) practically guarantee low correlations even for the "obvious" tests of psychophysiological parallelism, e.g., dream emotionality and heart rate.

During wakefulness there are obvious differences across individuals in the degree to which mental activity is associated with overt or external activation. For example, some individuals move their lips when reading while others do not. If we had information only about lip movement (analogous, say, to eye movements during REM), could we assume that the absence of such movement implied the absence of verbal cognition? Even if we had evidence of lip movement, could we say something about *what* the individual was reading, or why he was reading? This example illustrates the fact that not all dimensions of physiological activation are relevant to all subjects and that the information yield of such data is limited. A similar point has been made by Bem and Allen (1974), in the area of personality trait research; some personality trait measures are irrelevant to predicting the behavior of some subjects. Validation of a trait measure requires that we use subjects only for whom the measure is relevant. Likewise, heart rate variation may be a relevant variable only for some subjects, and even for such subjects, there may be a variation in the direction of the correlations. Ignoring individual differences in physiological responsiveness probably constitutes a major weakness in the research to be reviewed below (see Stegie, Baust and Engel, 1975).

A third issue is that of content specificity. Should we expect to find correlations between physiological variation and general qualities, e.g., affective tone, pace of dream events, clarity of recall, etc. more readily than specific events? It is my impression that to the degree that physiological activation determines dream content, it will influence the quality more than the specific content of the dream. The latter is far more likely to be determined by personality and presleep incentive-related events. For example, eye movement activity is more likely to be related to the pace and intensity, rather than the exact content of dream events. Even if it could be demonstrated that eye movements were related isomorphically to direction of gaze (a correlation which appears to be occasional) we can never deduce from those movements what it is that the dreamer is following. However, I must qualify my statement that physiological activation is more likely to be related to quality rather than specific content of dreams. It is possible that dreamed experiences are correlated, through classical conditioning or simply by contiguity, with certain patterns of physiological activity. Therefore, the activation of such patterns may indeed facilitate specific content sequences, or vice versa, specific sequences may activate such physiological activity patterns. We simply do not utilize the sophisticated methodologies that would be necessary to isolate and measure such psychophysiological complexities. In the final analysis, we cannot be sure of the statistical weighting to be given to physiological activation (itself affected through presleep behaviors) vs. psychological preoccupation in accounting for variance in specific dream content sequences. If I dream that I am hiking along snow-covered mountain ridges high above the timberline, can I attribute this dream to preoccupations with aspiration, tendencies toward introversion, and the like, or to events such as room temperatures or presleep diet (which affect, through the activity of neurotransmitters, physiological activity and its feedback to the central nervous system)? Are many of the specifics of dream content merely the phenomenological dramatization of sequences of patterns of physiological activation? To date, we simply cannot answer such questions. But they illustrate that dreaming, like waking experience, is embedded both casually and reactively in an inextricably interrelated psychobiological context. Our fundamental ignorance of these complex "mind-body" interrelationships probably explains why it is so easy to talk about psychological *or* physiological influences as though these were separate. Yet despite its limited success, psychophysiological research represents an attempt to demonstrate the valid assumption that dreaming is basically a psychobiological process.

A fourth point is that the failure to establish strong correlations between physiological activity and dream content may in part be a function of the operational definition of dream content. Typically, manifest dream content categories are isolated (e.g., number of characteristics, presence of verbalization, indoor vs. outdoor setting, etc.). But these manifest characteristics may be functionally noncomparable across subjects. That is, the meaning or intent (latent content) of a category may be as important, perhaps more important. For example, a dream about playing football may involve compensation for inferiority feelings in one subject, achievement strivings in another, dominance motivation in a third, etc. These different motivations will undoubtedly be related to different patterns of physiological activation even where these subjects are matched for individual response specificity. In the absence of knowledge about the personality dynamics and immediate and remote reinforcement histories of research subjects, even the most sophisticated of research methodologies must yield minimal information about dreaming. Scientific knowledge about dreaming must eventually come to grips with the biological foundation of symbolic thought, but at present, we are not even on the threshold of such knowledge.

Finally, it should be noted that much of the work on psychophysiological correlates involves an investigation of the relationship between dream content and peripheral physiological events. If thoughts or affects differentiable in the waking state are not found to be highly correlated with autonomic patterns, why should dream content/autonomic measures be expected to yield high correlations?

To summarize, what we can and cannot say about the biological context of dreaming from the perspective of psychophysiological correlational research is determined by (a) the quality of the dream report, (b) the adequacy of physiological measures, (c) recognition of individual differences (which also determine which variables are relevant), (d) knowledge about the effects of presleep and sleep events (experiences, personality, diet, sleeping conditions, etc.) on neural and physiological activity, and (e) use of manifest vs. latent content of dream reports.

Autonomic correlates of REM dream content

The best single review of the results from research on psychophysiological correlates is the masterly review by Rechtschaffen (1973). Much of what I will touch upon is based on that paper plus reviews by Snyder (1971), Koulack (1972), Wolpert (1969), and Hauri and Van de Castle (1973a). In spite of evidence that injections of epinephrine during NREM sleep increase the salience (vividness, emotionality, bizarreness) of the subsequent report (Hersch, Antrobus, Arkin, and Singer, 1970), it is unlikely that autonomic arousal *levels per se* can account for the sometimes striking difference in amount of quality typically observed between REM and NREM reports. First, there is only a small difference between REM and NREM autonomic *level*. Second, level of ANS arousal tends to decrease from earlier to later REM periods (Snyder, Hobson, Morrison and Goldfrank, 1964) while there is a corresponding tendency for dream reporting and dream content salience to increase during the REM periods of a night. On the other hand, although the relationships are modest, there seems to be a more pronounced correlation between *variability* in a number of these dimensions and dream content characteristics (Rechtschaffen, 1973).

A number of investigators have found, for some individuals, a significant correlation between cardiac and respiratory irregularity and dream salience but results have typically been modest and mixed (see Chase, 1972, p. 243). Hauri and Van de Castle (1973a, 1973b) reported significant relationships between GSR activity and dream emotionality, but there are at least two reasons for doubting the generalizability or importance of such a relationship. First, GSR fluctuation tends to occur during eye movement activity so that obtained relationships may be indirect or secondary to more fundamental central events largely initiated in the brain stem. Second, most GSR activity occurs in delta sleep which calls into question the psychological significance or importance of the relationship between GSR and content during REM sleep.

Penile erections occur during the REM sleep of infants, adults, and the aged. In the light of relative infrequency of erotic dream content, they are best not considered of great emotional significance. "One could argue from a psychoanalytic orientation that there is something intrinsically sexual in all dream content. . . . But unless one specifies reliable empirical criteria for inferring sexuality, then the designation of all dreams as sexual is made *a priori* on a theoretical basis rather than on observable distinguishing features of the dream content" (Rechtschaffen, 1973, p. 26). (Surely one would not want to generalize from the heightened peristaltic activity of the stomach during REM that there is something intrinsically "consummatory" about dream content.) There is evidence, however, that the presence of sexual content can facilitate penile activity (Fisher, 1966), and evidence that aggression or anxiety during REM dreaming can elicit detumescence (Karacan, Goodenough, Shapiro and Starker, 1966). The relationship between male genital activity and dream content has been studied in a somewhat different manner. Bell and Stroebel (1973) reported that anxiety dreams were significantly correlated with a diminution of the "scrotal complex response" composed of autonomic indicators of the activation of the smooth dartos and striated cremaster musculature. According to Bell, such a measure is probably a more sensitive external indicator of dysphoric dream content than is penile detumescence *per se* but as far as I know, no dream researchers have taken her up on the suggestion to use such a measure!

A few studies have reported a generally negative relationship between body temperature and dream salience. This relationship has been demonstrated in a number of different ways: first between REM periods that differ in rectal temperature; second, in comparisons between early (higher temperature) vs. later (lower temperature) REM periods of a night. Indirect support for this relationship comes from a study by Karacan, Wolff, Williams, Hursch and Webb (1968) who reported that under conditions of induced increase in body temperature, a markedly lower percentage of subjects reported dream activity than under baseline conditions. If it can be assumed that emotionally intense dreams are more readily recalled (the salience hypothesis), and if it can be assumed that there is an inverse correlation between body temperature and dream salience, then the recall findings of Karacan *et al.* are consistent with the other findings mentioned above. One final bit of evidence comes from a study by Ziegler (1973) who reported a negative correlation between room temperature (with corresponding vasodilation-constriction) and dysphoric dream emotionality. Considering the evidence (discussed in Chapter 1) that body temperature during REM sleep (more than NREM) is *positively* correlated with external temperature (poikilothermic characteristic), it is likely that external temperature and body temperature will have some effect on certain characteristics of the REM dream experience.

Given what is known about the powerful inhibitory action of brain stem centers, overt bodily movement probably represents momentary disinhibition. Thus, correlations between this aperiodic and fragmentary peripheral activity and dream content should be relatively general and nonspecific. Dement and Wolpert (1958) found a relationship between REM periods with frequent incidences of motor activity and reports of fragmented and discontinued dreams, while REM periods with little activity were associated with reports of long and continuous dreams. More specific relationships between body movement and dream content have been reported by Gardiner *et al.* (1975). They found a significant relationship between amount of limb movement during REM sleep and reports of dreamed activity in the corresponding limbs. Such relationships demonstrate the potential yield when attention is paid to the quality of dream reports. It might be interesting to speculate about how expressive humans would be during sleep were it possible to eliminate the action of pontine inhibitory centers during REM. Presumably, body movement, or even sleep talking, would be more readily expressed and we might be in a better position to evaluate both psychophysiological relationships and the validity of dream reports.

Eye movement and REM dream content

There has been more theorizing about the relationship between dreaming and rapid eye movement than any other physiological activity. Eye movements are hypothesized to be external manifestations of repression, information processing or rate of information flow, nonspecific indications of arousal, and dream imagery scanning. We will concern ourselves with the latter two hypotheses which have most often been tested within a correlational framework.

That features of dream content were associated with the presence, amount, and direction of eye movement did more than anything else to establish the scientific legitimacy of dream research. Dement and Kleitman's (1957) report that subjects spoke of dreaming about a ping-pong game or climbing a ladder after being awakened from a REM period characterized primarily by horizontal or vertical eye movements respectively was most compelling. Research on eye movement-dream content parallelism reached a new level of sophistication when Roffwarg, Dement, Muzio and Fisher (1962) demonstrated that eye movement patterns could be postdicted reasonably accurately from careful interviews of subjects just awakened from REM sleep. These kinds of findings lent support for the *scanning hypothesis* which holds that eye movements represent scanning of the dream scene.

In a sense, the Roffwarg *et al.* study marked the watershed of the so-called new experimental dream research. But as soon as it was established, the scanning hypothesis was in trouble. First, there were reports of failure to replicate the kind of eye movement-dream content parallelism demanded by the scanning hypothesis (Jacobs *et al.*, 1971; Moscowitz and Berger, 1969). In addition, "there is evidence which shows that the amplitude, density, velocity, stereotypy, predominant direction, sequential pattern, temporal distribution, or organization of eye movements during REM sleep is different from those of eye movements during wakefulness" (Rechtschaffen, 1973, p. 177; also see Jacobs *et al.*, 1971). Also, it is apparent that a distinction between isolated vs. burst eye movement should be retained since the former may be related to cortical activity while the latter may have more to do with nonspecific CNS arousal initiated in the pons. Finally, the fact that mentation, often very much like that of REM, can be elicited from NREM sleep while, on the other hand, the congenitally blind have eye movements but no visual imagery and thus no scanning (in the sense implied by the hypothesis) tended to cool enthusiasm for the hypothesis. This is not to say that, occasionally, hallucinated events elicit appropriate (conditioned?) eye movement or scanning. This may even be more frequent than recent research indicates since anything but the most thorough assessment of well-recalled dream material will create an enormous Type II bias. The point is that scanning is not necessary and therefore, its significance beyond that of validating the dream report can be questioned.

An alternative to the scanning hypothesis is the hypothesis that eye movement activity indicates fluctuations in general arousal level. If this latter hypothesis is true, and if there is a kind of nondirectional psychophysiological parallelism, there ought to be an association between eye movement activity and dreamed activity. Dement and Wolpert (1958) found a correlation between eye movement activity and reports of activity by the subject during the dream. Of 58 reports from eye movement-active REM periods, 38 (66%) were blindly rated as showing a high degree of dreamer activity. Of 49 eye movement-quiescent REM period reports, only 10% were so rated. This statistically significant parallelism was essentially replicated in a different study (Berger and Oswald, 1962), though in a more recent study (Firth and Oswald, 1975) the relationship was found to be extremely weak: hardly the results that powerful theories are built upon. There have also been some reports that eye movement activity tends to correlate with the salience of dream content (e.g., vividness, affect) but the correlations, on the whole, are rather weak (Cohen, 1974d).

Perhaps we need to pay closer attention to individual differences in both waking and sleeping eye movement as well as to the adequacy of the categories of dream content that are used to assess the relevance of eye movement activity to the phenomenology of REM sleep. Eye movement density is one of the few sleep measures that appears to be reliable within subjects across nights (Clausen, Sersen and Lidsky, 1974; Jacobs et al., 1971). There is evidence that certain kinds of highly altered presleep environments affect eye movement density. For example, some investigators have found that deprivation or radical alteration of sensory input increases REM density (Baekeland, 1970; Baekeland, Koulack and Lasky, 1968; Potter and Heron, 1972; Prevost, DeKoninck and Proulx, 1975; Zimmerman, Stoyva and Metcalf, 1970) while others have reported that there is no such relationship (Allen, Oswald, Lewis and Tagney, 1972; Bowe-Anders, Herman and Roffwarg, 1974). These inconsistent findings provide little comfort to those who believe that eye movement patterns are external manifestations of information processing rate during REM, *and* that such patterns should reflect significant sensorimotor adjustments such as those imposed on the subject in these experiments (de la Peña et al., 1973; Dewan, 1969).

Of course, it may be that there are important individual differences in the importance of REM, and in the role of different REM parameters (eye movement, REM duration, number of REM periods), which typically go unassessed in these kinds of studies. De la Peña et al. (1973) found highly significant positive correlations across subjects between waking measures of eye movement activity patterns (e.g., eye track length, fixation rate, etc.) and related REM measures (eye movement intensity, number of bursts, etc.). These results were interpreted in the context of a sensory control for information processing or SCIP hypothesis which assumes that eye movement activity is an external manifestation of sensory/cognitive information flow inherent in CNS activation. There is a further assumption that for a given presleep environment of known complexity/surprise value, more experience/developed individuals (for reasons both organic and experiential) will experience relatively more "sensory deprivation". This will be compensated for during REM sleep by increased information flow (i.e., more eye movement rather than longer REM periods or higher REM percentage). This homeostatic model, which predicts a negative wake/REM eye movement correlation within subjects, has recently obtained experimental support (Prevost et al., 1975). The SCIP hypothesis is concerned with individual differences that are usually ignored in sleep research. But it also suggests the potential importance of focusing on certain aspects of dream content which would reflect CNS activation hypothesized to indicate increased information flow.[3]

---

[3] A preliminary report of EEG-dream content relationships suggests a possible approach to this question. Moiseeva (1975) has reported that "complex dreams with simultaneous actions in different aspects ... with disturbed temporal and spatial relations, take place against a background of polymorphous EEG. ... The correlation between the bioelectric processes occurring in different structures is lower than during dreams with a logical structure."

The findings that eye movement density is related to dream activity or excitement do not go far enough. More attention needs to be paid to the rate of events in the dream, the variety of experience, the novelty of experience, etc. The relatively low correlations obtained between eye movement measures and dream content variables again suggest the importance of improving measures and assessing individual differences. The SCIP hypothesis provides an opportunity to assess certain properties of dream content from a psychobiological perspective.

Molinari and Foulkes (1969) originally reported that dream narratives elicited from REM periods with eye movement activity were richer in what they called "primary visual experience". On the other hand, they reported that dreams elicited from REM periods with no eye movement activity were richer in "secondary cognitive elaboration" (thinking, problem solving). However, follow-up studies *predicting* such a relationship were more or less unsuccessful (e.g., Foulkes and Pope, 1973). The original Molinari and Foulkes finding appeared to be due largely to an artifact of the reporting process rather than an important indicator of dream content. That is, REM active (with eye movements) reports did contain secondary cognitive elaboration but tended not to be reported. Under conditions calling for more complete reports (asking about secondary cognitive elaboration rather than obtaining merely spontaneous reports), differences between REM quiet and REM active reports largely disappeared.

Dense eye movement activity during REM is *not* necessarily an indication that visual, dreamy, or emotionally intense experiences are predominating over more rational or logical or verbal forms of thinking. Let us for the moment assume that there is a correlation between eye movement activity and waking mentation that can be used to predict from REM eye movement patterns something about REM mentation. Such an assumption is supported by recent findings that there is a correlation across subjects between density of waking and REM eye movement activity (de la Peña *et al.*, 1973). However, there is evidence that the intensity of waking imagery is *inversely* related to eye movement density (Klinger *et al.*, 1973; Lavie and Kripke, 1975; Marks, 1972). Also, one of my former graduate students, Merrill Hiscock, found a sharp and discrete *increase* in eye movement activity when subjects shifted from 10 trials of imagining mostly static images (e.g., how many windows are there in the U.T. tower?) to 10 trials involving verbal constructions (e.g., what is the meaning of the proverb, "one swallow doesn't make a summer"?). This marked increase in eye movement activity from the tenth (imagery) trial to the eleventh (verbal) trial was sustained throughout the 9 subsequent verbal trials and was relatively constant for all subjects tested. This finding is consistent with other published data. For example, Weiner and Ehrlichman (1976) found that questions of a visuo-spatial nature were associated with fewer eye movements than were questions of a verbal-conceptual nature. They interpreted these results as being inconsistent with the idea that visual imagery is necessarily associated with scanning eye movements. It is likely that had Hiscock used kinetic as well as static imagery, he might have found more eye movement for imagery (Antrobus, Antrobus and Singer, 1964). But the point is that eye movement during REM cannot, *a priori*, be assumed to indicate a change from more thoughtlike to more hallucinatory modes of mentation unless the dynamics of eye movement during sleep are quite different from those of wakefulness (Foulkes and Fleisher, 1975). In fact, Lairy (1975) has reported that the extremely dense REM periods of chronic paranoids belies the "mental 'void', apparently existing in chronic psychotics, even during REM sleep, which is richer in phasic events than controls' REM sleep . . ." (p. 130).

Central events: PGO, PIPs, and dream content

During REM sleep in cats, eye movements are accompanied by spiking discharge activity that originates in the pons and which can be recorded in the lateral geniculate and occipital areas. According to Benoit and Adrien (1975), "it seems that at the time of the PGO wave, there is a simultaneous enhancement of the internal excitatory phenomena, and of the blocking acting on the sensory afferences and motor efferences. The effect of this double phenomenon is an increased isolation of the individual from the environment, and so prevents the state of 'internal excitation' from being transposed to the behavioral level" (p. 25). Brooks (in Webb, 1973, pp. 79-80) develops a psychophysiological hypothesis regarding the functional significance of PGO:

> I suggest that PGO waves have to do with a mechanism which enables the visual system to make an orderly transition from the analysis of one visual image to the next. According to this idea, when the analysis of each image is about to end, a stimulus of brainstem origin prepares the visual system for the arrival of an entirely new image, and this process manifests itself as a PGO wave. The nature of the transient events which must take place in visual structures at the point of discontinuity between analysis of successive images is uncertain. For the sake of argument, let us say that the role of the brain stem input is to erase existing patterns of neuronal excitation and inhibition at all levels of the visual system. As a result, the next image will be perceived as a new one, rather than as an initially blurred or displaced version of the preceding image. The erasure process must be active, involving increased neuronal discharge rates somewhat analogous to the whirring of gears one hears when the "clear" button removes stored data from a calculator before a new computation is started. ... This general hypothesis, like one of those cited above, implies a relationship between PGO[REM] and the imagery of dreaming, but it differs in suggesting that the neuronal events associated with the imagery occur in the intervals between PGO waves. That is, during both wakefulness and REM sleep PGO waves signify the transition from the analysis of one image to the next.

This proposal is a variant of the hypothesis that eye movement activity is an important component of the process by which perceptual and memory imagery is generated and reactivated. Additionally, it assumes that the brain stem, more specifically pontine nuclei, are integral aspects of this as yet largely unknown process. I have already mentioned the work of Ornitz et al. (1973) which supports their hypothesis that vestibular dysfunction underlies the eye movement anomalies observed during the experimental manipulation of the REM sleep of autistic children. In addition, there is research (Noton and Stark, 1971) strongly suggesting the crucial role of successive eye movements which, during perception, trace out the outlines of objects such that they are built up *sequentially* into gestalt schemata.[4] Perhaps during REM sleep there is a "read out" of information composed of

---

[4] That images (schemata) of objects are built up through sequential eye movement tracing rather than holistically is suggested by the fact that it takes longer to recognize that a target ("correct") stimulus compared to a nontarget stimulus is a match for a remembered (stored) object. That is, one searches sequentially through each segment of the stored image, comparing each with the perceived stimulus until all segments are tested. If the stimulus is nontarget, a subject will, on the average, recognize a mismatch earlier than if the stimulus is the target. In the latter case, he has to go through all the segments of the memory trace, and realize that all segments are congruent with those of the stimulus. If visual perception were merely holistic, there should be no difference in reaction time to decision for target and nontarget stimuli.

schemata made up partially of eye movement patterns. Or, as Paivio (1971) suggests, "eye movements may facilitate the generation of imagery in some circumstances by providing proprioceptive retrieval cues, acquired through conditioning" (p. 70). (Note that this does not require the assumption that eye movement is *necessary* for all vivid imagery.) Thus, PGO/REM activity might have two properties, one more or less representative of the decoding of (motorically encoded) information, the other functional in the sense of actively modifying that "read out" process. Brooks' proposal suggests one kind of active modification, that is the sharpening of the boundaries between imagery events. We will see shortly that Rechtschaffen (1973) had a similar notion, suggesting that PGO may serve to break up the flow of information. These two variants of the psychophysiological approach to PGO suggest that the informational flow during REM sleep is neither random and unrelated structurally or temporally to prior experience, nor is it merely a simple read out of information exactly as originally experienced. PGO theory, like REM dream research data in general, is consistent with the Bartlettian view of memory as reconstruction (Bartlett, 1932) rather than reproduction.[5]

PGO spiking cannot be directly observed through standard surface recordings. However, Rechtschaffen (1973) has described the evolution of a technique involving the recording and integrating of electrical activity near the extraocular muscles of humans. The result is a credible equivalent of PGO, namely periorbital *p*hasic *i*ntegrated *p*otentials or PIPs. The advantage of recording PIPs is that they occur during NREM as well as during REM. Thus one can assess central activation independent of eye movement, and its relationship to dream reports. In addition, PIPs seem to be an external manifestation of a more fundamental biological activity than are eye movements.

Preliminary data on PIP-dream content relationships (Rechtschaffen, Watson, Wincor, Molinari and Barta, 1972; Watson, 1972) suggested that, regardless of the presence or absence of eye movement, PIP activity appears to be related to distortion and bizarreness of the dream content of REM or NREM sleep. One hypothesis, not unlike that proposed by Brooks (in Webb, 1973) to account for his PGO data, is that PIPs are the sign of fragmentation or loosening of cognitive associations initiated in the pons. However, more recent attempts to replicate this relationship have not yielded findings as clear-cut as the initial ones (Watson, personal communication, June, 1976). Thus, speculation about the role of PGO activity in the biological regulation of "creative" reorganization or reprogramming during REM dreaming may be somewhat premature. This speculation could be given firmer scientific respectability were it possible to establish a relationship between the quality of "solutions" to problems during dreaming and the quantity and quality of PIP activity. Jouvet (1974) speculates that "some genetic coding could initiate the complex succession of PGO events. The synaptic organization of the hardware (and the hypothetical long-lasting modification which takes place during learning) would be subjected during [REM sleep] to a genetic coding. Thus, there would be two different possibilities for evolution to improve the brain. Mutations could affect either the organization of the hardware or the genetic coding of the software ... paradoxical sleep (and dreaming) would represent the

---

[5] It should be noted that not all researchers are as enthusiastic about the theoretical implications of the PGO phenomenon. For example, Morrison and Bowker (1975) have reported evidence that PGOs indistinguishable from the spontaneous kind were elicited by auditory signals. The results suggest that PGO spikes may be a sign of a startle response due to the "neural turmoil" of REM. The authors say that "this conception is a novel one and bestows far less importance on PGO spikes than is common in the sleep literature".

interactions between some system of neurons whose anatomical organization is genetically programmed (the hardware) and another system of neurons having much more plasticity (some MA neurons). These latter neurons would be responsible for some genetic coding through a functional system whose final electrical expression is the PGO activity" (p. 228). What Jouvet is suggesting is that dreaming may be the phenomenological expression of both nature (genetic coding) and nurture (learning) mediated by the interaction of neuronally distinct areas.

Research on PIP correlates suggests important distinctions among (a) the organization and processing of recent and remote information arising from CNS activity during REM sleep, (b) attention or consciousness during sleep and the translation of information processing (latent content) into manifest cognitive characteristics (verbal, visual, affective), namely, the creation of a dream, and (c) retention of experienced information during sleep and during the transition to wakefulness. There is evidence that these different aspects of the dreaming process are controlled and mediated by different but interrelated parts of the CNS. Activation (low voltage fast EEG) in the cerebral cortex seems fundamental to the generation of a well-organized flow of information which, through largely unknown mechanisms, gets translated into a dream experience (Kleitman, 1967). Inhibition of thalamic and hippocampal influences may be important in heightening consciousness during sleep (Jouvet, 1975; Torda, 1968, 1969) and in turn may influence dream recall. Limbic structures and temporal cortex are undoubtedly crucial in determining the affective quality and the recallability of the dream (Brazier, 1967; Greenberg et al., 1968). When we speak of the effect of personality or environmental situation on dream content and dream recall, we undoubtedly are speaking about effects that are mediated through changes in CNS activity that directly affect the production and accessibility of the psychological phenomena. Unfortunately, in the absence of information about the specifics of such mediation, we must rely on manipulations of variables (traits, presleep conditions) of relatively unknown biological reference and significance. This is not to say that we cannot learn a good deal about dreaming from such manipulations. My disposition toward reductionism in things nonsymbolic is not all that doctrinaire. It simply means that we need to be aware of the limitations of our explanations.

2. THE TEMPORAL FACTOR IN REM DREAM CONTENT

REM dreams are embedded within a shifting pattern of physiological activity and therefore have somewhat different characteristics depending on the time of night. With no abrupt changes immediately prior to the termination or reestablishment of wakefulness, there is a gradual diminution during sleep in oxygen consumption, respiration rate, rectal temperature, skin temperature (after rising during the first two hours). Conversely, there is an increase in body movement and (after an initial decrease during the first two to three hours) an increase in systolic blood pressure. REM periods participate in these changes. However, note that there is a marked increase in variability of these measures both after transition from NREM to REM and from one REM period to the next (Snyder, 1971). This REM-to-REM physiological variability tends to increase across the night. In addition the duration of REM periods increases until about the third one after which it tends to average about 30 minutes (though some REM periods may last as long as an hour).

Temporal factors and sleep quality

There are marked individual differences in the levels and changes of some of the physiological characteristics just described. For example, in his now "classic" study of good vs. poor sleepers, Monroe (1967) obtained evidence that poor sleepers were physiologically more active; they had significantly higher rectal temperature, more frequent vasoconstrictions per minute, more body movements per hour, higher skin resistance, and trends toward higher heart rate per minute and pulse volume. These differences tended to obtain throughout the night and in REM, as well as NREM (though the REM differences were not statistically significant in all cases). In addition, the poor sleepers had significantly less REM time and lower REM percentage of total sleep. In addition, they had significantly higher elevations on MMPI scales.

Monroe's (1967) data provide the framework for speculation about the nature of good vs. poor sleep and its relationship to long vs. short sleep. Individual differences in habitual sleep time can, broadly speaking, be thought of as a reflection of two general events: (1) *Normal* individual differences in the "setting" of a (probably brain stem) instinct requirement. (2) Individual differences in primary (e.g., narcolepsy, encephalitis, etc.) or secondary (e.g., neurotic) disturbance or *abnormality* of circadian cycles. For example, some people have a short sleep requirement and thus sleep only a few hours. Others have a normal sleep requirement but, because of some disturbance that is external to the process that determines sleep duration, cannot attain sufficient sleep. *Hypo*somniacs (the former) should be distinguished from *in*somniacs (the latter). It may be, as Hartmann (1973) has argued, that long sleepers tend more often to be emotionally disturbed while short sleepers tend to be emotionally healthy. Attempts to replicate this observation on college student populations have largely been unsuccessful (e.g., Webb and Friel, 1971). Perhaps there is a greater association between long sleep and emotional problems than there is between short sleep and emotional health.

Let us consider relatively healthy individuals who differ in sleep time. Is it possible to think of short (noninsomniac) sleep as relatively more efficient than long sleep? What I would like to suggest is that, to be efficient, sleep must be as physiologically *different* as possible from wakefulness. That is, if sleep has a specialized function that is in some sense different from the function of wakefulness, then one requirement for efficient or good sleep is biological distance from wakefulness. Distance would be presumably measurable along a number of dimensions, both physiological and psychological. For example, efficient sleep might mean a relatively large percentage of delta sleep (electrocortically "deep"), high auditory arousal threshold (behaviorally "deep") and relatively more unconsciousness (phenomenologically "deep"), *especially early in the night*. Presumably, individuals who can sleep few hours with no ill effects should show patterns of "deep sleep" along these dimensions. Evidence from Hartmann (1973), Monroe (1967), and Coursey, Buchsbaum, and Frankel (1975) is commensurate with these speculations. In addition, in commenting on the Monroe (1967) data, Rechtschaffen and Monroe (1969) propose an explanation for individual differences in sleep characteristics that is not unlike the psychobiological concept I am suggesting. The relatively better NREM recall and sense of being awake prior to early NREM awakenings observed in poor sleepers suggest that "they are physiologically closer to wakefulness than good sleepers, although both are behaviorally asleep. Rather than unimportant epiphenomena, the subjective reports of sleep mentation and light sleep in

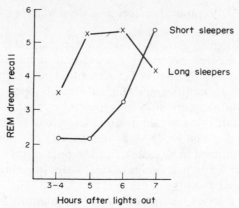

Figure 7-1   REM dream recall for seven short and seven long sleepers as a function of the temporal position of the REM period.

poor sleepers may be sensitive indicators of the incomplete and nonrestorative quality of their sleep" (Rechtschaffen and Monroe, 1969, pp. 168-169).

Recently, I was able to select some dream recall data from a small group ($N = 7$) of habitual short (less than 7 hours) sleepers and a small group ($N = 7$) of habitual long (more than 7.5 hours) sleepers. Figure 7-1 shows the distribution of dream recall (seven point scale composed of a four point "amount" plus a three point "clarity" scale) for REM sleep awakenings at four points during the night after. These differential distributions appear to support my speculation that sleep efficiency may involve greater depth or "psychobiological distance" between sleep and waking states. I have already discussed in some detail the relationship between dream recall and psychobiological depth (or boundaries between states) in Chapter 6. Suffice it to say here that perhaps the reason that *some* long sleepers need more sleep is that they have to make up via quantity what they lack in quality. This would presumably not apply to those long sleepers whose circadian setting is determined by instinct rather than by disturbance.

I have just suggested the concept of psychobiological depth as one way to talk about sleep efficiency, a quality presumably characterizing the sleep of short sleepers. A behavioral approach to the question of sleep efficiency would be somewhat different. Under conditions of gradual reduction of sleep, would individual differences in adaptability (differences in fatigue, performance, mood, etc.) be another indication of sleep efficiency? My guess is that some combination of large amounts of delta *and REM* during the first half of sleep typical for an individual would be positively associated with the capacity for sleep reduction proportional to baseline without behavioral deficit.

Temporal determinants of REM dream content

The role of temporally constraining physiological factors in cuing and modifying dream content is largely unexplored. Consider the following observation from a study by Trossman, Rechtschaffen, Offencrantz and Wolpert (1960). Certain dream elements (e.g., fat woman) recurred across two nights at identical positions (third period of the REM-NREM cycle or at the same time of night). One subject dreamed of the same male friend during the third REM period of five different nights. On the sixth night, the subject arrived at the laboratory later than usual so that his first REM period on this night occurred about the time that his third REM period normally occurred. On this night, the friend appeared in the dream of the first REM period! Such a phenomenon, if replicated, might indicate an important role for some temporally-keyed physiologically mediated factor (e.g., hormonal, neurological), and would clearly contradict the assumption that physiological variables have no influence on the specific content of dreams. Dreams may be as capable of representing somatic as well as psychological events; that is, dreams may be cognitive representations of important *organismic* events. If psychological preoccupations are correlated (say, through classical conditioning) with somatic events, then patterns of somatic activity during sleep may act as conditioned cues for psychological preoccupations.

Increase in physiological activation, presumably mediated by those limbic structures which influence emotional behavior, ought to manifest itself in changes in dream content. Indeed, there are reports that during the night, REM dream content tends to become more dreamlike (more vivid, emotional, active) (Snyder, 1970; Verdone, 1965). From the perspective of nonspecific psychophysiological parallelism, such findings make a good deal of sense. However, I am beginning to think that the relationship between temporal position of the REM period and dream content is more complicated, perhaps even more interesting. I have carried out some preliminary analyses which suggest that there may be a gradual increase in left cerebral hemisphere dominance or control over dreaming across REM periods during the night. This hypothesis, which I hesitantly call GILD (gradual *i*ncrease in *left d*ominance), is based on eye movement, EEG amplitude, and dream content data obtained from different samples of male subjects.

The rationale behind the series of analyses which I will describe below is derived from two interests, one related to the idea that dreaming can be adaptive, the other that lateral specialization of brain function mediates behavior and experience. If the adaptive properties of dreaming bear some resemblance to those of waking cognition, then dream content analysis ought to reveal some evidence that the dream experience is at least influenced by the left hemisphere. Changes in such influence across REM periods might tell us something important about the evolution of brain function during the night. Our approach to the problem of dream content and adaptation starts with the assumption that dreams reflect underlying neurological characteristics. However, ultimately we are interested in the implications of such events for hypotheses about the effect of dreaming on postsleep behaviors, i.e., the adaptation hypothesis (discussed in Chapter 10).

An interest in lateral specialization of function led me to question its relevance to the dreaming state. Goldstein, Stoltzfus, and Gardocki (1972) had reported that during shifts from NREM to REM sleep there is a change in the ratio between left and right EEG amplitude. The result is a relatively lower left amplitude during NREM and a relatively higher left amplitude during REM sleep. Such findings suggested that the onset of REM sleep was associated with relatively greater right hemispheric activation, which fits with assumptions about the role of the right hemisphere in the mediation of spatial coding and imagery (dreaming).

There are two problems, however. First, the results were found not only in human subjects, but in cats, rabbits, and rats, organisms not known to be cortically specialized to any significant degree. Second, these findings were not assessed with regard to changes from one REM period to another during the night, and therefore could not be related to data on changes in dream content across REM periods. In addition, these results did not jibe with some preliminary results from our lab suggesting that there is a gradual and modest change in the percentage of right vs. left REM eye movements. These changed from about 50-50 for the initial REM periods to about 54-46 favoring right looking during the last few REM periods. This would indicate a tendency toward left hemispheric dominance. Our data on direction of eye movement are relatively weak because they were based on scoring a.c.-recorded EOGs (electrooculograms) that are inherently more ambiguous with respect to direction than are d.c. recordings. Also we found tremendous differences within individuals across REM periods, and between individuals, within REM periods. These difficulties prompted me to focus on dream content as a potential indicant of changes in hemispheric dominance. When available, eye movement direction and left vs. right EEG amplitude data could be used to supplement the dream content data.

I started with REM dream reports produced by 22 college men each of whom spent a single night in the sleep laboratory. Each subject was awakened five to ten minutes into each of the REM periods of the night to obtain dream reports. Adequacy of dream recall was estimated on the basis of a seven point (0-6) scale reflecting amount and quality of material. The subject was asked about affective experiences during the dream (e.g., mild affects vs. strong emotions), and then rated the adequacy of his ego functioning (e.g., concentration, judgement, competence, etc.) on seven 3-step scales (poor, fair, good). These ratings were later combined and averaged to yield a 3-step scale of general ego functioning (1 = poor to 3 = good). REM dream content was then assessed by two judges who achieved acceptable levels of reliability for categories that seemed relevant primarily to left and to right hemisphere activity. The decision to categorize a dream category as "left" or "right" was made on the basis of the cortical lateralization literature (e.g., Bakan, 1971; Kinsbourne, 1972; Sperry, 1968). Only ten subjects provided REM dream data during each of the time periods selected to represent early, middle, and later REM periods (Cohen, 1977a).

Table 7-1 shows evidence of a gradual increase in the percentage of subjects whose REM reports showed signs of left categories and an apparent lack of change in right categories. The decision to use good dream recall as indicative of left activity was based on two assumptions. First, it was assumed that the left hemisphere mediates consciousness, i.e., awareness that can be verbalized (Albert, Silverberg, Reches and Berman, 1976; Eccles, 1973). If the *recallability* of a dream experience is partly determined by consciousness of the

TABLE 7-1.   Percentage of Subjects ($N = 10$) with Left- and Right-hemispheric REM Dream Content at Three Points During Night

Dimensions	Hours since lights out			p (Change[a])
	3–4[a]	5–6	7[a]	
Left hemisphere				
Good ego function	10	30	70	0.05
Verbal activity	30	90	100	0.05
Good recall	20	70	80	0.05
Right hemisphere				
Music	10	20	10	
Spatial salience	30	40	30	
Strong emotion*	56	44	67	
Bizarre events	30	40	30	

*$N = 9$.

TABLE 7-2.   Percentage of REM Dream Reports with Left-
or Right-hemisphere Content

| Category | REM period | | | |
	1st	2nd	3rd	4th
Left hemisphere				
Verbal activity	57	65	77	93
Positive affect	9	17	33	40
Right hemisphere				
Negative affect	23	22	19	7
Bizarreness	45	32	20	29

Note: *N*s (reports) vary from 15 to 23.

dream experience (salience) then conscious experiences should be more readily recalled than unconscious experiences. Second, it was assumed that the left hemisphere mediates *reportability* because it contributes to the verbal encoding of material to be decoded via the same mode. Thus, an increase in left-mediated information processing should be associated with a corresponding increase in the probability of good dream recall. This expectation is fulfilled by our data. Nevertheless, in the light of the complexities of dream recall determination, and in the interest of focusing on content, I decided to ignore the dream recall factor in the analyses of data from other studies. Changes in content which we have found are, in my view, sufficiently impressive without recourse to additional variables like dream recall which might be considered as artifacts that could bias our results in the desired direction. It should be noted that additional analyses (e.g., using only well-recalled reports) suggested that recall quality was *not* a major factor in the differential results based on content categories.

The reliability of the findings shown in Table 7-1 was assessed by considering REM content data from two other studies that had been carried out earlier (for purposes other than that which concerns us here). Categories which had been scored in those studies and which seemed relevant to the left vs. right hemisphere distinction were selected. The results of these two analyses are shown in Tables 7-2 and 7-3. They constitute two conceptual replications of the initial results.

I then went back to the eye movement data which were obtained from the 10 subjects in the first study. Although there is some evidence that right looking is a relatively crude indication of left dominance (e.g., verbal rather than spatial thinking) (e.g., Kinsbourne, 1972), there are many reasons for caution when applying such findings to REM data. First, a.c.

TABLE 7-3.   Percentage of Subjects (*N* = 11)
Whose REM Dream Reports Show Evidence of Left-
or Right-hemisphere Activity

Content category	Early REM	Late REM
Left hemisphere		
Verbal activity	36	73
Positive affect	45	91
Right hemisphere		
Negative affect	36	18
Bizarreness	73	45

EOG recordings are inherently ambiguous. Second, much eye movement activity is mediated by cortically nonspecific brain stem activity (Rechtschaffen, 1973). Third, there is no evidence that directional data implying cortical specialization during wakefulness can be generalized to sleep. (This was one of the questions that I was interested in because it related to the more general issue of continuity between waking and sleep characteristics of the individual.) And fourth, there is some question as to the adequacy of direction of gaze as an operational estimate of cortical dominance (Hiscock, 1977). With these qualifications in mind I made the following predictions based on the hypothesis of a gradual change toward relatively more left hemisphere control during later REM periods (GILD).

First, with respect to *temporal effects*: there should be a tendency for the percentage of right eye movements (R/Total = R%) to increase from earliest to latest REM period. Of ten subjects whose REM dream data appear in Table 7-1, eight showed an increase, two a marked decrease, in R%. A question of individual differences was clearly indicated by these nonsignificant but suggestive results. Second, with respect to *psychophysiological correlation*: changes in left (but not right) REM dream categories should correlate with changes in R% across the REM periods. A composite left score was given to the early and late dreams of the ten subjects of Table 7-1. The correlation between change (from first to last REM period category) in left composite score and corresponding change in R% was .79 ($p < .01$). Note that the correlation between change in R% and change in *dream recall* quality was only .20, suggesting that the overall relationship cannot be dismissed merely as an artifact of dream recall. Note also that the correlation between R% and a composite right hemisphere score was only .07. Thus, despite the inherent ambiguity of the eye movement data, results consistent with the GILD hypothesis were obtained. Fortunately, I was able to obtain EEG amplitude data on subjects from an earlier study (Cohen and MacNeilage, 1974) whose dream data are shown in Table 7-2. On the assumption that EEG amplitude is inversely associated with activation, I made the following two predictions. First, with respect to *temporal effects*: there should be a tendency for left over right EEG amplitude ratios (L/R) to decrease (i.e., relative increase in left hemispheric activation/control) during the night. Six of the nine subjects from the Cohen and MacNeilage (1974) study, for whom we had computer scored EEG data, showed the predicted decrease in L/R from the first two REM periods to the last two (averaging over nights). The mean difference was marginally significant ($p < .10$), again suggesting the importance of individual differences. Second, with respect to *psychophysiological correlations*: there should be a tendency for L/R decreasers to show a greater increase in verbal activity compared to L/R increasers. For the five decreasers, mean change in verbal activity was +23%, and for the increasers, 0%. Though not a significant difference, it is in line with expectation.

There is growing evidence that left-handedness is associated with less cortical specialization (Levy, 1972). Thus, handedness is an obvious factor that could attenuate results predicted by a hypothesis about hemispheric specialization during sleep. Fortunately, we had asked the subjects in the Cohen and MacNeilage (1974) study to fill out a handedness questionnaire composed of 23 items. There was a —.59 correlation between left-hand preference and L/R decrease; sinestral tendencies were associated with no change or an *increase* in L/R. In fact, the subject with the strongest sinestral tendency was the subject with the greatest L/R increase.

In the process of following up these preliminary analyses with more attention to the changes on dream content across REM periods, a new set of results can now be added to the initial findings. Dream content was obtained from male subjects from each REM period during an eight hour night. Subjects were awakened either during the estimated midpoint of each REM period (Middle condition) or at the estimated endpoint of each REM period (Late condition). In order to have sufficient number of subjects producing scorable content from both the early and later parts of the night, content from REM periods occurring from the second through sixth hour after lights out was compared to the content of the same subject from REM periods occurring during the seventh and eighth hours after lights out.

Five left hemisphere-related, and four right hemisphere-related categories were used.[6] The former consisted of (a) significant verbal activity (not just isolated words), (b) high activity or energy output (e.g., running), (c) active participation in dream events (rather than passive participation or merely looking), (d) affect such as surprise, curiosity, apprehension, sympathy, etc. (rather than raw emotion), (e) ego strength defined as a rating of "good" for *both* the capacity to evaluate what is going on during the dream and the capacity to respond intelligently and competently to the challenges of the dream situation. The right categories consisted of (a) hearing music, (b) salient spatial configurations (e.g., unusual shapes of spaces within which the dream takes place), (c) bizarre or impossible events, (d) emotion, i.e., raw, high arousal experiences such as anxiety, euphoria, excitement, depression, anger.[7]

The percentage of *subjects* whose dreams during the earlier and later parts of the night were characterized by each of these qualities was assessed. In addition, a composite score for left and for right categories was derived to indicate the "saturation" of left or right hemisphere influence during the dream experiences. This score was derived by counting the number of check marks indicating the presence of characteristics satisfying the criteria for each of the five left and four right hemisphere categories and dividing this number by the number of categories on which the dream could be scored. For example, if during the early part of the night a subject achieved three "high" ratings (e.g., significant verbal activity, high activity and high ego strength) and two low ratings (e.g., no affect, passive participation in the dream), his composite left score would be 3/5 or .6.

Table 7-4 shows the results for the subjects in the late condition, and Table 7-5 shows the results for the subjects in the middle condition. It is apparent that the percentage of subjects producing strong expression of left categories increases from early to later REM periods; the percentage of subjects producing strong expression of right-related categories changes little. The composite scores indicate a greater "saturation" of left-related experience later in

[6] There are basically two reasons for the differences across studies in the lists of hemisphere-related categories. First our ideas about what constituted the best representatives tended to change. There was virtually nothing in the dream literature to guide us in this exploratory enterprise. Also, with respect to the studies that had been carried out earlier, we were limited to the categories that were available.

[7] The importance of distinguishing between affect and emotion became more apparent during this series of studies. Affect is here defined as a phylogenetically and ontogenetically more advanced kind of "emotion". Affect is conceived to be different from emotion in a number of ways. Affect is the product of a "filtering" process that is controlled by the neocortex, and thus reflects a wider range of physical and symbolic stimuli, is more subtle in expression, and is associated with a lower level of autonomic, cortical, and behavioral arousal. The assumption that affect in general, or positive affect in particular, is relatively more determined by left-hemisphere than right-hemisphere control (Dimond, Farrington and Johnson, 1976; Myslobodsky and Weiner, 1976) is admittedly more speculative than the assumption that it reflects degree of neocortical inhibition/filtering of subcortical activity. In any case, the data presented here suggest that a distinction be made between affect and emotion expressed in dreams. If the primary feelings expressed in later REM dreams tend to be affective rather than emotional, then researchers who lump both kinds of experiences into an "emotion" category will find a trend toward greater expression of "emotion" in later REM dreams. This will give the erroneous impression that dreaming becomes more "primitive" during later REM periods. That this is an erroneous conclusion is suggested by the fact that no one has reported an increase in bizarreness.

TABLE 7-4.   Percentage of Subjects Whose REM Dreams Show Evidence
of Definite Left vs. Right Hemisphere-related Content: Late Condition

Dimensions	N	Hours since lights out	
		2–6 hr.	7–8 hr.
Left hemisphere			
Significant verbal activity	15	40	67
High ego strength	11	27	55
High activity (energy)	8	38	75
Active participation	15	67	87
Affect (subtle feeling)	12	67	92
Composite left score (saturation)	15	0.50	0.75*
Right hemisphere			
Music	15	20	7
Spatial salience	15	33	20
Strong emotion (high arousal)	14	21	14
Bizarreness (impossible events)	15	0	20
Composite right score (saturation)	15	0.19	0.15

Note: Subjects rated their own dreams on affect, emotion, ego strength.
All categories were reliably rated by judges. Also, the Ns refer to subjects,
not to dream reports, and vary depending on whether subjects produced
scorable data at both early and late points during the night.
*$p < 0.01$, $r_{bis} = 0.61$.

the night than earlier in the night, and this appears to be true regardless of whether the
dreams are obtained at the midpoint or at the end of the REM periods.

The distinction between positive and negative feelings was not replicated. That is, within
either the affect or the strong emotion categories, there were no consistent differences
between early and later REM periods in the positive or negative valence of the experience.
Also, as is apparent from the two sets of data, there was no consistent change from early to
later REM periods in the percentage of affect regardless of valence of the affect.

TABLE 7-5.   Percentage of Subjects Whose REM Dreams Show Evidence
of Definite Left vs. Right Hemisphere-related Content: Middle Condition

Dimensions	N	Hours since lights out	
		2–6 hr.	7–8 hr.
Left hemisphere-related			
Significant verbal activity	18	44	67
High ego strength	17	12	59
High activity (energy)	15	27	47
Active participation	17	17	94
Affect (subtle feeling)	17	94	76
Composite left score (saturation)	18	0.49	0.67*
Right hemisphere-related			
Music	18	11	28
Spatial salience	18	11	0
Strong emotion	17	24	29
Bizarreness (impossible events)	18	17	11
Composite right score	18	0.15	0.17

Note: See explanatory note for Table 7-4.
*$p < 0.06$, $r_{bis} = 0.45$.

Combining the results of Tables 7-1, 7-2, 7-3, 7-4, 7-5, there appears to be a consistent pattern in the following: (a) an *increase* in left categories of verbal activity and ego strength (general competence) vs. (b) a *decrease* or *no change* in right categories of music, spatial salience, and strong emotion.

That the change in the dominance relationship of left and right hemisphere may be a general characteristic of sleep rather than specific to REM periods is suggested by a study by Myslobodsky, Ben-Mayor, Yedid-Levy and Minz (1976). Spindle activity of NREM sleep was more prominent over the right than over the left hemisphere. Also, slower activity in certain properties of the visually evoked potential was observed on the left side. These findings support the hypothesis that the dominance relationship shifts from wakefulness to sleep. More interesting, from the perspective of the GILD hypothesis, is the finding that the relative prominence of spindling over the right hemisphere *decreased* in linear fashion across each successive third of the night, and that the change was due to a relatively greater increase in left than right activity.

The hypothesis that these apparently reliable differential change patterns in REM periods really do reflect, albeit rather indirectly and crudely, a change in lateral organization (GILD hypothesis) may be tested in the context of a variety of experimental paradigms. For example, subjects could be given a series of tasks designed to exercise either right or left hemisphere functions. To provide right hemisphere exercise, subjects could be exposed to and asked to engage in a continual flow of nonverbal events and tasks, e.g., involving uncomplicated music, form recognition, and responding with the left hand. Other subjects could be given analytical verbal tasks to be answered verbally or with the right hand. Would right hemisphere exercise reduce the discrepancy between left and right dream categories? Would this effect be especially noticeable for right-handers? What would be the effect of these manipulations on REM pressure induced by REM deprivation? If the compensatory influence of right hemisphere is an important property of REM sleep, would REM deprivation have less effect on behaviors mediated by that hemisphere under conditions of right hemisphere exercise? Would REM deprivation adversely affect performance, especially on right hemisphere tasks of individuals for whom it is hypothesized that REM sleep is more important?

Another question raised by the GILD hypothesis regards the responsiveness of the sleeping individual to discriminate stimuli. If there is an initial dominance by right vs. left hemisphere over dreaming which is *relatively* greater during early REM periods, does this dominance relate to the processing of *external* events as well? Or is the right hemisphere relatively more preoccupied during the early REM periods with its dreaming function? If so, then a tactile cue presented to the right side of the body and requiring a right-hand movement should be less effective during early REM periods than during later REM periods. A left side stimulus requiring a left movement response should not show as great a differential reliability during early vs. late REM periods.

While it is too soon to evaluate the status of the GILD hypothesis, the initial findings may have some important implications for research concerned with the psychobiological basis of dreams. First, more attention needs to be paid to the potential artifact of dream recall. While preliminary analyses suggest that it is not an insurmountable problem, the fact remains that differences among individuals and differences across the REM periods of the night need to be taken into consideration. Second, changes in dream content may be artifacts of scoring. Results may be quite different if they are based on the judgments of those other than the dreamer. This point has been ably made by Van de Castle (in Chase, 1972, pp. 249-250). Third, evidence for the GILD hypothesis does not contradict other observations that REM dreams become more intense and vivid and active later in the night (Foulkes, 1970; Van de Castle, 1970).[8] Neither does it contradict the hypothesis that the right hemisphere, even later in the night, enjoys a special status with respect to the generation of the manifest dream (Bakan, 1976). What is asserted tentatively here is that the left hemisphere will play a *relatively* more important role in organizing REM dreaming processes later in the night, and that this growing influence will be most readily detectable in normal, right-handed individuals whose dream content is carefully assessed.

The GILD hypothesis refers to changes in *REM* dreaming. It has no obvious relevance to the "dreaming" or dreamy experiences of the hypnopompic period. As I suggested in Chapter 6, I believe that popular ideas regarding the regressive qualities of dreaming are largely derived from experiences that are associated with the *transition* from sleep to wakefulness (thus the frequent reports of dreams recalled after awakening from afternoon naps which rarely contain REM sleep). The gradual transition from sleep to wakefulness may be a poorly defined state, a loose combination of neurological and phenomenological events compared to the well-organized state of REM. In short, the phenomenology of NREM or transition state (stage 1-NREM) does not constitute evidence against the face validity of a hypothesis that pays special attention to the role of the left hemisphere in mediating REM periods near the end of the night.

Giving way to the temptation to speculate on the implication of these psychophysiological changes during the night, I suggest two possible factors that could account for the data. First, the two hemispheres might be governed by temporally distinct biorhythms during the nocturnal phase of the circadian cycle. Perhaps the left hemisphere, more than the right, gives up a certain degree of control during the early REM periods, undergoing a phase of neurophysiological rest and reorganization. This phenomenon could be conceptualized with the framework of reprogramming or creative incubation. Second, it is possible that the left hemisphere requires a more varied "diet" of subcortical (pontine, reticular, limbic?) stimulation which we have already seen tends to increase across REM periods during the night. We might even say that the increase in left hemisphere activation is a sign that the organism is "closer" to wakefulness when left dominance (at least with respect to adaptation in the conventional sense) is relatively complete. Intensification of the dreaming process would then be seen as a reflection of this neurophysiological preparation for wakefulness.

Fromm (1951) suggested that "dreaming is a meaningful and significant expression of any kind of mental activity under the condition of sleep" and that "if we can find out what the specific effect of sleeping is on our mental activity, we may discover a good deal more about the nature of dreaming" (pp. 25, 26). Since dream symbolism is a function of neocortex, Fromm's statement is a call for more precise information on the state of neocortical functioning during sleep, or more specifically, given the emphasis in the present work, the state of neocortical functioning during REM sleep. In Chapter 1, I discussed the evidence that the right hemisphere has a predominant influence, relative to wakefulness; in the present chapter, I provided evidence that this relative dominance tends to wane during the latter REM periods. The shift toward right hemispheric dominance of information processing could be important to an understanding of the biological basis of certain properties of REM experience, or dreaming, as emphasized by numerous clinical investigators. REM dreaming, relative to waking mentation, tends toward the personal and the subjective (according to C. Hall), the affective and the intuitive (according to Hall and Fromm), the

---

[8] There is some evidence that methodological artifact (i.e., multiple awakenings by the end of the night) may account for much of the apparent increase in dreamier quality of later REM compared to earlier REM dreams (Cartwright, 1975).

aesthetic and the insightful (according to Jung and Fromm). In addition, the dream tends to be passively received as though from some unknown (unconscious) source (according to Jung). These characteristics appear fully congruent with what is known about waking thought when under the increased influence of the right hemisphere. There is even a hint in the data presented in this chapter of a biological basis to the hypothesis that later (REM) dreams might be "better" in that they would combine the qualities of creative flexibility given by right hemispheric influence with the objectivity given by the increasing influence of the left hemisphere. While it is only tentative, this hypothesis is not without historical precedence. According to Fromm (1951), Talmudic tradition has it that "the sleep in the morning is less deep than in the early night, and the sleeper is closer to his waking consciousness. Rabbi Jochanan apparently assumes that in this state of sleep rational judgment enters into the dream process and permits us to have a clearer insight . . ." (p. 128).

In this and prior chapters I have discussed some of the highlights of research on neurological, physiological, ontogenetic, and phylogenetic characteristics of REM sleep. Wherever possible, I have tried to develop implications for a biological perspective on the dreaming process and dream content. The influence of events typically defined as "psychological" (e.g., personality characteristics, presleep experiences) on both REM and NREM dream content will be developed in more detail in Chapters 8 and 9. This alternative approach requires a brief commentary.

Most experimental research on dream content has been characterized by group comparisons, situational manipulations, or their combination. Effects of these on dream recall and dream content have been explained on the basis of variables such as needs or traits whose expression in the biological properties of REM sleep are unknown or, at best, barely understood. While it is true that much can be said about dream content and dream function from such studies, a full explanation must eventually take into consideration the effect of these variables on the biological context within which the dream takes place. For example, there is evidence that individuals with a larger REM percentage have somewhat elevated scores on the MMPI and Eysenck Personality Inventory neuroticism scale (Beaumaster, 1968; Rechtschaffen and Verdone, 1964). Individuals with elevated neuroticism scores may have more REM periods (Beaumaster, 1968) which are marked by relatively frequent awakenings (Schubert and Jovanović, 1973). There are undoubtedly other, virtually unexplored, individual differences in REM characteristics at the electrophysiological, biochemical and neurological levels. A most obvious example is the case of schizotypes, and of schizophrenics in premorbid, clinical, and remitted conditions. High heritability of psychoticism clearly indicates a role for biochemical and physiological mediation in both wakefulness and sleep, though the details of such mediation lie more in theory than in empirical fact. Surely much of the nonsymbolic characteristics of REM dreaming will require an understanding of such biological mediation (not likely to be revealed by the relatively crude methods that yield electrophysiological statistics like REM time).[9] Thus, while we will speak about the influence of normal and abnormal personality

---

[9] The validity of conclusions about dreaming and the relationship between dreaming and biological factors drawn from dream reports of chronic psychotics may be seriously questioned. The usefulness of dream reports is largely dependent on (a) the verbal capacity of the subject (e.g., chronic schizophrenics are typically of less than average IQ), (b) motivation (e.g., in chronic schizophrenics, typically unreliable), and (c) memory capacity during the transition from sleep to wakefulness. In addition, the potential utility of data from psychotic individuals in revealing possible biological foundations of dreaming is compromised because studies of dreaming in psychotics typically do not emphasize nosological distinctions that are known to be biologically (genetically) distinct. For example, it seems no longer reasonable to combine the data of reactives (and some paranoids) with those of nuclear (process) schizophrenics (Abrams, Taylor and Gaztanaga, 1974; McCabe and Stromgren, 1975); likewise, unipolar and bipolar psychotic depressives need to be separated.

variations on dream characteristics, these "independent variables" must be thought of as theoretical conveniences with as yet largely unknown immediate biological referents during REM sleep. The relationship of a category like neuroticism to dreaming must eventually be understood to affect both the meaning (symbolism) and the quality of dreams.

Finally, it should be noted that empirical research on biological and psychological factors related to the dreaming process and dream content has revealed relatively little about the symbolic meaning of dreams. There is virtually no experimental psychological research on dream symbolism (as opposed to content analysis). I have already mentioned the limitations regarding a biological perspective on symbolism. The symbolic approach requires intensive knowledge about subjects as individuals, and a belief in one's theory of dream meaning (through which translations of manifest content into latent content are affected) that have not characterized experimental research. Thus, despite the wealth of information about dreams and dreaming that has emerged during the last 20 years of sleep research, dream symbolism remains largely the province of clinicians and literati.

CHAPTER 8

PRESLEEP DETERMINANTS OF DREAM CONTENT

Given what we know about the organismic fluidity, spontaneity, and autonomy of brain activity and dream experience during REM, the title of this chapter is somewhat presumptuous. It would seem more to reflect a scientific ideal and empirical goal than the actual state of affairs. In fact, dreaming is *never* a reproduction of presleep events. Rather, it may be *about* those events, but it is always much more. While those events may sometimes influence the content of dreaming, they have very little effect on the process of dreaming, its spatial and temporal organization, and its function. Presleep events can be thought of as "releasers", influencing the probabilities associated with the occurrence of preoccupation and the rules which determine the organization of those preoccupations. What I am proposing is that the relationship between environmental events and dreaming is similar to that described by Lenneberg (1967) for the development of language. "The situation is somewhat analogous to the relationship between nourishment and growth. The food that the growing individual takes in as architectural raw material must be chemically broken down and reconstituted before it may enter the synthesis that produces tissues and organs. The information on how the organs are to be structured does not come in the food but is latent in the individual's own cellular components" (p. 375). Lenneberg's view of language as realized structure resulting from the releasing of latent language structure by exposure to the cultural environment is an organismic analogue of Freud's view of the dream as manifest content resulting from the releasing of latent content. In both models, the relationship between specific behaviors (a sentence spoken, or dream experienced) and social events cannot be understood without recourse to a theory of species-specific, organismically-mediated processes which are the product of the maturation of the nervous system. Since our theories of linguistic and nonlinguistic deep structure are in a primitive state of scientific elaboration, our views about the relationship between environment and the products of knowledge are at best imprecise.

1. METHODOLOGICAL AND THEORETICAL CONSIDERATIONS

In contrast to the interpretive approach which is really an art form, an empirical approach to dream content attempts to establish orderly relationships between categories of experience and external events (e.g., presleep events, personality characteristics, physiological events, etc.). The meaning and function of dreams are therefore basically statistical generalizations derived from reliable nomothetic associations. In this chapter I will draw attention to some of the research on presleep experience-dream content relationships, and reserve for Chapter 9 a discussion of research on the effects of personality, and personality × situational interaction, on dream content. To provide some orientation to the data, it is desirable to say a few things about the nature of both dream content and presleep conditions. First dream content.

Defining categories of dream content

There are at least three descriptive aspects of dream content. The first is the *manifest* vs. *latent content* distinction. The goal of empirical approaches is to achieve better-than-chance prediction, e.g., that individuals tend to dream about affiliation in one situation, relaxation in another, aggression in a third. While individual experiences may symbolize something quite different, the fact that predictions from situation to dream events can be made is a valuable first step. This is not to say that investigators are uninterested in what the dream "really" means. Rather, it is to say that empirical methods are preferred in attempting to reveal situation-content and content-content interrelationships from which meaning is inferred. For example, we may never be able to predict *specifically* what the individual will dream about no matter how precise our information about the presleep situation. This is given by the complexity and spontaneity of the brain and mind. But we may be in a position to predict that certain *classes* of content will have a high probability of occurring.[1] On the basis of such relationships it is possible, in principle, to derive meaning and significance (latent content) that goes beyond the given manifest content of the dream report. However, the empirical approach to inferences about dream meaning is generally more conservative than that of the clinical approach.

A second distinction, *literal* vs. *symbolic representation*, has to do with the degree of informational transformation. Assuming that an individual has dreamed about an aspect of the presleep situation, to what extent is the dream imagery a literal reflection (or replication) vs. a symbolic expression of the event(s)? This question is more than rhetorical because it has serious methodological implications. If a man's propensity for symbolic thinking continues during dreaming (Hall, 1966), if "he is *schematizing* rather than photographically recording" (Murphy, 1947, p. 419), and if, especially in dreams, his symbolism is individualistic and idiosyncratic, then relationships between situation and dream content will be difficult to ascertain. These connections will not be revealed by the rather crude dream content categories and scales typically employed in dream research.

Suppose that a subject is run in a presleep condition defined by the experimenter as "positive". Suppose further that the subject dreams that the experimenter comes into the sleeping area to obtain a dream report and is wearing glasses with Y-shaped slits in the lenses. (I borrow this example from Bonime, 1962.) It is possible that the dream is a symbolic expression of the subject's feeling that the experimenter's "positive" attitude is forced and artificial, that he is demonstrating merely "token kindness". This interpretation presumably would be a function of our knowledge that the subject is cognitively complex (given to symbolic elaboration), rather suspicious, insightful about the "real" attitude of the experimenter, and born and raised in New York (where people often use subway tokens which are round metal objects with a Y-shaped slit cut out of the middle.) This

---

[1] This distinction between specific content vs. classes of content is merely an application to the area of dream psychology of the principle that brain function, mind, and behavior are statistical in nature.

hypothetical example illustrates two basic limitations in empirical research on dream content. First, we usually know next to nothing about the remote history or immediate details of the subject and situation; our relatively crude estimates of personality (when they are used at all), and the rather artificial manipulations of situation which we typically impose on the subject, provide only minimal information. (They do provide the illusion of experimental control.) Second, we know next to nothing *empirically* about how dreams transform information, and how the transformations are expressed in the various sensory and cognitive modes of the manifest content.

During the first night in the laboratory, subjects (especially those who are interested in, or threatened by, the situation) often dream about the laboratory setting (Whitman, Pierce, Maas and Baldridge, 1962; Dement, Kahn and Roffwarg, 1965; Hall, 1967). A dream about the experimenter adjusting the polygraph or putting on electrodes raises few interpretive problems. But what if the subject dreams that he is the catcher in a world series baseball game? Is this dream a literal rendition of a recent preoccupation? Or is it an inventive recreation of the experimental situation? Does the pitcher symbolize the experimenter? Should we interpret "baseball game" as a dream pun for base "ballgame", i.e., a commentary on the underhandedness of the subject-experimenter relationship, a relationship with possible homosexual implications for the subject? If the pitcher is wearing the same kind of sneakers as the experimenter, we might feel more justified in scoring this dream as a symbolic reflection of the presleep situation. It is also possible that the image of sneakers merely elaborates upon the discomfort of the subject who must accommodate to the "sneaky" experimenter. If two independent judges rate this dream as an incorporation of presleep events, we are even more confident that there is a real connection (though interrater agreement is no guarantee of the validity of a specific interpretation of meaning). Thus, by virtue of having some control over, and knowledge about, the situation, we have made headway toward an empirical understanding of the meaning of the dream.

To some, this approach is too superficial since we are saying nothing about the real meaning of the dream, e.g., its reflection of dependency needs or repressed hostile impulses. However, the apparent superficiality reflects the limitations of our knowledge rather than the inherent limitations of the method. If we had additional information about the individual, we might be able to say more about the meaning of the dream. For example, certain types of individual (e.g., selected for immaturity) might be found to have classes of dream imagery of which the catcher dream is one example. Other individuals might be found to have quite different kinds of dream imagery in the same situation. If this were so, a hypothesis about the reflection of dependency needs could be derived (and tested in subsequent research).. The point is that such a derivation of meaning would be based on reliable and replicable relationships rather than *a priori* assumptions.

The problems of literal vs. symbolic expression of presleep events is a methodological can of worms. Most research on dream content is not designed to deal with symbolism, and the insensitivity of content categories or scales to symbolic transformation may severely affect both the results and interpretations. For example, Cartwright, Bernick, Borowitz and Kling (1969) reported that dreams experienced after exposure to an erotic movie had less heterosexual erotic content and more allusions to the laboratory than the dreams they experienced on other nights. However, these dreams appeared to be replete with *symbolic* allusions to sexuality. Data from Cohen and Cox (1975) suggested that laboratory references in dreams were more literal and less symbolic under positive presleep conditions. Clearly then, implications for hypotheses about the continuous or discontinuous relationship between waking and dreamed experience (discussed below) will depend on presleep events as well as the dream content analyses that are employed. For example, it might be predicted, on the basis of the *p* hypothesis, that there will be a positive correlation between presleep challenge and degree of symbolic transformation (rather than literal reproduction) in dreams. Challenge would be defined independently of the dream data in terms of emotional importance, degree of difficulty, etc. The prediction follows from the assumption that current concerns require (or at least benefit from) reprogramming (thinking *about* the problem) and that reprogramming is reflected in symbolic or transformed content. This prediction would represent an alternative interpretation to symbolic process from that given by the repression hypothesis.

A third distinction regarding dream content is that of *open* vs. *disguised* expressions. Again, this distinction has to do with what the dreamer is preoccupied with, and whether the preoccupation is associated with the presleep situation which the experimenter has controlled. Open dream content is defined here as dream content which reflects a straight-forward relationship to an event; disguised dream content is content which may seem to be about one thing but which is actually about another thing. Both open and disguised content may be expressed literally or symbolically. For example, a dream about taking a series of tests might be scored as a literal (nonsymbolic) representation of the presleep situation which the subject is openly preoccupied with. A dream about swimming against a strong current might be scored as a symbolic representation of the same presleep situation. That is, in both cases, the dream is openly about a presleep event, though in one case it is literal, and in the other it is symbolic. (Whether a dream is a literal or a symbolic expression of a pre-sleep preoccupation will presumably depend on many factors such as the stressfulness of the situation and the capacity or readiness to think in symbols.) On the other hand, the test-taking dream might be scored as a literal expression of presleep events that disguises a motive to outperform or show off in front of the experimenter, while the swimming dream might disguise in more symbolic fashion a similar motivation. The empirical approach has, as yet, virtually nothing scientific to contribute to the distinction between open vs. disguised content; the distinction is largely clinical and hypothetical. I bring it up here to emphasize the difference between it and the distinction between literal vs. symbolic expression.

The assumption that dreaming is largely symbolic is *not* equivalent to the assumption that dream symbols serve to disguise "real" meaning (Hall, 1966). For Piaget, dream symbolism "extends far beyond the field of what can be censored or repressed, and rather than being a disguise or a camouflage, seems to constitute the elementary form of consciousness of active assimilation" (Piaget, 1962, p. 191). Again, "the essential point is that the field of unconscious [dream] symbolism is wider than that of repression, and consequently of what can be censored. The question which then arises is whether its unconscious character, i.e., the subject's ignorance of its meaning, does not merely result from the fact that he is incapable of direct and complete consciousness of it. For Freud, censorship is a product of consciousness, and symbolism a product of unconscious associations, which elude censorship. In our opinion, it is worth considering whether these two terms might not be reversed, censorship being merely the expression of the unconscious, uncomprehended character of the symbol, and the symbol itself being the result of a beginning of consciousness assimilation, i.e., an attempt at comprehension" (Piaget, 1962, p. 191).

Reliability in observing dream content categories

Interpretation of dream content can be discussed in the abstract. But the scientific investigation of dream content requires that, at minimum, we have events or categories that are reliably observable. That is, prior to the question of validity (e.g., does the category in fact relate to something external such as a personality characteristic, a presleep event, a sleep-physiological process?), we must demonstrate that the category does in fact exist in the dream report. In order to establish the reliability of a category, a minimum of two judges must *independently* agree on the presence of the category. For categories that are "nominal" (either present or absent), some form of concordance estimate is desirable. For ratings along a prothetic dimension such as amount of bizarreness or number of characters, etc., some kind of interrater reliability coefficient is desirable. In the typical research report, the specific method of estimating interrater agreement for a particular category or dimension is not specified. Since validity data are usually based on nominal dream content categories, I will address the problem of concordance estimates.

What determines a judge's rating that a dream content category is present in a dream report? Of course there are the obvious factors like (a) amount of material, (b) quality of the report (detail), (c) motivation and sensitivity of the judge. It is axiomatic that the more material available, the more likely that a category will obtain (Van de Castle, 1969). Less obvious is the salience or concreteness of the category. For example, the presence or absence of music reported in dreams is sure to be reliably detected by two judges working independently despite the rarity of the category. However, a category like "hostility" or "anxiety" which requires a certain degree of inferential leeway will be more difficult to observe reliably. The result of all of these kinds of factors is a different *base rate* between judges in rating a particular category. And base rates along with *chance* will affect concordance. Yet the typical estimate of interjudge concordance does not directly take these two factors into account. Let me give some examples to illustrate what I believe to be a tendency to report inflated interjudge concordance rates, and which, at the same time, will exemplify a major difficulty that any investigator faces when doing research on dream content.

Spitzer and Fleiss (1974) describe a statistic that takes base rate and chance factors into account. The following illustrations are based on their formula. First consider the problem in the abstract. Assume that judge A and judge B are asked to determine independently the presence or absence of a category in the dream reports of a set of subjects. Assume the simple case of a single report of good quality per subject. "Presence" will be symbolized by "P" (for category present), while "absence" will be symbolized by "Q".

Table 8-1 represents the dichotomous situation for the two judges. Note that one cell (top left) represents the number of times that *both* judges independently detect the presence of the category. This number is represented by n_{AB}. The number of times judge A detects the presence of the category (regardless of what judge B says) is represented by the marginal n_A. Likewise, the number of times judge B detects the category (regardless of what A says) is represented by marginal number n_B. The symbol, n'_{AB}, represents agreement between the judges that the category is *not* present, while the number N represents the total number of pairs of judgements (the number of dream reports judged). Symbols in the other cells are omitted.

TABLE 8-1

Judge B	Judge A		
	P_A	Q_A	
P_B	n_{AB}		n_B
Q_B		n'_{AB}	
	n_A		N

Now the usual estimate of concordance, what is called the *proportion of overall agreement*, can be thought of as $(n_{AB} + n'_{AB})/N$, or the proportion of total judgements representing agreement that the category is present *or* is absent. The problem with such an estimate is that it disregards both the base rate of category use for each judge (n_A or n_B) and chance agreement, which, for "presence", is $(n_A \times n_B)/N$.

Consider the following rather trivial example. Suppose that both judges have a high base rate, that is, they each detect the category in 70% of the dream reports. (Whether they are "correct", that is, whether their judgements are valid, is another issue.) The chance that they will agree if they are *randomly* assigning the category to 70% of the reports is .49. Even if they agree 80% of the time, this agreement represents a gain over chance of only 31%. What about two judges each of whom uses the category for only 20% of the reports? If they also agree 80% of the time, their performance represents a gain of 76% over chance (since they will both use the category by chance on only 4% of the reports). It is readily apparent that high concordance in the sense of overall agreement can be misleading both with respect to the quality of the judgements and the utility of the categories.

In order to control for base rates one can compute the *proportion of specific agreement* (p_s) that the category is "present". (Note that we are focusing on the judgements regarding the presence of the category, and ignoring judgements on the "absence" of the category.) This represents mutual agreement on the presence of the category *relative to average base rate*. In terms of Table 8-1,

$$p_s = \frac{n_{AB}/N}{\frac{1}{2}(n_A/N + n_B/N)} = \frac{p_{AB}}{\frac{1}{2}(p_A + p_B)}$$

In many cases this will be sufficient to express the "real" concordance of agreement between judges, given their base rates (or more precisely, an estimate or average of their base rates). However, to compare agreement estimates across studies, it is useful to take chance agreement into consideration. In the terminology of the table, the chance proportion of specific agreement, p_c, is:

$$p_c = \frac{n_A \times n_B}{N \times N} = p_A \times p_B$$

The statistic that represents concordance, once base rates and chance are taken into consideration, is called *kappa*:

$$\kappa = \frac{p_s - p_c}{1 - p_c}$$

Kappa can be interpreted as the actual *nonchance* agreement relative to the expected or possible *nonchance* agreement. It can be directly interpreted as percentage of variation in performance due to "real" agreement, i.e., agreement based on something like skillfulness or aptitude.[2]

To illustrate the problem of representing concordance of judgement, consider some data from a recent study (Cohen and Cox, 1975). The problem was to assess interjudge agreement that a subject was dreaming about the presleep laboratory testing situation. The judges were familiar with the presleep condition, and were asked to determine (on the basis of any number of REM and NREM dream reports per subject) whether the subject was

TABLE 8-2

Judge B	Judge A		
	P_A	Q_A	
P_B	9	1	10
Q_B	3	31	
	12		44

dreaming about the situation. Table 8-2 shows the distribution of ratings of direct preoccupation (P) or not (Q). The proportion of overall agreement was .91. However, the proportion of specific agreement (taking average base rates into consideration), i.e., $1/2$ $(10/44 + 12/44)$, was .80. (Kappa = .79.)

However, consider the case where judges are asked to detect a relatively rare phenomenon whose definition is relatively vague. Table 8-3 shows the distribution of judgements for the presence (P) or absence (Q) of "spatial distortion or unusualness" determined for data from another study. This category refers to peculiar shapes or volumes, e.g., a very long or angular room. Note that the proportion of overall agreement (the presence or absence) for this category is a healthy .8 while the proportion of specific agreement is only .42. However, note that the fact that a category is rarely detected is not necessarily an indication that the proportion of specific agreement will be low. If the category has clear referents, e.g., the presence of music, both judges are likely to detect it when it does appear. The basic point is that when a category is rarely used, or used quite frequently by judges, it is likely that the proportion of overall agreement can be spuriously high. One of the most difficult problems

[2] Readers with some familiarity with behavior-genetic methodology will recognize the formal similarity between kappa (κ) and the Holzinger estimate of heritability [h^2]. The latter is derived from behavior concordance (C) observed for MZ and DZ twins: $(C_{MZ} - C_{DZ})/(1 - C_{DZ})$. In the language of kappa, the numerator represents "agreement" due to that degree of gene similarity *beyond* the "chance" gene similarity represented by DZ twins, i.e., *actual nonchance* similarity. (The environmental factors of MZ and DZ are assumed to be equally similar and thus are removed by subtraction.) The denominator $(1 - C_{DZ})$ represents the *possible* range of "real" nonchange agreement. Specifically, there is a genetic component and two environmental components (one for each type of twin pair) represented by "1". Subtracting the DZ genetic component and DZ environment still leaves a genetic component (the extra gene component of MZ beyond DZ) plus the environment of MZ. Thus, h^2, like κ, represents an estimate of the relationship between observed nonchance agreement (or concordance) and possible nonchance agreement. In one case validity refers to some kind of real "skill", in the other, a genetic substrate.

S.D.— P

TABLE 8-3

Judge B	Judge A		
	P_A	Q_A	
P_B	1	3	4
Q_B	0	11	
	1	14	15

in dream research is achieving high proportions of specific agreement. The more categories, and the more these categories are interpretive in nature, the more difficult the problem.

Assessing the situation

Problems of reliable recognition and categorization of dream content are easily matched by problems of classifying the boundless variety of presleep manipulations used in empirical research on situation-content relationships. These include manipulations of sensory, perceptual, and cognitive information, organismic deficits (e.g., sleep deprivation, food deprivation), and various kinds of psychological stress (e.g., scary films, failure, threat, sexual arousal). Manipulations vary along so many dimensions: duration, frequency, affective arousal, psychological importance, complexity. All too often, there are too few data per category of manipulation to assess the reliability of a finding when a significant result is obtained. In addition, it is not always clear that a manipulation is either (a) psychologically significant, or (b) of sufficient duration to affect dream content. At minimum, the effectiveness of a presleep manipulation should be established *independently* of the dream content. This is especially important to interpretations of a failure to find a significant situation-content relationship. But it is also true when we do obtain a statistically significant event-content relationship which appears to support a prediction. Of course, a "sleeper-effect" might operate, especially if our measures of event effectiveness are too crude to pick up the effect; that is, dream content may, under certain conditions, be a *more sensitive* indication of the effect of a manipulation than are measures of waking behavior. But this is a rather weak argument. Let us take two examples that illustrate the problem.

Cartwright *et al.* (1969) found less dream recall and more symbolic allusions to sexuality on the night when an erotic film was shown to a group of male subjects. These results were tentatively interpreted as reflecting defensive processes (dream recall failure and symbolic disguise). However, there was no independent assessment of the stress characteristics of the film, and no attempt to select subjects for susceptibility to defensive behavior. In addition, there was evidence that the sleep characteristics of the film night were "more normal" (deeper?, more relaxed?). A reasonable alternative inference is that dream recall reflected the deeper quality of sleep, and that the symbolic allusions to sex (assuming their validity) were open rather than disguised. Other interpretations are possible. The point is that consideration of sleep quality and cognitive style may yield more parsimonious and valid interpretations than considerations about anxiety and defense when independent evidence of the latter is either not available or contradictory.

Consider another example from one of my early studies on dream recall (Cohen, 1972b).

Subjects in the stress condition expected to participate the next day in a threatening learning situation. Each subject watched an accomplice "subject" attempt to learn a task which included "shocks" for errors. The observer subject was told that the next morning he would perform the task while being observed by new subjects. The bogus situation included a realistic apparatus and performance by confederates with consummate acting skills. Also the subjects appeared to be quite attentive to the problems of the learner (presumably so they could learn the task and avoid the shocks). However, it was thought desirable to test formally the psychological impact of the situation. I quote from the original paper. "Immediately after viewing the accomplice's ordeal, S was given Card III of the Rorschach. Another group of Ss was given Card III without having been in the stress condition. It was felt that in addition to the above-mentioned behavioral indexes, assessment of the effect of stress on fantasy material generated by the Rorschach would be relevant, since the study was concerned with the effect of stress on content and amount of fantasy dream material generated by the waking situation. A group of six clinical psychology graduate students was given the responses of each S one at a time. They discussed the material, and voted whether to call it 'experimental' or 'control'. The Rorschach responses of those Ss who had been in the stress condition received a total experimental vote of 48 and a control vote of 11. For those Ss who had not been in the stress condition, the vote was 19 for experimental and 35 for control [Chi square = 24.901, $p < .001$]. Though graduate students were using many kinds of clues, they were helped by the fact that many of the stress group responses contained dark, eerie, bloody, and threatening imagery not seen in the responses of the control group Ss. One S in the control situation said 'the red blotches at the side look like blotches on the wall . . . maybe flower arrangements.' An S in the stress condition said, 'the red blobs look like a bad wound on, say, someone's forehead as the blood trickles down.' Another control S perceived 'someone dribbling some basketballs' and, 'a couple of girls pulling on something' as well as other relatively benign imagery. Another stress condition S perceived 'a frog stabbed with a knife. This is blood pouring over the sides.' He also saw 'a madly excited boar.' After providing some surrealistic imagery, he responded with the percept of an X-ray of a 'bad throat condition'. Another S in the stress condition saw 'a fly with his head chopped off. Then the body cut off. The red spots are bleeding'" (Cohen, 1972b, pp. 124-125).

This study was not primarily done to assess dream content, and the dream reports were rather limited in this respect. Nevertheless, there was an association between the stress condition and *both* elevated hostility content in the dreams and elevated hostility toward the experimenter on the postexperimental questionnaire. The findings suggest that testing hypotheses regarding the relationship of presleep events and dream content can best be done in studies that use hypothesis-relevant manipulations, subjects selected on personality variables relevant to the manipulation, and *independent* assessment of the immediate and long term impact of the manipulation. Good examples of studies which include such design considerations are too infrequently reported (see Goodenough *et al.*, 1974; Witkin, 1969).

There are two other points which require some discussion, one regarding presleep stress manipulations, the other regarding dream content analysis. Stress manipulations are popular in sleep research, presumably because dreaming is believed to mediate stress. But it is not clear that different kinds of stress are functionally equivalent (Auerbach, Kendall, Cuttler and Levitt, 1976). For example, scary movies or threat of shock are often used to create emotional discomfort. However, dreaming may have far less to do with adjustment to what is basically an external or physical threat than with internal or ego threats. Scaring a subject is quite different from threatening his self-esteem. Higgins and Marlatt (1975) have made the same point with respect to stress and drinking. I think that Garfield is quite right to question the usefulness and relevance of many of the threat manipulations that are typically used in laboratory research:

"One of the problems of trying to study behavior in the laboratory, however, is that the experimental situations or laboratory analogues created tend to lose their resemblance to the living situation they are supposed to represent. In essence, they become *artificial representations of reality*, and the applicability of results obtained in the laboratory to the life situation outside can be questioned. For example, there have been numerous studies performed on stress and the effect of stress on various intellectual or emotional responses. The stress situation in the laboratory, however, although it may have the benefits of an operational definition, may be of real significance only to the experimenter. The experimental subject may see it as an artificial or forced situation with which he must comply for the time being. It is in no way comparable to the stress which the individual experiences when he is taking a final examination, the acute discomfort he has when he is told he is on the verge of being dropped from school for poor grades, or the distress he feels when his best girlfriend tells him she no longer cares for him. As a result, generalizations derived from stress situations in the laboratory may have little carry-over to the stress experienced by normals in difficult life circumstances, to say nothing of neurotic and psychotic patients" (Garfield, 1974, p. 375).

If Garfield is basically right, then results from studies using quite different stress manipulations are at best not comparable, at worse, irrelevant (Greenberg and Pearlman, 1974; Pearlman, personal communication, October, 1972).

My second point has to do with dream content analysis. The relationship between presleep events and dream content, and inferences which are derived from these relationships, will depend on decisions about which aspects of dream content are selected for study. When a particular hypothesis-derived prediction is tested, decisions about what variables are relevant are more obvious. However, *post hoc* analyses probably introduce selective biases toward findings which, at a minimum, require replication. The problem of selecting variables brings up one final issue regarding general assumptions about the relationships between content and presleep events, i.e. situations and personality characteristics.

Continuity vs. discontinuity between wakefulness and dreaming

The relationship between waking experience and sleeping experience can be characterized as *continuous* (similar in frequency, duration, content) or *discontinuous* (unrelated, dissimilar, or opposite), or both, depending on the person, situation, method of dream content analysis, and assumptions about dream function. Dream content may bear an especially striking resemblance to waking preoccupations in individuals who are relatively open to inner life. According to Cartwright (1974), "the healthier the individual, the more access he has in waking life to his affective responses and therefore the more parallel his waking and dreaming mentation" (p. 338). Of course, the same might be said for anxiety neurotics whose fears perseverate during dreaming. Continuity is likely to be revealed in dreams if we focus on what the dream is about and how it is organized rather than on the specific events. This is essentially the trait hypothesis of Adler and C. S. Hall.

According to Hall, "each person dreamed about much the same sort of thing from year to year even when there were radical changes in his waking life. We attribute this consistency to the unchanging character of the unconscious. . . . Dreams appear to be variations on a few basic infantile wishes and fears that have not been fulfilled or resolved" (Hall, 1966, p. xvii).

An important contribution to the concept of traitlike invariance despite major situational and behavioral changes is the recent work of Hauri (1976) on the dream content of remitted unipolar depressives. Hauri obtained evidence that, despite major changes in clinical status, former depressives still produce dreams characterized by (a) "masochism" and (b) "covert hostility out". "Masochism" refers to events like crying, being abandoned, rejected, blamed. "Covert hostility out" refers to hostile events involving others rather than the dreamer. That is, "the remitted dreamer sees the world as a generally hostile place, but this hostility neither emanates from him nor is it specifically directed against him" (Hauri, 1976, p. 8). On the basis of prior research on actively ill depressives, Hauri concludes that a consistent characteristic of the depressive *personality* is "masochism". That a view of the world as generally hostile may also be a traitlike characteristic of depressive personalities must also be considered a possibility. Finally, a past (rather than present or future) time perspective may also be characteristic of depressive, or more likely, sensitizer personality, as data that I will describe later suggest. Perhaps we may generalize from these kinds of data as well as from clinical wisdom about the implications of behavioral rigidity (Wachtel, 1973) to say that a reliably dysphoric view of the world manifested in dreams is a sign of vulnerability to various kinds of clinical disturbances. I am suggesting that an empirically based psychology of dream content will require more systematic knowledge about the continuity of sleep and wake experience, its temporal stability, and the affective and substantive content of experience.

On the other hand, there are numerous hypothetical factors which could make dream content appear to be discontinuous with the frequency, duration, and conscious emphasis of waking experience. Peripheral perceptions which are semipermanently encoded but given insufficient conscious attention because of distraction may be especially prominent during dreaming (Poetzl hypothesis). Dreams may portray conditions that are opposite to those created by situation-inducing drive states, e.g., the food-deprived individual dreams of eating. Dreams may demonstrate discontinuity by expressing motives that are defended against (repressed, minimized) during wakefulness. These motives may be revealed (C. S. Hall's view) or continue to be disguised (Freud's view) in dream symbolism. Alternatively, because of the flexibility of the sleep cognition, insights into self and others may be more prominent during dreaming. Thus, dreams may be more valid and creative than waking thought (Fromm's view).

The apparent discontinuity between waking and dreaming thought may in fact be an actual continuity. That is, a fleeting thought, perhaps suppressed out of a sense of social propriety, may be given great emphasis during a dream. Or, a suppressed motive, just as real as its substituted counterpart (defense, sublimation), may be given its due emphasis during dreaming. In both cases, the dream *complements* the waking thought such that the two, together, form a more complete picture of the individual. For example, Fromm describes a dream about an important and well-regarded person whom the dreamer had just met. The person is transformed in the dream such that he has a "cruel mouth and a hard face". In the dream, the person tells the dreamer how he has just cheated a poor woman. During the initial meeting with the person (prior to the night of the dream), the dreamer had noted a "fleeting feeling of disappointment" which disappeared immediately (suppressed?). Later, well after the dream, it turned out that both the dreamer and others learned "that there was in the man an element of ruthlessness" (Fromm, 1951, pp. 36-37). Thus we have a reasonably credible example of an insightful dream, one that demonstrates a hidden perceptiveness only apparently discontinuous with less insightful thoughts that are encouraged by the social situation. As Hall says, "dreams cut through the pretensions and deceits of waking life and lay bare the true feelings we have of people" (Hall, 1966, p. 13). I believe that this kind of social insightfulness is a product of right hemisphere intelligence which is normally suppressed during wakefulness but more readily expressed in dreams.

Consider another example given by Fromm (1951, p. 165). An "ardent anti-Nazi" dreams about having a pleasant and satisfying conversation with Hitler. The apparent discontinuity is resolved when one understands the basically authoritarian personality of the dreamer (e.g., a combination of rebelliousness against authority plus receptiveness to praise from authority figures). A discontinuity between dream and political views belies the continuity with basic personality.

At the risk both of belaboring the obvious and appearing to be naive about the scientific status of projective techniques, let me offer one last example. Many years ago one of my undergraduate students, who demonstrated an inordinate faith in the power of the Draw a Person (DAP) test, collected a set of drawings for the purpose of discovering who among the girls residing at the local dormitory was responsible for some rather bizarre slashings of clothes and other inanimate objects. Suffice it to say, she never discovered who it was. However, one of the productions is particularly interesting in the light of our discussion of continuity-discontinuity of wake-dream experience. The drawing of the comic strip type character, shown on the left of Figure 8-1, was done first. Then, as though expressing uncertainty regarding the degree of commitment to the figure (as a projection of self), the drawing is "cancelled" with a lightly and delicately (ambivalently?) drawn wavy line. On the back of the paper, a new drawing was made (right side of Figure 8-1). The initial childlike, wide-eyed, and open figure has been transformed into a more mature, less open, darkly shadowed, and gravitationally less stable character. The first figure has a hysteroid quality, the second suggests depression. Perhaps it is not too far-fetched to suggest that these are two sides of the same personality. On the basis of clinical experience, I have long suspected that if you probe the hysterical personality you will discover depression. I have since discovered that such a correlation was affirmed by some of the great psychiatrists (e.g., J. M. Charcot and P. Janet) at the turn of the century. So I am in good company.

Let us consider briefly some clinical material obtained on two individuals with similar hysteroid defensive strategies which were beginning to break down when these individuals sought clinical intervention. The first was a 22-year-old college female, the second a 21-year-old male. A few selected examples of TAT responses and information about the interaction between each person and the tester (me) will suffice to illustrate my point about the close relationship between hysteroid behavior (dramatization, childish attention-seeking, exaggeration, sexual repression/naiveté, and oedipal conflict) and the struggle with depression.

When given the first card, the female exclaimed: "I hate it, I just hate it. I can't tell stories. (Why?) I can't do it unless I am being cute. You'd better pamper me and tell me that I'm cute ... you don't know what you are doing to me." Her representation of the mother figure (the oedipal competitor) in the cards was most unflattering, indicating suspiciousness, lack of understanding, anger. Males were portrayed as appealing but undependable ("he'll probably make a relatively nonemotional exit from the relationship"), and somewhat

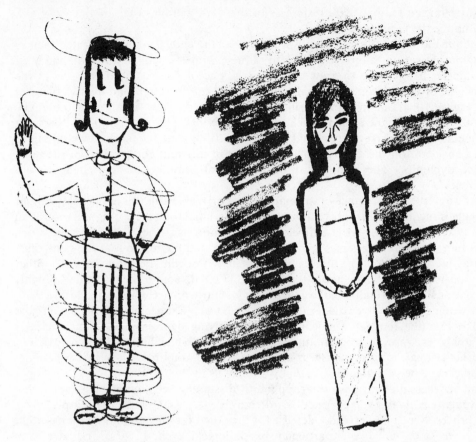

Figure 8-1   Two drawings made in response to the request to draw a person.

exploitive. Emotionally close relationships prove undependable; "these moments are very elusive and fleeting" . . . people try to "make some sort of human contact with each other, mentally and emotionally" . . . but they "go through most of their lives, just sort of living meaninglessly . . . until they die and rot" (a typically flippant and silly comment that neutralizes the impact of distressing fantasies and which at the same time allows communication of information that would otherwise be too distressing). The hysteroid quality of her personality was further revealed in the childishly seductive manner that she curled up in her chair with her shoes off.

The classical psychoanalytic view that oedipal conflict manifested in sexual naiveté and cognitive difficulties (perceptual blocks, disruption of thought) with sex-related content underlies hysteroid personality organization is supported by her performance on the cards. On one card she said: "How can I possibly tell you a story? . . . I can't think about anything that has to do with sex." On card 13 MF she completely failed to see the half-naked woman in the midground of the picture. It was not until halfway through her story, a story replete with comments like "I can't think" and "Don't look at me when I think", that, after much probing and finally the question "Is there only one person in the picture?", she exclaimed: "Oh, there's a female there, with a sheet over her or something . . . I'm sorry, I didn't see that at all." Any clinician familiar with responses to this card will be struck by the rarity of a failure to notice the female on the bed.

Throughout the series of cards, but especially near the end, she communicated themes suggesting an increasing failure to deal with sadness, hopelessness, depression, and even ideas of suicide. If one were to draw two pictures, one of the hysteroid and one of the depressive side of this person's personality, one could not do better than the two pictures shown in Figure 8-1. If one were to describe her behavior in different situations one might be tempted to speak of the "inconsistency" of behaviors across situations. Such an environmental view of personality would of course entirely miss the mark; it would fail to take into consideration the different manifestations of different components of the same personality dynamics. The same must be true of situation-dream and dream-dream "discrepancies".

In many ways, the performance of the male subject on these cards was remarkably similar (though suggesting more schizoid creativity). This individual took the testing situation as an opportunity to entertain the tester with clever and humorous stories, a playful style which permitted him to reveal his distress, generate sympathy and interest, but at the same time, maintain a safe "distance". The stories were replete with oedipal fantasies about mother figures, fantasies that were sometimes transparently sexual. Yet on card 13MF, this highly verbal, ideationally fluent individual was stymied, lost for words. He finally made up a story about the decline in morals of modern women (even though it began with the male figure trying to seduce the female!). Indications of underlying depression were more clearly manifest in his responses to a questionnaire about himself which he later filled out. In it he indicated his struggle with goallessness and retreat from ambition, all of which he hides from people since he is "gifted with the power of bullshit".

The point of these illustrations is that apparently dissimilar, even complementary psychological events (e.g., waking experiences vs. dream imagery), may reflect two aspects of a complex process. One may serve as a defense for the other, but this may not be the case. The problem is to find out why a particular psychological event occurs, or under what circumstances one rather than the other is likely to be experienced or expressed. For example, are apparently complementary dream images more likely to be expressed under defense-inducing stressful conditions?

In general then, apparent discontinuity between dream content and waking experience may be artifacts of (a) selecting the wrong scales, (b) inability to translate dream symbolism, (c) lack of knowledge about the individual, (d) insufficient control over presleep conditions, (e) selective recall. Whatever the apparent relationship between specific presleep events and specific dream content, most clinical theories assume that personality functioning continues during sleep despite (a) altered quality of mental functioning, and (b) compensatory reactions to unusual conditions (e.g., organismic deficit) that may be irrelevant to personality. Finally, it should be noted that there is no necessity to assume that dreams must be continuous or discontinuous with observable behavior and with experience: complementary or compensatory images may function to satisfy or express continuing habits, motives, skills, and feelings.

The best example of a dream that represents the operation of both continuity and discontinuity is the famous Irma dream reported and analyzed by Freud in his *Interpretation of Dreams*. The dream is too long and complex to describe here. Suffice it to say that it includes two kinds of events: (a) those expressing a continuity of a conscious, presleep preoccupation with a particular patient named Irma, and (b) the representation of peripheral or even suppressed hostile thoughts about a colleague. The latter are gratified through the dream events in which that individual, who constitutes professional and an intellectual threat, is portrayed as a bungler. From the perspective of personality, the dream clearly represents the continuity of what may be loosely called a "paranoid" style: the tendency to defend against insecurity or vulnerability via projection of blame as well as general suspiciousness. In short, the dream is a good example of the continuity of presleep preoccupation and major personality characteristics, as well as compensatory emphasis for thoughts that are not given sufficient attention during wakefulness.

Table 8-4 summarizes issues regarding dream content, presleep events, their interrelationship, and the methodological and theoretical implications. Unfortunately, the data which I will review in this and the following chapter do not resolve many of the problems I have discussed. Rather, they constitute a beginning, a first step in the attempt to establish minimal connections between aspects of dream content and factors that influence it. Compared to the rather elaborate, often exotic interpretations and formulations available in the clinical literature, these empirical relationships seem paltry and superficial. In the short run, the disappointing yield from empirical investigation contrasts poorly with the rich harvest of clinical work. However, in the long run, these two approaches are not irreconcilable. More and better data will give way to better theories which will undoubtedly overlap with clinical assumptions. Clinical assumptions often guide empirical research. It is not merely a distinction between the simple-minded and the muddle-headed, but rather a mutually reinforcing influence that should characterize dream research. The beginnings of an integration of the science of content analysis and the art of dream interpretation have already been established (e.g., Cartwright *et al.*, 1969; Witkin, 1969).

TABLE 8-4.   Summary of Issues and Factors Related to an Empirical Approach to Dream Content

Domain	Issues, factors, problems
Dream content	Manifest vs. latent Symbolic vs. literal Open vs. disguised

Presleep events	Dimensions
	    frequency, duration, significance
	Types of manipulation
	    cognitive
	    organismic
	    stress (internal vs. external?)
	Individual (personality) differences and
	    person x situation interactions

Methodology	Assessing effect of manipulations independently from dream content
	Selection of dream content categories,
	    variables
	Controlling irrelevant variables that may
	    influence content (dream recall, sleep
	    characteristics)
	Scoring reliability (interjudge agreement)

Assumptions about event-
    content relationships
	Continuity-discontinuity (in personality and
	    experience)
	Defensive vs. homeostatic compensation

2. SOME EMPIRICAL FINDINGS

Compensatory relationship between presleep and dream events

While most studies employ rather salient and often stressful manipulations, some have used more subtle events. According to Poetzl's "law of exclusion", peripheral information that is excluded from conscious elaboration is more likely than focal information to saturate consciousness at a later time under conditions of altered ego functioning such as dreaming (see Fisher, 1960b). That is, we tend to be preoccupied in dreams with information to which we have not paid sufficient attention. The hypothesis does not assume that the excluded information is emotionally important. Initial evidence for the phenomenon (e.g., Fisher, 1954, 1956, 1957, 1960a) was later shown to be empirically weak and unsupportable when tested with adequate controls (Johnson and Eriksen, 1961; Waxenberg, Dickes and Gottesfeld, 1962). Interest in the Poetzl phenomenon has since diminished. However, for a number of reasons, I am inclined to believe that at times, and under certain conditions, we do appear to give more dream emphasis to *important* information that is peripheral to waking attention.

First, I question the relevance of tachistoscopic presentations of psychologically meaningless material whose duration of exposure is at or just below recognition threshold. That information of this sort, presented in this way, does not appear more frequently than chance in dreams the next night cannot, in itself, constitute definitive evidence against the hypothesis. After all, if we are looking for a kind of Zeigarnik effect, then information of at least some minimal significance to the individual could be presented briefly before the individual's attention is distracted to other things. Under such conditions, dreaming about the information might be more likely to occur than if the information were presented frequently and for long durations.

Second, none of the studies either supporting or refuting the hypothesis was carried out in the sleep laboratory and tested with REM dream material. It is therefore not surprising that the elusive phenomenon evades detection, especially in the context of studies designed to prove the null hypothesis.

Finally, there is abundant anecdotal evidence that occasionally we dream about events that seem to be trivial or to which we have paid too little attention. (Recall the first example from Fromm discussed on p. 217.) Foulkes (1966, pp. 150-152) gives an example of a subject who dreamed about an abstract painting, the only definite detail of which was blue shoes. Later, it turned out that in her office at work there was a calendar picture containing blue shoes. The subject had presumably seen the picture many times but had never really paid careful, conscious attention either to the details of the picture or to the fact that it was of an erotic nature. Similarly, I recently had a dream about long cylindrical objects. Was it an erotic dream, or rather, did it have something to do with the fact that the previous evening I was in a restaurant that had long cylindrical sugar sticks in a bowl, something I had never seen before and which only momentarily caught my attention and interest? The point is that whatever the meaning of the dream, a compensatory process like that hypothesized by Poetzl could affect the probability of certain dream events. Admittedly, anecdotal evidence is insufficient, but I agree with Foulkes (1966) that a sleep laboratory study of the phenomenon would be desirable. Foulkes' example of the blue shoes dream raises the question of individual differences. Recall the data which I discussed earlier which showed that individuals who indicate that they are not affectively involved in the laboratory situation are more likely to dream about the laboratory situation during more REM periods. Perhaps there are important individual differences in the degree of complementary dream emphasis on waking preoccupations. Perhaps repressors, who tend to avoid in consciousness and/or conversation certain kinds of (unpleasant) experiences, more often dream about those kinds of experiences. If this is so, it is likely that the dreamed experiences are transformed some way so as to rob them of affective significance. This could be accomplished either through elaborate symbolic transformation (disguise) or through dream solutions.

The Poetzl hypothesis is one variant of the larger hypothesis which holds that dreaming compensates for waking thought, that insufficient attention to, or systematic exclusion of, personally relevant experience is compensated for in fantasy to restore psychological balance (Jung, 1933). In a sense then, dreaming is a kind of reminder (or should I say, REMinder?). It is a process that often seems to induce a compensatory *intensification* of information (perhaps highly transformed) given insufficient attention during the day.[3]

If we accept for the moment the argument that dreaming (at least REM dreaming) is in some fundamental way a function of the dominant right hemisphere, then the compensatory hypothesis has some indirect neuropsychological support. Anecdotal data on split-brain behavior reported by Sperry strongly suggest that under certain conditions, the right hemisphere may impose a compensatory adjustment so that behavior mediated by the left hemisphere is altered. For example, there are occasions when emotional or gestural behaviors (mediated by the right hemisphere) are expressed during verbal performance mediated by the left hemisphere which is "incorrect" from the point of view of the right hemisphere. If a question mark is flashed to the left hemisphere while, simultaneously, an erotic stimulus is flashed to the right hemisphere, the split-brain patient (actually his left hemisphere) says he saw a question mark while at the same time he (his right hemisphere) shows signs of blushing or arousal which he (his left hemisphere) cannot explain. Perhaps he may dream about the erotic stimulus just as we may dream about suppressed or repressed information stored by the right hemisphere. In other words, to the degree that there is suppression or insufficient attention paid to right hemisphere-mediated information, the right hemisphere-dominated dreaming process may give compensatory emphasis to that information.

In fact, the compensation hypothesis may be considered a special case of the more general hypothesis that dreaming involves the integration of new information, specifically, the integration of right and left hemisphere-mediated information. If we accept Galin's (1974) suggestion that repressed information is, at the neurophysiological level, the storage of information of the right hemisphere, then the more (or the more important) the split-off information, the greater the motivation for integration during the dreaming process. Perhaps such a process is temporary, allowing for nightly re-experiencing in dream

---

[3] Eysenck (1976) has developed a classical conditioning model for anxiety which includes certain assumptions that are strikingly congruent with a number of ideas that I have been discussing in this book. He believes that the persistence and intensity of neurotic anxiety is determined by (a) a strong, frustrative UCS (comparable to ego threat), (b) short presentation of the CS (comparable to briefly attended or quickly repressed perceptions or ideas surrounding the frustration), and (c) certain personality characteristics, e.g., high neuroticism. The basic idea is that failure to work through (adapt to) information that is related to important personal concerns will induce an incubation effect, i.e., emotional, behavioral, and cognitive persistence. Emotional, intriguing, and repetitive dreams may be one class of such phenomena. This kind of phenomenon was discussed more fully in Chapter 5.

consciousness of right-hemisphere-mediated information which is again lost during wake-fulness but which to some extent modifies total personality organization for having been re-experienced at some time. Perhaps such a neuropsychological hypothesis provides a model for what Freud called the "regressiveness" of the dream. If it is true, as many have suggested (Gazzaniga, 1972; Neisser, 1962), that information about early childhood experience is lost to waking memory because it was largely coded in spatial or analogical forms (forms believed to underlie right hemisphere coding in the adult and expressed consciously in the form of imagery), then the dominance of the right hemisphere during REM dreaming would be associated with a higher probability of re-experiencing the quality and content of early experience (i.e., "regression"). Thus, the lateralization hypothesis for REM dreaming has the potential for integrating three hypotheses which have been important in the area of dream psychology: (a) Freud's regression hypothesis, (b) Jung's compensation hypothesis, and (c) variants of the metaprogramming hypothesis (e.g., Dewan, 1969).

The compensation hypothesis is typical of psychodynamic approaches. For example, Freud (1955) suggests that "if we wish to classify the thought-impulses which persist in sleep, we may divide them into the following groups: (1) what has not been carried to a conclusion during the day owing to some chance hinderance; (2) what has not been dealt with owing to the insufficiency of our intellectual power — what is unsolved; (3) what has been rejected and suppressed during the daytime" (p. 554). To these Freud adds another group of events, those impressions toward which we appear to be indifferent. Parenthetically, one might conclude that prominent impressions in a dream which appear inconsistent with attentional invest-ment during that day should be considered psychologically important. Alas, this conclusion does not take into consideration the hypothesized deviousness of dreamwork according to Freud. "We assume as a matter of course that the most distinct element in the manifest dream content of a dream is the most important one; but in fact (owing to the displacement that has occurred) it is often an *indistinct* element which turns out to be the most direct derivative of the essential dream thought" (1952, p. 53).

Thus, from a strictly classical psychoanalytic position, hypotheses about the compensatory processing of waking information do not readily lend themselves to straight-forward predictions regarding the importance or meaning of dream material. In fact, one has the impression that what is psychologically fundamental during *both* wakefulness and dreaming is what is either repressed or trivialized. This is not the case with other clinical views of dream compensation which consider important those aspects of dream content which are relatively prominent or discontinuous with respect to waking preoccupations or beliefs (e.g., Fromm, 1951).

Different presleep conditions have been shown to yield compensatory dream content. For example, Hauri (1968, 1970) employed three presleep conditions in an own-control design which included six hours of each of the following: relaxation, physical exercise, studying. These manipulations had surprisingly little effect on sleep characteristics during the first 3.5 hours of sleep (e.g., higher heart rate in REM and NREM sleep after exercise vs. other conditions; more GSR variability in delta sleep after exercise, less after relaxation compared to the studying condition). Correspondingly, he found little differential effect of the conditions on dream content. However, there was less physical activity in the REM and NREM dreams (combined) under the physical activity condition (compensation). Hauri tentatively concluded on the basis of these and other data that "under certain circumstances, dream life is complementary to waking experience" (1970, p. 274).

There are other scattered sources of evidence to support this contention. For example, Wood (1962) found evidence of an apparent compensatory increase of social interaction in REM dream content after a day of social isolation. Bokert (1965) found more thirst-related imagery on nights when subjects were water-deprived (and a negative relationship between evidence of such content and morning thirst!). Newton (1970) found evidence for an apparently compensatory role of dreaming in that recently paralyzed individuals reported more physical activity, long-term paralyzed individuals less physical activity compared to normals. These data are commensurate with the idea that *acute* conditions involving cognitive, physical, or organismic deprivation or over-stimulation are associated with psychological compensation during dreaming. This phenomenological evidence is also commensurate with physiological evidence for the hypothesis that information processing during REM sleep, as defined by eye movement activity, compensates for acute excess or deficiency in information processing during wakefulness (de la Peña *et al.*, 1973). The Newton study (1970) also suggests a hypothesis that *chronic* deprivation of sensory or organismic information would eventually be reflected in a diminution of dream preoccupation with such information, while chronic availability of such information would be reflected in continuity of dream preoccupation. Such a hypothesis is commensurate with the continuity assumption regarding the relationship between habitual temperamental and behavioral "styles" and dream content which reflects these styles.

Attempts to influence dream content

A favorite device used in the study of presleep event-dream content relationships is the "stress" manipulation, e.g., a scary or otherwise emotionally arousing film. Since much of this research is, and should be, done in the context of an assessment of individual differences (e.g., Breger, Hunter and Lane, 1971), I will devote more discussion of this approach in the next chapter. However, there is one well-known study that deserves mention here. Foulkes and Rechtschaffen (1964) studied the differential effect of a violent vs. a travelogue (control) film on the REM and NREM dream content of 24 male and female volunteer subjects who served as their own controls. Just as there was apparently little differential effect on sleep characteristics (only sleep and initial REM onset latencies were mentioned), there was relatively little differential effect on dream content. There was no difference in REM or NREM dream recall, but the violent film was associated with longer REM (but not NREM) reports which were more imaginative and more vivid. These findings are relatively inconclusive because no attempt was made to assess possible interaction effects of film and personality which appear to be important (discussed in the next chapter). Also, there was no independent assessment of the personal significance of the two films (the elements of which were virtually absent in the dreams) and only minimal information on the effect of the films on sleep.

Arousing films do affect sleep characteristics. For example, Baekeland *et al.* (1968) reported that a subincision film, compared to a travelogue film, increased the proportion of REM periods interrupted or terminated by spontaneous awakenings, and increased the density of eye movement activity. There was no such differential effect on NREM awakenings. While the violent film used by Foulkes and Rechtschaffen was probably not as arousing as the subincision film used by Baekeland *et al.*, a more modest differential REM vs. NREM sleep effect may account for the modest REM vs. NREM content effects reported by Foulkes and Rechtschaffen. The increase in eye movement density found by Baekeland *et al.* is particularly interesting in the light of my (1975) finding that presleep stress was associated with higher REM density in repressor subjects. It would therefore have been most interesting to know if there were differences in eye movement activity and dream content between repressor and sensitizer subjects in the Foulkes and Rechtschaffen study. The fact that there were correlations between TAT and MMPI measures and certain aspects of dream content (e.g., higher MMPI scale scores were associated with "dreamlike qualities") makes it all the more likely that film × personality interaction effects might have obtained. Thus, the Foulkes and Rechtschaffen study (1964) illustrates some of the problems and issues related to the empirical investigation of presleep event-dream content relationships: (a) assessment of the personal significance of the situation (mediated by manipulation-trait interactions) both in theory and operationally, (b) control over content-related sleep variables, (c) control over dream report quality, (d) selection of dream content categories and variables, (e) attention to possible symbolic transformations.

Symbolic transformation presents an enormous obstacle to the empirical study of presleep event-dream content relationships. A personal example may be illustrative. In 1971 a fire destroyed much of the second floor of the psychology building during an evening when subjects were supposed to be run for an experiment I was conducting. That all experiments had been cancelled for the time being came as a (stressful) surprise. After coming to campus, investigating the charred and gutted floor where the fire had been, and returning home to contemplate the effect of the incident on both me and my colleagues, I had the following dream. I was walking along a major thoroughfare across the street from my old elementary school. On my side of the street there were stores (this is accurate) whose brown and grey facades seemed to be in dire need of a paint job. I remarked that they had a seedy appearance, and that $20 worth of new paint would suffice to make them appear like new. It seemed to me at the time that the dream was symbolic of a rather egocentric wish to undo damages, and the rather naive belief (wish) that renovation would involve little expense (i.e., would be a simple matter requiring little time and inconvenience). Had someone else scored my dream for literal incorporation of fire themes, the connection between the presleep event and the dream content would have been lost. Literal scoring methods may be more reliable, and they may be more credible, but they will yield underestimates of the degree to which dream content reflects preoccupations with concrete events.

A variant of the presleep manipulation strategy is the attempt to gain control over dream content through suggestion. There is evidence that at least some individuals are capable of dreaming more or less about a topic suggested by the experimenter, and that this ability is not necessarily enhanced by hypnotic inductions (see Walker and Johnson, 1974, and Tart, 1965 for reviews of these and related studies.) For example, Tart and Dick (1970) reported that most subjects selected for hypnotizability and good dream recall were able to dream about either of two prose passages. This was indicated by a significant number of passage-specific content elements and by a high degree of judged thematic continuity. Barber, Walker, and Hahn Jr. (1973) carried out a factorial study of the effect of hypnotic induction vs. no induction and type of suggestion (authoritative, permissive, or no suggestion) on dreaming about the death of John Kennedy. Both hypnotic and nonhypnotic suggestions to dream about the topic were equally associated with significantly more Kennedy themes than conditions without the suggestion. Interesting interactions were also found. For example, there was a greater effect on REM dream content for hypnotic subjects given the authoritative suggestion, but a greater effect on REM dream content for nonhypnotic subjects given the permissive suggestion. For NREM content, there was no such interaction, but the hypnotic induction had a greater impact on NREM content than the condition without hypnotic induction.

The significance of this kind of study goes beyond the experimental determination of the complexities of the wake-sleep connection. Tart and Dick (1970) suggest the possibility and advantages of using self- or other-mediated control over dreaming as a resource for personal growth. They refer to reports of widespread and effective control over dreaming in certain cultures, e.g., the Senoi (see Garfield, 1974). The potential use of dream control in our culture will remain largely in the realm of academic speculation for at least three reasons. First, there is a tendency in our culture to ignore or underrate the usefulness of dreams. Second, even if we decided that dream control were in principle advisable, we would not know what kinds of dream content would be useful. This problem raises the question of the functional (adaptive, defensive) effectiveness of dreaming which I will discuss in Chapter 10. Research on presleep suggestions (e.g., Tart and Dick, 1970) and during-sleep suggestions (Berger, 1963; Evans et al., 1970) makes it clear that subjects can be induced to dream, in general, about a topic. But how specific an effect can we expect? And how do we decide what is best for the subject to dream about? The latter question requires evidence of a *change* in behaviour which is mediated by dream content, a change in a desirable or useful direction. Such evidence is marked by its absence in the sleep-dream area. And there is little doubt that such a hypothetical effect would be closely tied to the type of subject and the type of situation.

Finally, objective evidence that control of dreaming, through a conscious presleep decision on the part of the individual, is hard to produce. A recent study yielded very disappointing results, especially considering the highly motivated group of subjects tested (Foulkes and Griffin, 1976). That suggestions for change, mediated through dream content, may be difficult is illustrated in a preliminary study reported by Cartwright (1974). On the basis of actual-self and ideal-self descriptions, an actual-self adjective was chosen that was relatively discrepant with the ideal-self rating. Subjects were instructed to repeat to themselves while falling asleep a wish *not* to be like the actual-self characteristic. To assess the effect on self characteristics in the dreams, two control adjectives were selected; each was as representative of the actual-self as was the target actual-self adjective, but was either as discrepant or nondiscrepant with the respective ideal-self adjective. These, along with the target adjective used in the induction, were used to assess the characteristics of the dream. The results suggested that, rather than changing during the dream in the direction of the presleep induction, the subjects seemed to resist change through maximizing the apparent benefits of the *status quo*, denying or disowning the ideal characteristic. That some subjects may resist the apparent intentions of the experimenter is nicely illustrated by an example from Witkin (1969, p. 24). After viewing a particularly threatening film, one subject "turned the tables". "After the quite bloody birth film, he dreamed of an idyllic park scene; after the subincision film, in which all the men are naked, he dreamed about characters who were elaborately dressed." This kind of "compensatory resistance" seems consistent with the old chestnut that patients in psychotherapy (perhaps most people) really do not wish to *be* different in any fundamental sense; rather, they want to feel better!

Are there certain aspects of personality functioning which, especially for some individuals, are reinforced by dreaming? Is dreaming then a conservative, self-protective, "personal fiction-maintaining" process of self-deception as Adler thought? Perhaps dreaming is a wish-fulfilling process with the wish for maintaining personality organization having as much status as or more than other kinds of wishes. Under what conditions, and for what kinds of individuals, is this kind of compensatory resistance most marked? Further research is required to answer such questions, and to provide suggestions about the value or usefulness of induced change through dreaming.

The laboratory effect on dream content

No discussion of the effect of presleep conditions on dream content can be considered complete without mentioning the impact of the laboratory setting. Evidence of incorporation into dreams of laboratory elements will be influenced by (a) the salience or impact of the situation (especially stress situations, and initial experience in the laboratory), (b) type of subject (e.g., field-dependent subjects and females tend to incorporate lab themes more than field-independents and males), and (c) scoring of content (e.g., sensitivity to symbolic transformation, discussed below). In any case, a large proportion of subjects will, especially during the earlier part of the night, dream about the laboratory situation (Whitman et al., 1962; Cartwright et al., 1969; Cohen and Cox, 1975; Dement et al., 1965; Goodenough et al., 1965). Before I give some examples of some of the ways that the content of the presleep situation can show up in the content of dreams, I should mention the general impact of the laboratory, the effect of which is to make the dream more conservative, cautious, and perhaps overly symbolic. For example, consider the following example of a "sexual" dream segment from a male subject.

> I am in the elevator sitting by myself against the wall. Now this girl comes in, and I say "Come sit by me", and she sits by me (I didn't even know her), and I lean over and try to kiss her, and she says "*No don't* do that". I say "How come?", and she said something about her *acne*, and I said it didn't matter and she laughed and we ended up kissing and stuff on the elevator, and then these *parents* got on . . . and the elevator was real *shaky*, and I was thinking that the elevator would *crash* or get *stuck* . . . I asked her "Is the elevator always like this?" and she said, "Yes", . . . so we finally got off at *number 2* — I was trying to get off at number 11 — but we finally got off at number 2. It was weird; I was scared of riding it.

Perhaps I go too far in suggesting (by the use of italics) that this dream is about sexuality inhibited during the dream through a continuing process of REM sleep vigilance with respect to the laboratory situation. Perhaps, at home, this subject would indeed "get off" at number 11. Perhaps the reason that wet dreams are such rarities in the lab is that subjects rarely get past number 2!

Some examples of dream reporting by different kinds of subjects tested in the Cohen and Cox (1975) study will illustrate the variety of types of lab incorporation observed. A sensitizer subject run in the "negative" (presleep ego threat) condition was awakened from a REM period and reported:

> I was having some sort of psychology test done on me for the perception of chemicals, and it was a strange situation . . . there was a battered up truck set out . . . I was supposed to perceive some differences. The chemical he was testing was tetramethyl chloride. I don't even know if that exists[4] . . . I came up wrong. I couldn't tell the difference.

---

[4] It doesn't.

Compare this apparent expression of concern about the challenge of the testing situation and possible failure or inadequacy with the dream of a repressor subject, the gist of which was as follows. He was seated in a football stadium and had with him a strength-giving potion. It seemed natural to him to have it, and his intention was experimentation and the possibility of increasing his intelligence. We are tempted to infer a difference in these two kinds of individuals, one experiencing failure and uncertainty, the other adaptation and self-confidence. Now consider the following REM dream of another repressor subject.

> Something to do with a baseball game . . . real strange. The perspective is as if inside a baseball. All I got out of it was one scene of coming at, across the plate as a guy is swinging his bat. It's like being among giant people or something . . . I see the catcher (through the window in the ball) and I feel the motion through the air. . . .

This example seems to reflect another characteristic of repressors, that of relatively neutral affect. The subject admits to feeling small, confined, and definitely not in control of his action; but his only affective reaction is interest and curiosity. The laboratory situation has apparently had a definite impact on the dream, inducing a kind of symbolic transformation of the situation. Does this cognitive recreation indicate merely a play on imagery (sport, recreation), or is there an element of defensive elaboration which makes a potentially threatening situation "safe" through abstraction and repression? The limitations of the experimental procedures do not permit a resolution of this kind of question.

In an unpublished pilot study on problem solving and REM dream content, we noted an unusually high percentage of subjects dreaming either literally or symbolically about the experiment (86%) or more specifically, about the problem (72%). Experiment-related dreams were almost as likely to occur in the second half of the night as in the first half (though the poorer quality of early REM recall may have artificially attenuated the evidence of early dream preoccupation with the experiment). Two kinds of incorporation theme are worthy of illustration: that regarding the role of the subject, including the subject-experimenter interaction, the other regarding dreamwork on the presleep problem.

Dreams about the apparatus, electrodes, and the task of recalling dreams are fairly common in our one night studies (and probably should be considered, along with the sleep characteristics, an aspect of "first night effect"). For example, one subject reported:

> I was worrying about — I was taking some sort of test, and there was a condition that I had to qualify before I could take the test, and uh, I can't quite remember what the condition was — it was sort of a conflict about taking the test . . . maybe qualification is a bad word. There were some — like some questions that I had to get right or something before I could go on with the test.

This fragment from the first REM dream suggests both task difficulty and self-doubt or insufficiency. The latter again seems to be reflected in the next REM dream, a fragment of which is as follows:

> I was describing to somebody why I was sick . . . in my dream I had a cold . . . I remember telling him I got the Hawaiian Kollywambas playing doubles . . . I got sick playing tennis.

In the following dream, the subject says that he got hit in the head with a blackjack just before awakening. And just before that he recalls:

> I forgot to get you to sign my [subject pool participation] card . . . there was some room where I was going to come back to get you to sign it . . . so I called your house and I couldn't get you so I called this Randy M. [administrative coordinator for the experiment] and I couldn't get him, so I said, "What am I going to do?" So I called this

professor Cohen — I don't even know who professor Cohen is — but I called him and
he said something rather aloof like "what are you doing calling me?", and I said, "boy,
I gotta have this card signed", and I felt like a complete fool because what are you
doing calling a professor about something like this, you know?

Again, in the next REM dream, there is a sense of self-doubt and inadequacy with respect to
being a good subject:

I was dreaming that I wasn't — I dreamed that you came in and you gave me a pill to
make me dream something, and uh, it didn't have any effect, and I wasn't dreaming, I
was just sitting there. For some reason I wasn't coming up with anything to dream. And
you couldn't figure out why and you gave me this pill to make me dream more . . . You
said "we'll try it one more time". So you turned out the light, and I went to sleep, and
you came back in and I wasn't dreaming or anything, and you said, "I'm going to the
bathroom. You'd better have something to dream when I come back" or something like
that.

The subject's obvious concern about performance adequacy is clearly manifest in the
following fragment of the same dream at a point where the dreamed experimenter returns to
the subject's room:

I was sitting up here with my head up in bed and I guess there was a mirror, and I was
looking at me in the mirror. It didn't look like me. I remember my face was all puffy and
I looked like I had braces on, and I looked like a different person, and uh, it kind of
scared me . . . I wasn't doing what I was supposed to . . . it looked pretty weird, I know it
was me. . . .

Sometimes a dream will reflect an apparent eroticization of the subject-experimenter interaction. Consider the following fragments of a REM dream from another subject:

I was dreaming about you and what we were doing right now except we weren't here.
You took me outside. We were going to do some little test outside the building . . . you
gave me some stuff to keep for you for a little while while you were at a party . . .
we [then] walked out of the building we were in . . . and we ended up in a car that I use
— my father has an old car that he lets me use. And that's where the stuff was that you
hooked me up to. You were going to give me something to eat . . . some kind of
chemical, and you told me . . . to be prepared to be sick . . . I was still outside the car
and squatted down. You were sitting in the back seat with your feet outside the car . . .
part of what I was keeping for you was a dish of ice cream. I had problems because it
melted . . . you were gonna depolarize something which doesn't make much sense.
That's what you told me we were gonna do . . . all you wanted to do was give me some of
this little stuff with a plastic bag with the white powder. There was a lot of it but you
were only gonna give me a little bit.

Dreams about the presleep task were also quite apparent. The problem was presented to
the subject as memory for geometric shapes. Sixteen 3×5 cards with at least one geometric
shape per card were presented, one at a time for about five seconds, then covered while the
subject drew the picture from memory. Each shape was a variant of a "standard" pattern
that was never seen. The sixteen variant patterns were derived by taking the standard
pattern and transforming it in any of a number of ways, e.g., reversing the right and left
shapes, changing the size (e.g., from large to small), eliminating one or more shapes,
substituting a "new" shape for a standard shape, etc.[5] The standard figure, the four standard

[5] This procedure was taken from an undated manuscript by J. F. Franks and J. D. Bransford entitled Abstraction
of Visual Patterns (Experiment I).

(a)

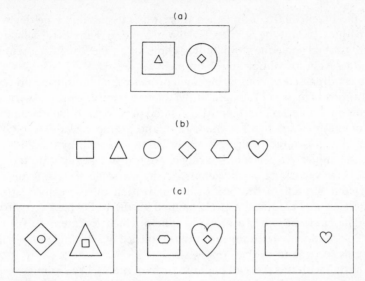

(b)

(c)

Figure 8-2   Standard figure (a), six shapes (b), and three examples of variants actually shown to the subjects during the presleep problem solving task.

shapes plus the two substitute shapes (heart and six-sided figure), and some examples of variant figures are shown in Figure 8-2. After going through the set of cards three times, the subject was told that the various figures that he saw and drew were variants of a standard shape, and were derived from transformations of the standard (as described above). His job was to think about the variants and try to come up with the best fit, that is, the standard figure. The problem was described as similar to the problem of inferring a basic personality characteristic from diverse behaviors of a person. The subject was told that in the morning he would be tested for his ability to derive the standard figure.

Many of the dreams reported by these subjects were literally and symbolically about this task. We estimated that 32% of all dreams were directly or indirectly about the presleep task. One subject dreamed about pouring from a bucket what seemed like separate ingredients of a substance, that is, separate components which, when combined, would yield the original substance. The subject spoke of a "whole being broken down unnaturally into its raw materials". This very unusual dream seems clearly to reflect an analytic-synthesizing cognition. Another example of such activity is a dream by another subject which involved individual words, meaningless by themselves, which suddenly came together to form a meaningful name.

> I remember being in prison, and there was one particular girl that was in prison . . . she kept making these songs, she would make these games . . . and we put them all together then they spelled Coca Cola . . . these odd syllables, these really odd words that she would think up and they all came together in Coca Cola. That was odd because it came as such a surprise.

The accent in this dream seemed to be on the synthesis of a meaningful whole out of meaningless parts. Another example of the process of organizing individual elements into a more meaningful whole is illustrated by the dream of another subject:

> It was a candy store or something. Sort of like conducting an experiment or a parable . . . and two little black boys came up to us. They had bags of licorice, you know the red

kind and the black kind ... and then there was this parable type deal — sort of an exercise in how to count the licorice. Say I put down so many here, can you tell me how many there is? And someone would put a whole lot on the floor ... it reminded me of a chapter in a psychology book on chunking.[6]

Another subject dreamed of comparing and contrasting communism and capitalism and drawing conclusions. This kind of cognition is relatively infrequently observed (at least in the reports from our subjects) and therefore may be presumed to have been elicited by the requirements of the presleep task. A more dramatic example of preoccupation with the geometric figures is illustrated in dreams about being assaulted by the shapes. In the first REM dream, the subject experienced trying to figure out something, trying to solve a puzzle. At first he was working on the geometric shape problem, putting answers in a box. Suddenly he found himself in the box (a dramatization of his really "getting into" the problem?). Once inside, he noticed a circle painted on the wall which starts to expand out into the box. The circle becomes a growing sphere which threatens to fill up the entire volume of the box. Suddenly it disappears and is replaced by a triangle which, in the form of a pyramid, begins to expand in the same way.

I was just sitting with this piece of paper in front of me ... I was going to try to solve the problem ... I remember writing down a square ... and then I write several other things and all of a sudden, before I get to put it into the box I just imagine myself in the box ... I try to head for one of the corners, but I never get there, and then I notice that there is something else in the box, and I turn around to look, and then I notice that there is a figure on the walls ... The first thing I remember when I turned around was a circle on one of the corners of the box ... at first it looks like a drawn figure on the wall ... then I look again and it starts getting bigger ... a solid taking up the volume of the box ... I start running, and I look again and it's gone. And I look at the other wall and I notice that there is another figure coming in, and I notice it's a triangle ...

In the next dream the subject dreams about police cars which are square-shaped. In the third dream, the subject again finds himself in the box, and this time, in addition to the circle and triangle, he experienced an expanding six-sided figure. Later in the dream, both the circle and the triangle come out together, the triangle on the left and the circle on the right. Note that this is the correct positioning of two of the shapes of the standard figure (which the subject had never seen, see Figure 8-2).

Other subjects represented the presleep task in unique ways. In his first dream, a subject recalled being preoccupied with a large slowly rotating square. In his third dream, part of which had to do with the experimental apparatus, the subject dreamed about being in a cottonwood grove and noticed the *heartshaped* leaves (see Figure 8-2). In his fourth dream, he and some friend were in pursuit of some ape-like australopithecine hominids who were seated in a circle on the snow-covered elementary school yard. (The subject had attended a lecture on evolution of humans the previous night.)

The asphalt of my old elementary school yard was covered with circles and squares — I didn't see — I just remembered they had four squares marked off and circles — sixteen different circles and squares ... the apes or whatever were sitting on the asphalt where the circles would have been under the snow. Where they were sitting there should have

---

[6] Chunking is a construct referring to higher order categories that organize numerous elements. Memory for elements is facilitated by "chunking" the elements and then remembering the chunks rather than trying to remember all the items individually. For example, older children and brighter adults (compared to younger children) tend to organize a series of items into their abstract categories (i.e., tend to chunk out information).

been a circle painted on the asphalt for a game we used to play . . . the old dodgeball circle.

The most delightful example of playful preoccupation with the geometrical shapes of the presleep task is illustrated by a long and complicated dream which included a football game on TV. Instead of real players there were animated triangles with spindly arms and legs running around the field. In the following dream, also quite long and complicated, the subject recalled working on the problem and visualizing a pattern which turned out to be a reasonably good approximation to the standard figure: a large circle enclosing a small diamond on the left, and a large triangle enclosing a small heart on the right. This dream appeared to express concern about performance and acceptance by the experimenter. The subject dreamed that the experimenter came in, and woke him up, and threw a newspaper at the subject saying that this was the subject's third and last trial, as though to indicate both the fact that the third trial was the final trial (in the presleep task) and some perceived annoyance on the part of the experimenter. The subject remembers that on the third trial (of the actual task) his performance was perfect except that he confused a small triangle for a diamond. In the dream, the subject wondered if he had done as well as another dreamed character against whom he was competing, a character of supposedly exceptional intelligence.

These examples make it clear how important it is to have information about the presleep situation in trying to make sense out of the content of the dream. Methodological problems in the study from which these examples come precluded an analysis of the role of motivation in determining the degree of incorporation, the role of personality and intelligence in determining the way that the incorporation was expressed, or the degree to which the presence of task-related themes (or the nature of these incorporations) was associated with postsleep performance (producing the standard figure). However, as we will see, these issues, especially that of dream content-postsleep performance, are of fundamental importance to an empirically based psychology of dream content.

CHAPTER 9

INDIVIDUAL DIFFERENCES IN DREAM CONTENT

1. INDIVIDUAL DIFFERENCES

Variation is a fundamental characteristic of living things. Psychobiological uniqueness is virtually guaranteed, even for "identical twins", by variation in genetic and nongenetic influences. Individual differences can be defined at the physiological, psychological, and experiential levels, and include categories such as age, sex, trait, intelligence, etc. These kinds of characteristics will inevitably affect the perception of events, and thus affect the influence of such events on dreams. In *The Descent of Man*, Darwin suggested that "the value of the products of our imagination depends of course on the number, accuracy, and clearness of our impressions on our judgement and task in selecting or rejecting the involuntary combinations, and to a certain extent on our power of voluntarily combining them." It is therefore remarkable how little empirical work on dream content and intellectual style and ability has been reported. (A happy but hardly sufficient exception to this deficiency is the study by Adelson, 1959.)

Notice that the research to be discussed is directed toward revealing the relationship between categories of individual differences (e.g., male vs. female) or dimensions of personality (e.g., masculinity-femininity) and categories of dream content (e.g., affects, settings, characters, etc.). This empirical approach can be contrasted with clinical revelations of the meaning of symbolic dream elements reported by individual persons at a particular time.

Validity vs. utility of dream categories: researchers vs. clinicians

Typically the difference between empirical and clinical approaches to the dream is reflected in (a) the way the dream is treated (e.g., as a correlate vs. as a symbol), and (b) a focus on average or statistical generalizations about groups vs. a focus on the individual. Consider the second distinction. The typical empirical approach to dream content includes a prior separation of groups or a manipulation of situations which is then related to differences in dream content. For example, the dream content of schizophrenics is compared to that of nonschizophrenics. Either *a priori*, or on the basis of some hypothesis about the nature of schizophrenic psychodynamics, the investigator expects a difference in the proportion of schizophrenics vs. the nonschizophrenics who dream about some topic. Following Wiggins (1973), the *validity* of that category (let us call it "s" for "sign") is the probability of s, given group membership, G. So, for example, if we use the dreaming of strangers as our "s", and schizophrenia as our "G", then the validity, $p(s/G)$, can be estimated from empirical data. As we will see, empirical research on the dream content of psychiatric groups is both scanty and of rather poor quality. Thus, we are not now in a position to extract a systematic, empirically based and *valid* set of dream categories that are associated with such groups. This is a remarkable and somewhat embarrassing state of affairs considering the amount of dream research done over the past 20 years.

However, the picture is even bleaker when we approach the problem of dream content from the clinician's point of view. More than validity, the clinician is interested in the *utility* of an s. The question the clinician would like answered by the researcher is: "Given an s, what is the probability that I am dealing with a G type person (or situation)? That is, what is the $p(G/s)$?" This is an entirely different kind of question for which the empirical literature on dream content provides little useful information. But this deficiency is not an exclusive characteristic of dream research. Reitan has noted that "some psychologists disdain an interest in individual human beings and prefer to direct their efforts to identification of abstractions and generalizations that have no demonstrable application to individual subjects" (1974, p. 21). Rae Carlson has developed this thesis in an important paper on the apparent scarcity of attention to the individual in personality research (1971b). While this chapter is oriented toward questions of validity rather than utility (i.e., which categories are related to different types of individuals) some comments about what the clinician does with dream content are in order.

In order to use a category (s) in the sense of "utility", the clinician needs three empirically derived probabilities or proportions: (a) the validity probability, or $p(s/G)$; (b) the proportion of G people in a specified population, or $p(G)$; and (c) the probability of detecting the s in the dreams of that population, or $p(s)$. Thus, a rational and empirically based best interpretation or diagnostic guess as to $p(G/s)$ is:

$$\frac{p(s/G) \times p(G)}{p(s)}$$

First, it is clear that there is no good basis in the empirical literature to estimate any of the probabilities involving s. Second, even if such information were available, it would be likely that any valid s for some group (G) such as schizophrenics would be sufficiently frequently observed in nonG groups to render the utility of s rather low. However, two things should be noted. Clinicians base diagnostic assessment on more information than a single sign. Second, there may turn out to be a group of dream content signs that are relatively rare (of "low validity") but of extremely high utility, even higher utility than an array of other more traditionally useful signs. Thus, a sign that is not particularly interesting to the researcher, who is interested in the validity of s, may be quite useful to the clinician.

This problem of validity vs. utility of categories is sufficiently important to require additional elaboration. Note that the distinction raises two interrelated problems, one about base rates and the other about the meaning of group comparison strategies. If one is interested in the *etiological* implications of a group difference, then the smaller the difference between a rare group and a control group, the more likely that inferences about etiology will be erroneous; likewise, a high rate of "false positives" will compromise the utility of a sign associated with a rare group. For example, suppose that we are interested in the utility of a dream content category (or its implications for etiology) associated with schizophrenia. Typically, a group of schizophrenics is compared to a group of nonschizo-phrenics with respect to the presence of the category.

Let us suppose that we have a very striking difference between the groups: 70% of our schizophrenics produce dream category X, while only 30% of our nonschizophrenics produce that category. We will even suppose that this is a statistically highly significant and replicable difference (a most generous supposition given the usual empirical state of affairs). What can we say about category X? Is it related in some casual way to schizophrenia? Is it a useful sign? The prevalence of schizophrenia in the general population is roughly 0.0085. If our groups are representative of normals and schizophrenics in the general population, then the chance of finding an individual, picked randomly from the population, who produces a dream with category X is .0085 $\times$ .7 or .006 (for schizophrenics) plus .915 $\times$ .3 or .275 (for nonschizophrenics) = .28. In other words, while category X is produced by roughly a quarter of the population, it is over 45 times more likely to be associated with *nonschizophrenia* than with schizophrenia. Of course, it is possible that the sign may still be of etiological significance; it may be a biological marker, an indication that the nonschizophrenic who produces it is a carrier of, say, schizophrenic genes. But this would be a very risky assumption.

A discussion of the theoretical and methodological pitfalls of group comparison strategies would take us too far afield. The point is that there is a danger when we generalize from truly valid signs (e.g., dream categories) that are associated with a statistically rare group of individuals to questions of utility and etiology. Thus, the meaning of differences in dream content across psychiatric and control groups will generally be more obscure than differences across groups of individuals who are found in roughly equal numbers in the general popoulation.

Dream interpretation

Dream interpretation, as opposed to content analysis, presents enormous difficulties to the researcher because dream interpretation is largely derived from theory or ideas about dream function held by the interpreter, and because meaning is as much a derivative of the innovative and artistic skills of the interpreter as the dreamwork. No phylogenetic or ontogenetic aspect of mental function has been ignored. Clinicians have described dreams as the symbols, on the one hand, of the regressive influence of infantile wishes and intrapsychic conflict (Freud, 1955; Hall, 1966), psychosocial conflict, and the need to perpetuate self-esteem through self-delusion (Adler, 1927; Bonime, 1962), and on the other hand, of the progressive influence of creative talent (Krippner and Hughes, 1970), and the capacity for insight and wisdom (Fromm, 1951; Jung, 1964). In virtually every case, the accent is on the very personal preoccupations of individuals which, when conditioned by the biological characteristics common to the human species, are the stuff of which art and myth are made.

One problem with these views is the tendency to interpret the dream as revealing something that is in some way more real or more true than the references of waking thought. There is a tendency in clinical writing to treat the impulse as somehow more real than the manifest content. It is like saying that homeostasis is more real than the reflex, the reflex more real than conditioning, conditioning more real than abstract thought. The former may be phylogenetically and ontogenetically older, prerequisite, and imperious characteristics of biological functioning, but they are no more real. A neocortex is no less biological than a brain stem. A full understanding of human functioning clearly requires as much attention to the capacity for adjustment, expression, and innovation as to the sources which elicit these processes. And it is important to remember that during sleep, there may be a shift in the focus and style of cognition. We may flatter ourselves during wakefulness, yet picture ourselves in quite a different manner during dreams. Both views are real, conditioned as they are by the context of thought. They are merely different perspectives that may appear to be, or may in fact be, in conflict. In short, I think it misplaced romanticism to conceive of unconscious processes as more real or more sinister or more wise than conscious processes.

Another problem with idiographic approaches to dream interpretation can be illustrated by comments made by clinicians who have rejected the idea that a particular dream element has a standard meaning. For example, Fromm rejects the Freudian notion that nakedness in a dream is always symbolic of the wish to expose the genitals. "Freud ignores the fact that nakedness can be a symbol of things other than sexual exhibitionism. Nakedness can, for instance, be a symbol for truthfulness . . . for being oneself without pretense" (1951, p. 90). Bonime (1962) argues for characterological rather than instinctual interpretations of symbols, and rejects the idea of a universal symbolism. Dreaming of a snake could mean any number of things depending on the context and, of course, depending on the particular individual having the dream: sinfulness, independence, competitiveness, courage. Dreaming of missing the bus could symbolize, for the rich person, snobbishness (unwillingness to travel with ordinary people), for the patient, the wish not to go to the therapy session, for the professor of Elizabethan literature (through the association of bus = kiss), the lost opportunity or failure to show affection toward his wife (Bonime, 1962, p. 33).

Empirical approaches to dream content will of necessity seem pale and insignificant in the dazzling light of the clinical artistry, symbolic inventiveness, and semantic wizardry of people like Bonime, Freud, and Jung. Nevertheless, "an *exclusive* devotion [to art], except in a professional, is almost surely hostile to intellect. For cultivating art out of fear or spite means preferring always what is ambiguous, what touches only the sensibility, what titillates through irony, what plunges the imagination into a sea of symbols, echoes, and myths, from which insights may be brought up to the surface but no arguable views. And this preference is at bottom love of confusion — confusion sought as a love of responsibility." "*Avant-garde* psychology, *avant-garde* art, and the philanthropy that coevals with them, alike cherish the warm confusions of animal existence" (Barzun, 1959, pp. 18-24).

On the other hand, exclusive commitment to the principles of scientific objectivity, reliability of assessment, replicability, predictability, construct validity has advanced only modestly our knowledge about the nature of dream content. Taking modern sleep research to task, Foulkes and Vogel (1974) ask, "Why is it that laboratory dream investigations have shed so little light on the crucial questions of dream psychology — e.g., the sources, organizations, meanings, and functions of dreams?" They suggest that the reason lies in part in an excessive emphasis on artificial conditions and "public or dictionary meanings of dreams rather than in terms of the dreamer's private meaning system as might be revealed through his dream associations". Perhaps the next major advance in content research will come from clinical researchers who are as comfortable with dream interpretation, even the "warm confusions of animal existence", as they are with issues of scientific control and objectivity (e.g., Foulkes and Vogel, 1974; Witkin, 1969).

Group comparisons of dream content

In this chapter, I will first discuss some of the research on categories of dream content associated with individual differences which are obtained in the absence of a formal consideration of differences in the presleep situation, and then discuss research on personality $\times$ situational interaction effects on dream content. The former type of research is typically based on group comparisons while the latter takes into consideration both the type of subject and the experimental manipulation. For purposes of illustration rather than comprehensive review, and because of the generally poor quality and/or dearth of research, I will focus on three types of individual differences: (a) normal vs. psychotic, (b) male vs. female, and (c) "masculine" vs. "feminine". Finally, it should be noted that most of this research is at least implicitly designed within the context of a continuity view; it involves an assumption that dream content will more or less reflect individual differences, or it involves an effort better to understand through dream content the nature of those differences. There is relatively little attempt to go beyond the manifest content or to interpret symbolism. Standard categories are used such as the presence of aggression, types of characters, affects and emotions.

A good review of the correlational research on trait-dream content relationships is given by Domino (1976a). This investigator set out explicitly to test the Jungian view of compensatory expression of traits, e.g., the extravert tends to express introversion during dreaming. On the basis of a large set of *positive* correlations between personality dimension scores derived from two tests and dream content ratings (e.g., for achievement, deference, dominance, change, heterosexuality, aggression), Domino opined that the study "does not support Jung, but is more in line with the theories of Adler, Fromm, and Hall who see dream content as not substantially different from conscious functioning" (1976a, p. 658). The problem with this inference is that it gives insufficient credit to the sophistication of the theories (e.g., Fromm spoke of compensation as well as continuity of dream theme) and no consideration of the importance of other factors which might elicit compensation. For example, it is unlikely that studies which ignore situational factors (e.g., which elicit suppression of thought, feeling, or behavior) will be sensitive to compensation (see Chapter 8). Also, it is possible that only a subset of individuals, those who often tend to suppress aspects of their functioning, will produce compensatory dreams. That is, compensation may simply be a largely irrelevant form of adjustment for many people, just as a particular trait measure chosen by the investigator may be largely irrelevant to a particular person (Bem and Allen, 1974). In short, I am suggesting that while trait-dream content correlational studies may be appropriate to testing the continuity hypothesis, they are largely *not* fair tests of the compensation hypothesis unless the latter is formulated in a rather simplistic fashion.

The adequacy of the assessment device is central to any test of the relationship between personality, or personality $\times$ situation interaction, and dream content, whether this relationship be hypothesized as continuous or compensatory. While a full discussion of the problem would clearly take us beyond the scope of the task at hand, some brief comments will be useful to sharpen our discussion.

What do we mean when we say, or assume, that dreaming is related to personality? From the perspective of empirical psychology, we mean that there are lawful relationships between what we would like to think of as measures of traits and categories of dream content. Since I have already discussed at length some of the major problems with the objective categorization of dream content, as well as the continuity-discontinuity issue

(Chapter 8), I will focus here on the problem of personality assessment. Typically, subjects are preselected on the basis of scores on some personality dimension. However, with few exceptions, such scores are ambiguous with regard to the following questions: (a) Are the scores reliable? How do we know that a subject scoring above the mean of some dimension will do so the next time the individual is tested on the same or comparable test? (b) How confident are we in the ability of the subject to estimate validly the presence (frequency, intensity) of the trait? There is evidence that only some subjects (e.g., those who are least concerned with their public image and/or subjects who are relatively conscious of their personal attributes) are capable of providing estimates that are, in fact, predictive of actual behavior (Fenigstein, Scheier and Buss, 1975; Turner, 1978). (c) Regardless of the reliability or validity of the score, does it say something about the importance or centrality of the dimension to the individual (Bem and Allen, 1974)? Again, possibly not, yet this ought to be important to any question about the relationship between personality and dream content. (d) Do the scores reflect merely above-average tendencies, or extreme dispositions? If the overall score reflects the sum of "true" responses, it is clear that the intensity and frequency (reliability) factors are confounded (Willerman, 1979). (e) Do the scores tell us anything important about the maximal capacity of the individual regardless of his or her typical behavior? If not, we may lose important information necessary for high-level predictions about dream content, especially if dreams have more to do with capacity or disposition rather than situation-induced behaviors. The reader may recognize some of the questions I have raised as those which are salient in current personality research (Willerman, 1979).

To demonstrate how dreams and traits are related, adequate assessment of both dream content and personality is clearly a prerequisite. I say this, not only to underscore the obvious, but to admit that the typically modest correlations between trait and content measures (Domino, 1976a) could lead the critically-minded to write off the utility of these relationships just as they have written off those between-trait measures and behavior (Mischel, 1968).

Critical tests of the relationship between traits and dream content will require that the trait score (a) is reliable, (b) represents a central dimension of the individual's personality, (c) derives from skilled assessment or self-assessment, and (d) represents a significant capacity or ability. It is my guess that a score which satisfies all these requirements will, other things (like the adequacy of the dream content measures) being equal, be more predictive of dream phenomena. I would like to emphasize my guess that dream content will reflect *abilities* (what a person is capable of and psychologically committed to) more readily and more clearly than habitual behavior (what a person tends to do, often for "extrinsic" reasons). Confirmation of this idea would do much to resolve apparent conflicts between continuity and compensatory hypotheses. Dreams may reflect what one does (typical behavior), and what one suppresses (compensation). But discontinuity between typical behavior and dream content may reflect an artifact of personality assessment. That is, if we were to focus on what the individual *can do*, and is fully conscious of, we might be impressed by the continuity of personality and dreaming.

Many interesting questions are raised by the potentially important distinction between habitual and maximal behavior. For example, we should expect different frequencies and kinds of dream content for two individuals who are maximal on some characteristic (e.g., the capacity for aggression) but who differ markedly on habitual measures. It appears to me that our ideas about the relationship between personality and dream content will profit greatly from studies which base their approach on these kinds of distinctions. Suffice it to say that the data to be described below constitute, at best, a modest and preliminary approach to an extremely complex problem.

Let us consider some of the findings with respect to dream content of schizophrenics. Carrington (1972) obtained five diary-recorded dreams per subject from 30 female *acute* schizophrenics some of whom were on medication and who tended to be above average in intelligence. Carrington characterizes the dreams as reflecting a "state of emergency or stress", the environment depicted as "overwhelmingly threatening". The dreams are replete with the aggression, bizarreness, "reflective of ego dyscontrol". They are "stark and tragic". For example, one dream was reported as follows: "I was decapitated. My ribs were picked clean, no skin, no muscle. My body was cut in half. I was just a pile of bones. They didn't know who it was, but I still knew who I was. I wanted to pull myself together, but I couldn't" (p. 348). In another nonlaboratory study (Kramer, Baldridge, Whitman, Ornstein and Smith, 1969), the most recent dream was obtained from 40 male paranoid schizophrenic, 40 psychotic depressives, and 40 VA medical inpatients. The percentage of dreams with hostility was 78 for the schizophrenics, 55 for the depressed, and 30 for the medical patients. Of these dreams, the direction of hostility was toward the dreamer most frequently (almost in all cases) for the schizophrenics while much less so for the other groups. Implausibility characterized the dreams of the schizophrenics (68%) more than those of the depressives (38%) or the controls (15%). Finally, and this is important because it has been replicated under different conditions, schizophrenics tended to dream about strangers while the depressed tended to dream about family members. The results of this study are somewhat ambiguous because there was no discussion of diagnostic procedures, age of subjects, drug status, nor was there any control for amount and quality of dream material.

A study of the REM dreams of 11 nonmedicated male paranoid schizophrenics (Kramer, Whitman, Baldridge and Ornstein, 1970) revealed a high proportion of aggressive to friendly events, a higher proportion of anxiety to other kinds of euphoric and dysphoric affect, and again, more preoccupation with strangers than with family or friends. These latter results tie in nicely with those of the earlier study but the absence of a control group and more specific information about procedure makes it difficult to evaluate the findings. The high percentage of dreams of schizophrenics with stranger vs. family occurs in yet another study (Kramer and Roth, 1973) in which the corresponding relationship tends to be reversed in the dreams of depressives. This study also obtained a higher percentage of schizophrenic dreams with more aggression than friendly acts. (Again there is insufficient information on age, diagnosis, chronicity, drug status, and no test of potentially important difference in the REM recall for the two groups: 71% for the schizophrenics, 51% for the depressives.)

The results of this set of studies are not generally commensurate with those obtained by a group of Japanese investigators (Okuma, Sunami, Fukuma, Takeo and Motoike, 1970). They collected REM dream reports from 21 male and female nonmedicated *chronic* schizophrenics and 34 college student controls. The controls had roughly the same REM recall percentage (68% for schizophrenics, 73% for the controls). However, the reports of the control subjects were longer, had a shorter response latency, and required less prodding and inquiry from the experimenter. Oddly, the dreams of the schizophrenic group were *less* bizarre, less affective (though dysphoric when affective) and relatively *more* often about family members than were the dreams of the control group. The authors interpret the less frequently bizarre content as a reflection of the loss of defense capability from which bizarreness in dreams originates. Such an interpretation, however, is contradicted by evidence that it is the dreams of individuals prone to anxiety and low self-esteem (presumably a reflection of defensive failure) who tend to have relatively more bizarre dream content (Cohen, 1974b; Foulkes and Rechtschaffen, 1964; Hersen, 1971; Pivik and Foulkes, 1968; Starker, 1974). One possibility is that the differences found across these studies (differences that are difficult to evaluate because of lack of sufficient information) are due to length of hospitalization, acuteness of the psychosis, and intelligence. Acute paranoid schizophrenics may be more preoccupied with the strangeness of their experience (symbolized by the stranger) while chronics might be more preoccupied with egocentric and regressive motives which may be mediated by associations to family. In addition, lack of bizarren.ss may in part be a function of the scarcity of the reports of chronics which in turn may be mediated by attitude, drug status, and low intelligence. In sum, we cannot conclude much from these kinds of studies regarding the relationship between psychological condition and dream content because there is a greater number of relevant variables of yet unknown influence operating in them than of group-content comparisons reported. These variables include diary (informal) vs. laboratory reports, age, sex, chronicity of disorder, length of hospitalization, drug status, acuteness of condition, diagnostic subcategory (especially those known to be of distinct genetic origin, e.g., bipolar vs. unipolar depression), intelligence, motivation, quality of report (including percentage of recall).

The best single review of nonlaboratory dream content differences between college males and college females of the early fifties is Hall and Van de Castle's book (1966). In terms of formal categories (e.g., settings, types of interaction, emotions, characters, etc.) there are remarkably few marked differences. One difference that has been replicated many times, and which can be considered a hallmark of sex differences in dream content, is the finding that females' dreams more often take place indoors (Brenneis, 1970; Hall and Van de Castle, 1966; Winget and Farrell, 1971; Winget, Kramer, and Whitman, 1972). Since these studies did not control for the duration and frequency of indoor to outdoor *behaviors* between groups, it is not immediately clear that the difference in content reflects something of general symbolic importance rather than merely a reflection of typical conditions. But evidence that male homosexuals also tend to set their dreams indoors (Winget and Farrell, 1971) makes the issue more interesting.

Another general finding obtained across studies is the predictable difference in aggression in dreams: males experience more aggression than do females (Brenneis, 1970; Cohen, 1973b; Hall and Van de Castle, 1966; Winget *et al.*, 1972). However, the differences are sometimes small, and in some samples (e.g., schizophrenic), not evident at all (Okuma *et al.*, 1970). In the dream, male dreamers aggress against male characters far more often than against female characters, while female dreamers tend not to show this preference or tend to show the opposite (Hall and Van de Castle, 1966; Okuma *et al.*, 1970). Thus, male characters in dreams are subject to much more frequent aggression than are female characters. This differential finding is clearly commensurate with laboratory data indicating that male subjects are less willing to aggress against (deliver shocks to) female subjects (Buss, 1966b), and therefore probably indicates a deep-seated (learned, instinctive?) inhibition which may be lost only in special cases, e.g., psychopathy, psychosis, and acute distress.

These sex differences in formal content, small and infrequent though they are, may reflect preferred as much as actual modes of behavior. Brenneis (1970) argues that a significant aspect of manifest dream content is the exercise of a wish for certain kinds of cognitive and behavioral action, that dreams about motion, extension, separateness reflect something basic about maleness. This view is derived from both Erikson's (1952) and Gutman's

(1965) views about the structuring of perception of reality in males and females. Although these ideas have a quasibiological ring to them, they can, in principle, be derived from what is known about differential socialization pressures on males and females.

A number of years ago, I decided to test the hypothesis that differences in sex-related dream content might be demonstrated (perhaps even more clearly) in samples differing in "masculinity" or "femininity". If comparable or greater differences were found, then it would seem reasonable to emphasize socialization factors since sexual biological variation within each sex is presumably less marked than variation between sexes. I propose this distinction with some caution because, while evidence for a biological explanation for psychological differences in men and women *appears* minimal (Maccoby and Jacklin, 1974), there may be a significant biological factor which interacts with socialization to produce differences in cognitive styles or "preferred adaptive ego modalities" (Brenneis, 1970, p. 440) that are reflected in dream content differences. For example, there is evidence that mesomorphic males are more physically active and aggressive in their dreams than are ectomorphic males (Van de Castle and Smith, 1972). Such a difference does not immediately resolve the biological vs. socialization issue. But it does suggest the importance of exploring *within-sex* variation in sex-relevant attitudes and behaviors which, covarying with biological sex, may account, more than biological sex *per se*, for more of the cross-sex variation in dream content. This was the initial assumption on which I based my study of the relationship of sex, and sex role orientation, to dream content. In addition, this is the only study on sex and sex role orientation that I know of that uses dream content categories which reflect theoretical concepts (e.g., "agency", "communion") regarding the general nature of maleness and femaleness as well as more traditional categories, e.g., aggression. It is possible that the use of general, theoretically relevant categories rather than a series of discrete, largely atheoretical categories constitutes a more powerful tool for assessing fundamental differences in the psychological experience of types of individuals. A similar problem occurs in personality research. Individuals may differ minimally if at all on any one of a number of scale items. Were individual comparisons between two groups made for each item, few differences would emerge. Yet, often, this is the kind of method employed in group comparison studies of dream content differences. Thus, out of 34 comparisons, Brenneis (1970) found only eight that reached statistical significance despite large sample size (72 males, 111 females). Had he employed more general, theoretically relevant factor-like categories, he might have obtained more powerful empirical support for his hypotheses regarding the fundamental differences in perception and cognition revealed in dreams of males and females. A factor analytic study of traditional dream content categories of male vs. female dreams would benefit theorizing about the nature of sex differences in dream content.

The study which I am about to describe (Cohen, 1973b) began with some general assumptions which suggested specific predictions. The major assumption was the continuity between waking experience as perceived by the individual and dream content. The validity of this assumption has been documented in a number of studies (Domino, 1976a). For example, Adelson (1959) reported some interesting differences in the dream content of bright college women who were categorized as more vs. less creative. The former group reported dreams that appeared to be more interesting, vital, innovative. The best study of creativity and dream content is probably that of Domino (1976b). He carefully selected, on the basis of teacher ratings and questionnaire data, two groups of high school students who differed on level of creativeness. The highly creative group produced dreams that were characterized by more "primary process thinking" (unusual or impossible events, bizarre material, condensations, inexplicable transformations, symbolic emphasis, etc.). Another finding commensurate with the wake-sleep continuity hypothesis was reported by Starker (1974). He found an association between daydreaming and dreaming styles. Individuals with a "positive daydreaming style" (pleasant and absorbing) tended to have more pleasant and less bizarre (diary-recorded) dreams than did individuals with "negative daydreaming style" (involving a preoccupation with guilt, fear, and conflict). Schechter et al. (1965) found the diary dream reports of art students to be more imaginative, and to be relatively more unpleasant than pleasant, than the reports of science and engineering students.[1] These differences may be a function of differences in cognitive style and/or emotionality. For example, it is now evident that social science majors as well as high school students intending to major in social science score higher on neuroticism than do science majors or even high school students intending to major in those areas (Horn et al., 1975).

Cross-gender biological differences and differential socialization pressure will tend to affect cognitive, experiential, and behavioral differences. According to the continuity assumption, these differences should be reflected in different dream patterns. However, within-gender variation in biological and socialization factors guarantees substantial overlap between the sexes in these characteristics. Therefore, it was predicted that differences in sex role orientation might be as important as or more important than sex difference per se, in accounting for differences in certain kinds of dream content. In order to capture the hypothesized essential quality of sex related experience, I utilized two categories derived from empirically tested (Carlson, 1971a) ideas of Bakan (1966). The first category, representing maleness, is "agency". This is characterized by self-assertion, separateness, instrumentality, mastery of physical environment, and libidinal sexuality. "Communion", the category representing femaleness, consists of interpersonal concerns and interests, connectedness with others, cooperation.

Each group of male ($N = 27$) and female ($N = 32$) subjects who produced at least two content-scorable home dreams was divided into a masculine or feminine sex role orientation subgroup by using the median of the California Personality Inventory (CPI) femininity (Fe) scale scores specific to each sex group. Fe is not a measure of effeminiteness but rather it is an estimate of the degree to which an individual subscribes to attitudes, interests, values, feelings supposedly characteristic of males or females in our society. It is an estimate of the fit between personality and stereotypical sex role orientation. A high Fe score denotes helpfulness, gentleness, moderation, sensitivity, sincerity, sympathy. A low Fe score denotes hard-headed outgoing ambitiousness, opportunism, robust activity, and impatience with delay. Each of the two dreams provided by each subject was scored for agency, communion, and aggression. Agency was composed of three subcategories including (a) "surgency" (e.g., self-expansion, assertiveness, etc.), (b) "instrumentality" (e.g., mastery, problem solving, etc.), and (c) "libido" ("raw" sexuality). Communion was composed of three subcategories including (a) "active social cooperation" (e.g., altruism,

---

[1] Schechter et al. (1965) also found a large difference in the spontaneous reporting of color perception in the dream reports (50% of the art students, 16% of the science students, and 0% of the engineering students). These differences tended to be maintained despite inquiry. The meaning of this difference is brought into question by a laboratory study of color in REM dreams. Kahn, Dement, Fisher, and Barmack (1962) found evidence of definitely colored dreams in 70.1% of the 87 reports, and evidence of "vaguely colored dreams" in 17.3% of the reports. The investigators conclude that color, while not readily noticed in dreams or wakefulness is commonly experienced, and "that it is the lack of color rather than its presence in dream recall which requires explanation" (p. 1055).

TABLE 9-1.   Agency Scores for Gender and Sex Role
Orientation

Gender	Sex role orientation		
	Masculine	Feminine	Combined
Male			
$\bar{X}$	1.87*	1.08*	1.48
SD	1.43	0.41	1.25
Female			
$\bar{X}$	1.40	0.82	1.11
SD	1.17	0.74	0.99
Combined			
$\bar{X}$	1.63**	0.95**	
SD	1.38	0.51	

*$p < 0.001$.
**$p < 0.01$.

helping, etc.), (b) "passive social connectedness" (e.g., reunion, receiving support, etc.), and (c) "eros" (e.g., expressions of warmth, sympathy, etc.). Each dream was scored for the presence or absence of each of these subcategories of agency and communion separately. A maximum score for either agency or communion was 6 (3 subcategories $\times$ 2 dreams). Since dream content may contain elements of both agency and communion, the scores should not be considered redundant measures. In addition to scoring these categories on which the two judges attained reliabilities of .77 for agency, .64 for communion, they scored the dreams for the presence or absence of physical and verbal forms of aggression.

Table 9-1 shows the results for agency, and Table 9-2 shows the results for communion. For both categories, the effect of sex role orientation was greater than that of sex. Male dreams were higher in agency than were female dreams but the difference was not statistically significant. Likewise, the effect of gender on communion was nonsignificant, with males slightly higher.[2] However, disregarding sex, masculine subjects had significantly

TABLE 9-2.   Communion Scores for Gender and Sex
Role Orientation

Gender	Sex role orientation		
	Masculine	Feminine	Combined
Male			
$\bar{X}$	0.67*	2.08*	1.38
SD	0.48	1.08	0.88
Female			
$\bar{X}$	1.33	1.00	1.17
SD	0.90	0.71	0.83
Combined			
$\bar{X}$	1.00**	1.54**	
SD	0.80	0.77	

*$p < 0.001$.
**$p < 0.05$.

[2] A recent study (Trupin, 1975) found higher agency in the REM dreams of boys, higher communion in the dreams of girls (median age 12 years).

TABLE 9-3.   Percentage of Subjects with Total
Agression in Their Dreams

	Sex role orientation		
Gender	Masculine	Feminine	Combined
Male	67	42	56
Female	47	35	44
Combined	57	38	

higher agency content than had feminine subjects while feminine subjects had significantly higher communion content than had masculine subjects. The interesting finding was that for both content analyses, it was the sex role orientation differences *within the male subjects* which accounted for the major effects. That is, masculine males had significantly higher agency and significantly lower communion scores than had their female counterparts.

Before I offer an interpretation of this pattern, consider the results from the aggression ratings. Percentage of subjects reporting dreams of aggression is shown in Table 9-3. Again there is a predictable trend indicating more males than females with such content, and a *somewhat larger* (but also nonsignificant) difference favoring masculine over feminine subjects which is largely the result of a greater *within-male* than within-female difference. When physical and verbal subtypes of aggression were separated, it was apparent that, while there was no clear relationship for verbal scores, physical scores were more clearly in the predictable direction. Thus, the masculine male group was highest in physical aggression content percentage (53%), feminine females were lowest (12%). Another prediction was tested: that subjects whose sex role orientation is contrary to stereotype (actually, that subgroup of subjects of unknown size whose personality reflects a resistance to, rather than an actualization of, socialization pressures) will tend to have dreams associated with dysphoric affect. Table 9-4 shows the results to be in the predicted direction, and again, the difference is greater (and statistically significant) for the males than for the females.

Aside from the obvious fact that sex-related personality characteristics tend to have as much or more influence than sex *per se* on certain kinds of dream content, what else do these results suggest? The most salient characteristic of the agency, communion, aggression, and affect data was the greater effect of variation in personality within the male subjects. This pattern of results suggested to me that, "because there is less toleration in our society for deviation from sex role stereotype in males, sex role orientation is a psychologically more salient commitment for males than for females" (Cohen, 1973b, p. 251). This hypothesis fits with other reported results suggesting that "young boys are discouraged from engaging in

TABLE 9-4.   Percentage of Subjects with
Unpleasantness Greater than Pleasantness
Associated with Dreams

	Sex role orientation	
Gender	Masculine	Feminine
Male	33*	67*
Female	60	47

*$p < 0.05$.

sex-inappropriate behaviors to a greater extent than are young girls" (Bem and Lenney, 1976), and that, especially for males, personality characteristics which are contrary to stereotype elicit negative reactions from both males and females (Bardwick, 1971; Hartley, 1959; Money and Tucker, 1975; Seyfried and Hendrick, 1973).

If these results are substantiated, then there may be two things to be learned from dream content about sex role orientation: (1) Males, far more than females, tend to maximize either agency at the expense of communion, or tend to cultivate communion while suppressing agency. (2) The male who develops a sex role orientation that is contrary to stereotype (especially when this occurs in apparent opposition to socialization pressure, e.g., from family) pays a psychological price in the form of susceptibility to anxiety, conflict, etc. By using some examples of dream reports, we can nicely illustrate both the clear discrepancy between masculine and feminine male personality, and the evidence of psychological disturbance that may accrue to the stereotype-incongruent male who does not have other sources of strength to draw upon.

Obvious examples of a feminine and of a masculine male dream are as follows:

I see G and L in Herman Park in Houston. I want G to go to the Winnipeg Royal Ballet with me that night. She already has tickets to go to some other club. I blow it off and am somewhat disappointed.

I dreamed that I was some kind of merchant dealing with both sides in the American Civil War. I took my payments in sex with northern and southern women.

I want to reinforce two points about the difference in the dreams produced by the masculine and the feminine males. First, the obvious difference in agency and communion, most clearly reflected in the two examples above, was more or less characteristic of many of the dream reports provided by the two subgroups. In order to demonstrate this, and to provide further support for the continuity assumption, a set of dream reports was selected. One was provided by masculine males, one by feminine males. The Fe scale scores of the feminine males were one standard deviation above (high Fe), those of the masculine males one standard deviation below (low Fe), the mean of the larger sample from which the original subjects were selected. Therefore, these two small samples of dream reports were derived partly from the subjects who produced the data for the major content analyses, partly from nonsubjects. For the following analysis, the disadvantage of using fewer reports of somewhat poorer quality per individual was offset by the advantage of having groups defined in terms of greater deviation from each other. Twelve feminine males (of whom 67% had been subjects) and 13 masculine males (of whom 62% had been subjects) provided at least a fragment of dream content. Each of 23 judges (first and second year graduate students taking a psychopathology course) received a differently randomized set of 25 dream protocols, one protocol per subject. Each judge was also given a description of the characteristics associated with high or low Fe scores. The descriptions were derived from the CPI manual. Of the 12 high Fe protocols, 77% received more "feminine" than "masculine" votes (a total of 177 "feminine" vs. 99 "masculine" votes); of the 13 low Fe protocols, 77% received more "masculine" than "feminine" votes (a total of 212 "masculine" vs. 87 "feminine" votes). Interestingly, the ability to label the protocols correctly was unaffected by the sex, theoretical bias (psychodynamic vs. behavioral), or confidence of the judges.

The second point that requires some discussion is that, especially in males, sex role orientation contrary to stereotype carries a greater risk for psychological conflict. This assumption has recently attained support from some rather novel data reported by Gur *et al.* (1976). They observed a tendency for higher psychopathology scores to be associated with males who habitually sit on the right side of classrooms (from their perspective) and females who sit on the left side. The association between seating preference and pathology was *somewhat greater for males* than for females. The basic argument is that one tends to seek out a seating arrangement that will maximize preferred direction of gaze. Direction of gaze preference supposedly indicates a dominance of the cerebral hemisphere *opposite* to the direction of gaze. The left hemisphere (analytical, mathematical, etc.) is "masculine" while the right hemisphere (analogical, intuitive, emotional, etc.) is "feminine". Males who prefer sitting on the right and who therefore tend to look left (toward the lecturer) are demonstrating a tendency toward right hemisphere dominance, and females who sit on the left demonstrate a tendency toward left dominance. Each of the characteristics is incongruent with stereotypical sex role orientation and thus is associated with a tendency toward more emotional disturbance. Thus, from left field as it were, we have additional support for the hypothesis which was supported in my dream content study (see Table 9-4).

A major problem with the dream content study was that I used the bipolar Fe scale which forces subjects to *choose* either a masculine or feminine preference when both or neither may apply. This criticism is supported by evidence (e.g., Block, 1973) that individuals scoring high on *both* masculine and feminine preferences (androgynous types) appear to be more mature and "self-actualized" than either masculine, feminine, sex-incongruent, or other types. The use of Fe-type scales precludes the separation of such individuals. Therefore, in follow-up research, we will make the following two predictions. First, individuals, especially males, who demonstrate significant sex role preference that is contrary to stereotype will show signs of psychological disturbance in their dreams (will be less well-adjusted). Of course, such a prediction would presumably fare better were we able to select those individuals showing such a preference despite socialization pressures in the sex-congruent direction. Second, individuals who show preference for masculine and feminine characteristics (androgynous types) will show maximal agency and communion and relatively little unpleasantness or misfortune in their dreams. A more interesting variant of this hypothesis is that individuals who show androgyny (agency and communion) and pleasantness in their dreams will more likely be happy and satisfied with their lives than individuals showing other combinations of dream content. Finally, it might be interesting to explore the relationship between the fit between dream and questionnaire-derived characteristics on the one hand and other kinds of behavior (e.g., personal or marital adjustment). For example, are the most enduring and successful marriages those composed of individuals each of whose dream and waking characteristics are congruent (continuous) or complementary? Likewise, is the incongruity between, say, dream emphasis on communion vs. waking emphasis on agency in a feminine activist an indication that her activities constitute a rebellious ("neurotic") phase, perhaps a desperate attempt to reject middle class values? The utility of dream content *vis-à-vis* waking behavior in testing the validity or stability of that behavior goes virtually untested in the dream content analysis literature: this, despite the possibility that dream-behavior disparity might provide a useful vehicle for the empirical assessment of conflictful vs. conflict-free behavior.

Let us return to the issue of sex-role preference contrary to stereotype as it is manifested in the dreams of male subjects. Consider the first dream reproduced above (p. 146). Aside from the obvious communional quality, there is a quality of sensitivity and nonassertiveness bordering on the helpless. Other feminine male dreams expressed these and other qualities suggesting disturbance, conflict, identity uncertainty. For example, here is a dream report of another high Fe male:

> J comes home with her parents in a convertible. She has *dyed her hair* red and cut it in a long shag. Her house is next to mine. C is present but *turns into B*. Apparently J's parents have gone to Colorado to get her. It is a *very awkward* situation. Her stepfather *doesn't remember* B or *me*. Mrs. S, J's mother, introduces us to Mr. S. B is wearing a bathing suit. He is turned on by J. He gets an erection which is very visible. His *penis falls out* of his bathing suit and starts *bleeding and deteriorating*.

I have added italics to emphasize what appear to be signs of identity uncertainty, vulnerability, helplessness. This kind of thing is seen in other reports of other subjects, for example, "turning into a woman", "a dog with its head cut off". It is tempting to hypothesize that there is a large subgroup of high Fe males who, despite socialization pressure to the contrary, have committed themselves to a personality style for which they pay a significant psychological price. This price may include the more frequent occurrence of psychological (e.g., fantasies suggesting "castration anxiety") and psychophysiological (e.g. impotence) problems. (Recall the findings of Beutler *et al.*, 1975 on the association between psychogenic impotence and high Fe scores.) Another subgroup, those males who have developed a feminine orientation out of a combination of temperamental and socialization influences both of which facilitate and encourage such an orientation, would presumably not be as adversely affected. In fact there is evidence that, in highly intelligent male individuals, a degree of femininity is associated with creativity (Kanner, 1976).

A similar distinction between what might be called a normal (or healthy) and neurotic organization of ostensibly similar behaviors was suggested by Hampden-Turner and Whitten (1971). They describe two different motives for antiwar feelings and activity during the Vietnam conflict: "the stage-6 man whose conscience shrieks at the barbarity of the Vietnam war perceives *himself* as an "active, creative, thinking, desiring, loving arbiter of right and wrong . . . [while] . . . the stage-2 radical objects to the war because it threatens to delay satisfaction of his own personal needs and impulses" (p. 41). Perhaps the dream content of these two kinds of activist, like that of the two kinds of high Fe male, could provide information beyond waking behavioral differences for a more extensive understanding of the motivation, attitudes, cognitive style, and temperament of these kinds of individuals.

2. PERSONALITY-SITUATION INTERACTION EFFECTS

I have been discussing some of the situational and individual difference influences on broad, nomothetic categories of dream content. Clearly, these cannot be considered to operate in a truly independent fashion either in or outside of the laboratory. Let us consider the interaction effect of personality and situation on dream content. The assumption is that the same conditions will be perceived and reacted to differently by different sorts of individuals. For example, a stress condition orchestrated in the laboratory will not have the same meaning or importance for all individuals. "The same fire that melts the butter hardens the egg" (Allport, 1937, p. 102). In addition, some kinds of stress (e.g., physical threats) are psychologically more salient for some individuals than other kinds of stress (e.g., ego threat). But even if we randomly assign individuals of differing personality characteristics to varieties of presleep manipulations, and even if we can demonstrate interaction effects, we have not necessarily reproduced in microcosm the nature of personality-by-situation effects in the real world. That is, we may artificially magnify interaction effects and minimize correlational effects.

By not giving subjects a choice of situation, we distort the nature of person-by-situation dynamics. In our experiments, situations "choose" individuals (through the process of random assignment to conditions). However, in the real world, the reverse tends to be true; individuals tend to choose situations in order to maximize needs and to exercise talents. Experimental personality research usually follows a paradigm which assumes the individual to be a kind of billiard ball pushed around by the effects of situation. We characterize the individual as a "dependent variable", *subject* to the situation-as-independent variable. The person has been lost in personality research (Carlson, 1971b), which artificially conceives of the normally active, environment-influencing individual as a passive recipient, a subject of external and independent events (Wachtel, 1973). However, individuals actively *choose* environments, selectively attend to environments, even influence those environmental events which then affect them (e.g., Bell, 1968; Harper, 1975). Thus, the so-called "independent variable" represented by the experimental treatment and generating a situation main effect *must* be an artifact. It will be artifactual, i.e., ecologically unrepresentative, when it does not give sufficient recognition to correlational events. Thus, the interaction effects obtained in the research I will be discussing below will to some unknown extent be an artifact of a paradigm which can only approximate the person-situation dynamics of the real world.

Individual differences in dream content associated with stress are easily demonstrated, though the selection of an isolated dimension of content may not yield large differences. For example, in an early study of presleep mood and dream recall (Cohen, 1974b) I separated into two groups those individuals with high or low mean self-confidence presleep ratings (made over a five day recording period). Individuals were then selected to form a set of pairs of subjects, one from each group, who were matched on the basis of an equivalent and low self-confidence rating on a single night and who produced a dream affect rating the next morning. This procedure yielded 14 pairs, each composed of a generally confident or generally nonconfident subject matched with respect to a relatively low mood rating on a particular night. For the confident group, mean unpleasantness of the dream experience associated with that night was significantly less than for the nonconfident group; that is, despite similar presleep situational nonconfident ratings for the two groups (typical for the nonconfident group, atypical for the confident group), the dream reported upon awakening the next morning was clearly pleasant for the confident group and somewhat unpleasant for the nonconfident group. A superficial content analysis carried out *post hoc* revealed very different dream characteristics in the two groups. The confident group produced dreams of shopping, studying, singing, partying, repairing, traveling, playing, and driving. The nonconfident group reported dreams about looking into a mirror, searching, smuggling, watching a funeral, lying down and being attacked, trying to revive a suicide, and feeling the imminence of death. While not directly testable, these findings are consistent with the continuity assumption and with the hypothesis that there are individual differences in the capacity of the dreaming process to work through problems. Thus, it would appear that some individuals (those *generally* feeling self-confident) are more capable than others of "bouncing back" through the active coping process of dreamwork.

In the subsequent study (Cohen, 1974a), an estimate of personality, independent of mood

TABLE 9-5.   Distribution of Subjects for Trait and for State Conditions

Trait	State	
	Highest self-confidence	Lowest self-confidence
Repression		
N	14	14
Mean repression–sensitization	30.9	30.1
Mean self-confidence	1.9	4.8
Sensitization		
N	15	15
Mean repression–sensitization	60.9	60.9
Mean self-confidence	1.7	5.4

ratings, was made by using repression-sensitization scores. Individuals above and below the mean were divided into two subgroups on the basis of either a highest or lowest self confidence presleep mood rating (on the 7-step bipolar scale from —3 through zero to 3). Fifty-eight subjects with scorable dream affect ratings were selected so that level of presleep confidence (on a high or low "target" night) and level of repression-sensitization were uncorrelated. Table 9-5 shows two subgroups of repressors differing markedly on level of presleep mood but not on level of repression, and likewise, two subgroups of sensitizers differing markedly (and similarly to repressors) on presleep mood but not on level of sensitization. Figure 9-1 shows a significant trait-by-mood interaction effect on dream affect. That is, there is a significant ($p < .01$) positive association between valence of dream affect and presleep mood in sensitizers, but a nonsignificant *negative* association between presleep mood and valence of dream affect in repressors. This differential pattern of results was interpreted as supporting the idea that individuals "who rate themselves low on

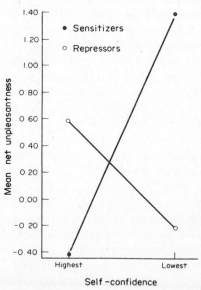

Figure 9-1   Mean net dream unpleasantness as a function of highest and lowest levels of self-confidence in repressors and sensitizers.

measures of coping effectiveness are more at the mercy of presleep mood. They are emotionally more 'field-dependent', that is, more apt to respond with negative mood to negative feedback, with positive mood to positive feedback. Likewise, during sleep, they are more apt to resonate with negative (unsuccessful) dreams in response to negative presleep mood and to resonate with positive (successful) dreams to positive presleep mood" (Cohen, 1974a, p. 153). These results provide additional support for the continuity assumption. They also support the hypothesis that sensitization (neuroticism) reflects a tendency to respond to certain characteristics of the environment with affective reactions which are stronger and more lasting than are the responses of repressors (Eysenck and Rachman, 1965). An additional test of the continuity assumption was carried out in a follow-up laboratory study of college males (Cohen and Cox, 1975).

Subjects who scored above 33 or below 17 on the Neuroticism scale of the Maudsley Personality Inventory (whom we will refer to as sensitizers and repressors respectively) were randomly assigned to a negative or positive presleep condition. There were 11 sensitizers and 11 repressors in the positive condition, 12 sensitizers and 11 repressors in the negative condition. The negative condition included nonfriendly or perfunctory treatment of the subject, little subject-experimenter interaction (including 15 minutes of subject isolation during the set-up of the apparatus), little information about procedures, and "failure" of an IQ test (induced by using some of the hardest items on the WAIS and artificially short durations for timed items). The positive condition was generally the obverse of these manipulations. Each subject was run individually on a single night. Both REM and NREM awakenings were made. Prior to lights out, the subject filled out a mood rating sheet which included three bipolar, seven step (—3 through zero to 3) affect dimensions (happy-depressed, angry-affectionate, nervous-relaxed). The ratings on these were combined to form a single affect mood rating. The subject was informed in the morning that another set of mood ratings was required. Finally, prior to debriefing, a postexperimental questionnaire was filled out to assess the perceptions of the subject regarding the experimental situation and to provide an estimate of the validity of the manipulations independent of the dependent measures.

The results of that questionnaire are shown in Table 9-6. The important thing to note is that there are marked and highly significant differences due to conditions, but no interaction effects. That is, both repressors and sensitizers had similar assessments of the situations.

Presleep, dream, and postsleep affect ratings provide the obvious theoretically relevant dimension to assess the condition-by-sensitization interaction effect predicted on the basis of both the continuity assumption and the sensitization-emotionality hypothesis. Figure 9-2 summarizes the results. The abscissa represents both the type of measure and the time since manipulation. The ordinate shows the *degree of association* (represented by point-biserial correlation) between type of presleep condition (positive vs. negative) and valence of affect (derived from presleep and postsleep affect ratings and REM and NREM dream affect ratings). Notice that for the sensitizer group, the association between condition and valence of affect is relatively strong both presleep (in the mood ratings) and during sleep (in the dream experiences), and then tends to diminish by morning. On the other hand, for the repressor group, the initial association is relatively weak (though positive), and drops precipitously during dreaming and upon awaking. The differential pattern of these curves fits rather nicely the prediction of a stronger and more lasting affective reaction in sensitizers than in repressors. The differential pattern for the two groups is consistent with data

TABLE 9-6.   Subjects' Perception of Experimental Conditions on Postexperimental Questionnaire

Question	Experimental condition		Effects		
	Positive	Negative	t	$p<$	r_{pb}
Amt information					
$\overline{X}$	1.50	3.27	7.265	0.0001	0.75
Summary	more than enough	not enough			
Amt interaction					
$\overline{X}$	1.77	3.68	12.259	0.0001	0.88
Summary	enough	less than little			
E Characteristics					
$\overline{X}$	1.32	2.86	11.938	0.0001	0.88
Summary	quite friendly	almost indifferent			
Quality of information					
$\overline{X}$	1.23	2.57	8.449	0.0001	0.80
Summary	quite satisfactory	less than satisfactory			
Quality of interaction					
$\overline{X}$	1.73	2.86	7.224	0.0001	0.74
Summary	quite pleasant	almost neutral			
Belonging					
$\overline{X}$	2.05	3.15	5.497	0.0001	0.66
Summary	part of group	somewhat isolated			
Personal treatment					
$\overline{X}$	1.52	2.95	8.314	0.0001	0.79
Summary	treated personally	treated impersonally			
Data be useful?					
$\overline{X}$	2.45	2.64	<1	n.s.	–
Summary	guess so	not sure			
Be subject again?					
$\overline{X}$	2.27	3.09	2.993	0.005	0.42
Summary	guess so	not sure			

reported by Goodenough et al. (1974). They found higher anxiety in dream content recalled by subjects run in a stress condition who had reported higher anxiety in the presleep situation.

The differential effect of conditions on the two groups was assessed in a somewhat different manner. The "meaning" of the dream was operationally defined in terms of the *correlation* between net unpleasantness of affect (unpleasantness minus pleasantness) and other formal properties of dream content that had been chosen prior to the experiment. Using affect as the major correlate was based on the theoretical relevance of this dimension to the types of subjects used in the study. Table 9-7 shows correlations, obtained separately for each group, between degree of negative affect and the following dimensions: bizarreness, total affect, excitement, personal significance (of the experience to the subject), and noncontemporaneous temporal setting. An interesting differential pattern of correlations is evident for the two groups. For the sensitizers, there is a *positive* correlation between dream unpleasantness and bizarreness, excitement, personal significance, and noncontemporaneous setting. On the other hand, for the repressors, there is a *negative* correlation between dream unpleasantness and bizarreness, excitement and personal significance. It is particularly noteworthy that sensitizers rate unpleasant dreams as

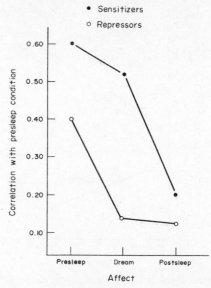

Figure 9-2 Correlation between presleep condition and affect ratings obtained during the evening (presleep mood), at night (dream affect), and during the morning (postsleep) for sensitizers and repressors separately.

personally more significant while the repressors rate those unpleasant dreams as personally less significant. A relatively straightforward explanation of this difference lies in the attitude of repressors and sensitizers toward dysphoric experiences. The differential pattern of correlations shown in Table 9-7 clearly demonstrates the limitations inherent in group comparisons of mean values of a particular variable. We have already seen how such comparisons often yield weak and nonreplicable findings in the psychophysiological correlate area of sleep and dream research (Hauri, 1975; see also Engel, 1975).

Of seven content dimensions, only one showed a trait-by-condition interaction effect that reached the .05 level of significance. This effect is shown in Figure 9-3. The sensitizers had a significantly greater proportion of dreams cast in the nonpresent (mainly, the past), and this was especially true under the negative condition. There are at least two explanations for the differential findings on temporal setting. One possibility is that the sensitizers are generally a more "creative" group. This explanation would be consistent with the following line of reasoning. Sensitizers tend to *report* higher dream recall frequency, and in some samples,

TABLE 9-7. Correlates of Dream Affect (net unpleasantness)

Dimension	Sensitizers		Repressors		Comparison	
	n	r	n	r	Z	$p<$
Bizarreness	22	0.17	18	−0.39*	1.688	0.10
Total affect	22	−0.21	18	−0.19		
Excitement	22	0.47**	18	−0.25	2.195	0.05
Personal significance	21	0.28	18	−0.48**	2.295	0.05
Temporal setting (nonpresent)	21	0.49**	17	0.09	1.267	

*$p < 0.15$.
**$p < 0.05$.

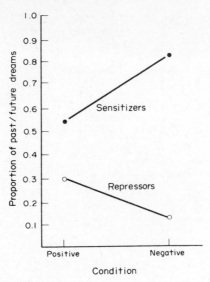

Figure 9-3   Temporal setting of the dream as a function of presleep condition and personality.

this tendency reaches statistical significance. Frequent recallers have been shown more often to be liberal arts- rather than science-oriented, and have dreams that are more creative and more often cast in the past or future (Cohen and MacNeilage, 1974; Schechter *et al.*, 1965). Thus, to some extent, sensitization, interest in "inner life", and creativeness will be associated. Noncontemporaneous dream settings would then be an indication of an innovative cognitive style.

The second possibility is that noncontemporaneous dream settings (especially past settings) indicate immaturity, instability, "regression". This notion would fit with what is known about sensitizers, the fact that noncontemporaneity was greater for sensitizers in the negative condition. It also fits with Hauri's (1976) finding that remitted unipolar depressives continue to cast their REM dreams more often in the past than in the present (or future) compared to controls. Unipolar depression is frequently associated with elevated neuroticism and neuroticlike behavior. Therefore it is not surprising that noncontemporaneity of setting is elevated both in unipolar depression and in high neuroticism subjects under stress. Perhaps under stress (e.g., separation, rejection, failure, etc.) sensitizers are more subject to the reactivation of thought process relevant to earlier satisfaction of anxieties. Perhaps they are more susceptible, under these kinds of condition, to the reactivation of "regressive" or infantile schemata which are dramatized by the dreamwork.[3]

It is particularly interesting that while both repressors and sensitizers tended to dream more *symbolically* (creatively?) about the laboratory situation under the stress condition, the sensitizers more often dreamed about the past while the repressors more often dreamed in the present. That is, for sensitizers, increased presleep stress seems to be associated with a

[3] On the basis of some empirical work reported by Van de Castle (1969) suggesting a correlation between "immaturity" (e.g., youth, late onset of menarche, primitive society vs. adult, early onset of menarche, industrialized society) and animal content in dreams, we predicted that sensitizers would have more animal content, especially in the negative condition, than would repressors. However, only six subjects had animal content, and there was no apparent trend in the data to support the hypothesis.

correlated increase in both symbolic activity and noncontemporaneous setting while for repressors, a corresponding change induces a negative correlation between the two kinds of content. It is tempting to hypothesize that a sign of maturity or ego strength is that capacity to adjust to presleep ego threat by an increase in symbolic activity which deals primarily with the "here and now" (rather than with past gratifications or obsessions) so that adaptive adjustments can be made in preparation for awakening.

Of course, the creativity and immaturity hypotheses proposed to account for the observed differences in temporal dream setting are not necessarily mutually exclusive. These characteristics have long been thought to appear together and to be influenced by a common genetic source (e.g., McNeil, 1971).

CHAPTER 10

DREAMING AS A DETERMINANT OF ADAPTATION

1. ANECDOTAL EVIDENCE

In Part A of this book, my intention was to develop inferences about the psychological properties of dreaming from biological properties of REM sleep. In this chapter, my intention is to develop the hypothesis that dreaming is a psychological process with adaptive properties that can be investigated from the phenomenological perspective. This hypothesis implies two things: (1) Dreaming may be a problem-*solving* process, not merely a problem-reflecting process. (2) Some dreams are "better" than other dreams, because the better dream has the *effect* (cognitive, affective, etc.) of "moving" the person closer to a desirable, useful, adaptive state. The dream is thus conceptualized as a mediating variable, a psychological event with causal as well as dependent properties.

Broadly defined, the concept of adaptation refers to behavior that promotes species survival through adjustment to ecological pressures (Ayala and Dobzhansky, 1974). In the present context, I use it to describe something more limited. Adaptation will denote a change, through information processing, in the relationship between an individual and some problem or challenge either presented by the environment or invented by the individual. For example, the dreaming process can be considered adaptive if an individual goes to sleep having failed to solve an intellectual or interpersonal problem and, after having dreamed about it, is in a better position to solve the problem upon awakening. Naturally, in the absence of systematic empirical examination, a single observation such as this is a rather poor demonstration of adaptation, since one could argue that the correlation between dream event and change in status of the problem may be fortuitous rather than functional. Anecdotes that cannot be substantiated through empirical, and particularly through experimental, test remain anecdotal. Therefore, it is incumbent upon the dream researcher to demonstrate that (a) there is a definite relationship between a presleep problem and a dream experience, and that (b) there is a definite relationship between the dream experience and a measurable increase in the capacity of the individual to deal successfully with the problem. The latter may be in the form of a higher probability of arriving at a solution, attainment of a better solution, or at least, an affective accommodation to the problem. While the laboratory demonstration of adaptation will tend to focus on dream-mediated psychological changes with respect to a specific problem, this must be thought of as a microcosmic representation of events that are more vague and amorphous. In the real world, problems are often less specific (e.g., general adjustment required to learn socially appropriate behaviors, values, attitudes, etc.), and adaptive changes may be more gradual and thus more difficult to identify.

A few points need to be made. First, I am suggesting that to demonstrate that dreaming is adaptive, it is necessary to show that positive or desirable changes are mediated by the specific, problem-relevant focus of the dreaming process. Second, not all dreaming will be adaptive in the sense of promoting measurable improvement in the condition of the individual *vis-à-vis* some challenge or problem. Third, recall of the dreaming experience is not required for adaptation. However, at some point in the research enterprise, it is necessary to demonstrate, on the basis of verbal reports, that dreaming of a specific sort has taken place. Fourth, it is neither necessary nor statistically likely that a solution occur in a dream. Rather, it is sufficient that the dream prepare the individual to be in a more advantageous position with respect to the problem. Fifth, there are situational and dispositional factors which affect the variability in adaptive responsiveness of the dreaming process and in the receptivity of the individual during wakefulness to changes wrought by the dreaming process. That is, a solution arrived at during the REM dreaming state may be available (part of LTM) but not accessible during wakefulness.

Formal properties of dreams and the adaptation hypothesis

The adaptive significance of dreams is not by any means universally assumed. According to Shakespeare's Mercutio, dreams "are the children of an idle brain . . . thin of substance as the air, and more inconstant than the wind". Par Lagerkvist's dwarf, a dyspeptic character of limited insights and cruel sentiments — a creature known for statements like "Love is always disgusting . . ." and "I know of nothing more detestable than music" — says of dreams: "I do not bother about dreams; they mean nothing and make no difference" (Lagerkvist, 1945). According to Murphy, the view that dreaming is a waste of time is a characteristic of modern, industrialized societies. Sleep "is a sad psychological waste that has no economic value except as a hostage to tomorrow's toil; its psychological product is industrial waste, occasionally salvaged by the psychoanalytical chemist, but for most people most of the time, so gross that it is not commercially worth the cost of claiming it." "Nobody wants a 'dreamer'. Let's get down to business. This attitude has resulted, I believe, in one of the greatest instances of myopia to be found in contemporary psychology" (1947, p. 416).

Kleitman, the founder of modern sleep research, and presumably receptive to the scientific investigation of dreams, nevertheless offers the following view:

> To those who insist that because dreams occur they must serve a particular purpose, it may be pointed out that not all processes have a teleological explanation. Vomiting, for instance, when it is elicited by some irritating matter in the stomach, serves a good purpose in evacuating the stomach and removing the irritant. The same vomiting act, when resulting from motion sickness, serves no physiological purpose. The explanation of the latter type of vomiting is that the vestibular centers in the medulla were unduly excited from the unusual motion of the body, and this excitation has spread to the neighboring vomiting center. This explanation is correct, but it is not teleological. Dreaming may be considered a crude type of cortical activity associated with a recurrent appearance of stage 1 EEG in the course of a night's sleep. Because this is an emergent stage 1 EEG, rising from a lower level of cortical function, it is less effective in furthering analysis, integration, and recall than the initial stage 1 EEG. As such, dreaming need not have a special function and may be quite meaningless. The effects of dream curtailment, discovered by Dement, may be due to interference with an acquired

habit. When one develops a craving for sweets — no vital nutritional necessity — and the supply is temporarily cut off, one may resent the curtailment and may overindulge, for a time, when the supply is restored (Kleitman, 1963, p. 107).

These views, collectively, can stand for the null hypothesis regarding adaptive significance, namely that, even if dreams have symbolic meaning, dreaming *per se* has no instrumental value. That the recall of dream content may occasionally elicit insightful solutions postsleep is not evidence for the rejection of the null hypothesis. That dream content may represent a *solution* to a problem which was unsolvable prior to sleep *would* constitute evidence for the rejection of the null hypothesis.

There have been three general methodological approaches employed by investigators who ,are more or less committed to the rejection of the null hypothesis regarding adaptive function. One is the comparison of the effects of REM deprivation and NREM interruption on learning, memory, and information processing. The problem with this strategy is that the data are more amenable to hypotheses regarding the physiology or psychophysiology of REM sleep than to the content of dreaming *per se*. In addition, the adaptive hypothesis may be better served by looking at different kinds of dream content rather than by trying to prevent dreaming, just as the exploration of the adaptive properties of thinking are better served by manipulating or noting differences in the problem-relevance of thoughts rather than by trying to prevent thinking altogether. In short, the question addressed here is the relevance, not the presence or absence, of dream content.

The second method for testing the adaptive hypothesis for dreams is basically one of inference from either the formal or substantive properties of dream content. Regarding the former, assume that an analysis of the formal properties of dream content reveals a chaotic, disorganized, sequentially fragmentary jumble. (I discussed in Chapter 6 some of the sampling and recall factors that could influence dream reporting so as to yield such an impression.) We could hardly infer from such characteristics the capacity to adjust in an adaptive manner, if not to solve problems.

A somewhat less radical view of the organization of dreaming is that it is neither chaotic and random, nor organized rationally in the service of problem solving, but rather that it is characterized by sequential packages of information, one cuing off the next and so on: a "ballistic, not guided" process (Klinger, 1971, p. 181). I believe that a purely ballistic view of dream sequencing is essentially incorrect. Paivio (1971) has offered a statement regarding imagery and the relationship between verbal and imagery processing that is congruent with my views about the nature of dreaming:

> Despite the supporting evidence, the conditioning model encounters general difficulties that must be recognized. Granted that sensations can be conditioned and that this might occur to a limited degree in the case of verbal stimuli, classical conditioning seems inadequate to explain the productive quality and flexibility of imagery as an associative reaction to language. The images aroused by verbal cues often appear too complex and creative for them to have been acquired on the basis of actual contiguities in experience. Thus one can imagine objects and events that have never been experienced as percepts. The elements may be familiar, but their combination as images may be quite novel, not explainable in terms of actual associative experiences as demanded by the conditioning model. Something analogous to primary stimulus generalization might further such an explanation, but it would be strained and lacking in empirical support. In this respect imagery is similar to language, which is characterized especially by its productivity — one can say things that have never been said

before, using old and familiar elements. Both imagery and verbal processes seem to require some kind of generative mechanism that will construct the content of the imagery or the verbal output from stored schemata, as emphasized by Bartlett (1932) in the case of memory, and more recently by Neisser (1967) in the case of cognitive processes generally. The nature of such a mechanism is unknown, although a neuropsychological theory such as Hebb's may eventually be sophisticated enough to cope with the phenomena. In any event, conditioning as it is presently understood in the laboratory setting is probably insufficient as a thoretical explanation for language-evoked images (p. 71).

If Klinger's (1971) ballistic concept were more valid than Paivio's "productivity" concept, we could hardly infer problem solving activity during dreaming. We could accept the idea that dreaming is about our current concerns and may, fortuitously, yield an idea or image that might be of some use to the individual once he is awake. But dreaming, like fantasy, would be relatively incapable of the instrumentally useful work that characterizes the directed thought of wakefulness. The two are seen as complementary though they may influence each other: dreams and fantasy providing raw material, directed thought providing the actual creative integrations. This view is more or less compatible with what, according to Hartmann (1973), REM dreams typically lack: subtle affects, a sense of free-will, changes in behavior due to feedback from others, concentration, reality testing. Surely, if these ego functions are mediated by catecholamine systems requiring "restoration" during REM sleep, and if they are solely the product of a fully functioning left hemisphere, and if dreaming is largely the product of information processing by the right hemisphere, then it is not surprising to find deficits in ego functioning that are represented in REM dreams, deficits which would make it more difficult to adhere to a hypothesis that REM dreaming is a period during which significant adaptations occur with reasonable frequency. However, as we have seen, our view of dream content is seriously affected by numerous subject, situation, sleep, and recall factors. In addition, Hartmann's own theory of the catecholamine restoration function of REM sleep supports the hypothesis that dreaming should become more and more reflective of good ego functioning, and thus more capable of supporting adaptive processes, as the night wears on and the catecholamine depletion is reversed by successive REM periods. Perhaps this is a major implication of the GILD hypothesis proposed earlier (see Chapter 7, section 2): that dreaming becomes more and more dominated by the left hemisphere, and that this results in a better balance between the intuitive and rational, subjective and sensible, impulsive and cautious. The result might be thought of as regression in the service of the ego, or in the language of the GILD hypothesis, a better integration of right hemisphere with left hemisphere functioning. The point is that inferences from formal properties of dream content about the limitations of the adaptive capacity of dreaming are subject to many sources of bias.

Dream content and the adaptation hypothesis

In addition to formal properties, substantive characteristics of dream content can be used to infer that problem solving occurs in dreaming. For example, Foulkes (1967) collected REM dream material from four preadolescent boys, and inferred a kind of problem solving process which he calls "anticipatory socialization". The child "is looking forward to what he would like to be in terms of his physical, social, and psychosexual development, or, perhaps even more accurately, to what he would like to *do* in the world about him — and he is doing so with a generally realistic appraisal of the difficulties involved". Foulkes suggests that "dreams of the preadolescent male may also profitably be viewed in terms of attempts at anticipating and mastering contemporary problems which arise in the social world. In this respect, there appears to be a considerable continuity between the child's play and his dreams, both as to content and as to function" (Foulkes, 1967, p. 97). Many dreams collected in our laboratory appear to contain elements of challenge (problem) and efforts to respond (solve), though obvious examples of solutions are extremely rare.

This is not to imply that mental work during dreaming in the laboratory is always interesting. Many of the dreams are relaxed, passive, hedonistic, narrow, simple-minded, two-dimensional, dull, mundane, parochial, shallow, egocentric, unenviable experiences that challenge the belief that the unconscious always merits our rapt attention. However, as with waking thoughts, there are other kinds: more complex, effortful, intellectual, suggesting that one of the basic characteristics of organized neural protoplasm in the head of the average undergraduate male is response to challenge. This problem solving activity comes in many forms both crude and lofty, self-serving and altruistic. In one dream, a subject successfully prevents a man from suiciding over the drowning of a young girl in a swimming pool. Another subject tries unsuccessfully to save a father from drowning after he hits his head against some object when he jumps into a river to save his little girl. Another subject runs after and catches the thief who removed some geological samples from a classroom. Alarm clocks sometimes have a focal role in the dreams of our subjects. In one, the dreamer unsuccessfully explains to the experimenter how a complicated radio-alarm clock works while in another dream, another subject tries without success to figure out how a giant six foot high alarm clock works. For many subjects, different aspects of the laboratory situation and sleeping arrangement create problems to be worked on during the dream. One subject dreamed that the reference wire (attached to the ear) was too short. His attempt to solve the problem was both noninnovative and unsuccessful; he asked the experimenter if it could be lengthened. The experimenter declined, saying something about possibly "messing up the frequency". The experience was so vivid and realistic to the subject that he says, during the actual interview subsequent to the dream: "Oh boy! It seemed like you came in here and we were talking about this stuff. I can't separate what's happening now from what was happening in the dream. I might be in the dream right now!" We are immediately reminded of Chuang-tsu's man who awakens from a dream of being a butterfly, only to wonder if a butterfly is now dreaming of being a man!

Sometimes both the problems and the solutions are more challenging, complicated, and unsuccessfully handled. For example, after dreaming (during the third REM period) about an unsuccessful attempt to teach his younger brother some piano exercises through demonstration, remonstration, and explanation, the subject has a dream (during the fourth REM period) which proves him to be a master at problem solving:

"... may have been about a test and about blocks. I guess you couldn't make a circle with those blocks, could you? (Describe the test.) OK, the test was on a sheet of paper and pencil ... I was not the only person taking the test — there were a lot of people like at the university level — in a large room, and, uh, the only thing I remembered about it was a circle ... just a large circle ... [something about] testing. I think I wrote the block. I drew in the circle on the sheet of paper, and I think that was the correct response. I was real elated ... I just understood, I just understood ... I got the feeling that I was the only person in the room that would get it right ... that it was very unique to get the right answer ... I knew intuitively that that was the correct answer."

Of course, the validity of this kind of "solution" cannot be evaluated against some external criterion as in the examples to be given below. In this case the subject had worked on the block design of the WAIS IQ test prior to sleep. Blocks may have been on his mind though there is no solution. Perhaps the subject was dramatizing, during the dream, some kind of insight about the similarity or comparability of square and circular forms, some passing thought he might have had and suppressed during the presleep task.

Sometimes the impoverished and disorganized quality of the recall process gives one the impression that much of the cognitive effort characteristic of some dreams is illogical at best, pedestrian at worst. One subject reports about a dream where he debates with fraternity members the best way to improve the finances of the fraternity; the subject argues in favor of investing in certificates of deposit, others argue the merits of stocks and bonds. This dream, notable for its rather pragmatic, mundane, and undreamlike quality, is all the more remarkable coming, as it does, from the 14th REM period of a night of rather severe restriction of REM sleep! Now consider the following example of nocturnal "logic" in what we might call "the prisoner's riddle":

It was about a proof — a logic problem . . . this guy is sitting in prison thinking about it . . . the problem is the guy is sent to prison and he is a murderer or something, and the judge convicts him, and he's gonna be hanged . . . on Monday, Tuesday, Wednesday, Thursday, or Friday of the next week at six o'clock in the morning — but he won't know which day till that morning. This guy is just sitting — this is actually in the dream — he is sitting on the bed thinking about it . . . hands on his chin. . . . Anyway, so the guy says that he can eliminate Friday cause if they haven't come to him by Thursday, he'll know Friday — that he will be hanged, and it wouldn't be a surprise in the morning. If you can eliminate Friday, then Thursday is the last day, so you can eliminate Thursday cause if they didn't come Wednesday morning he'd know they were gonna come Thursday cause Friday was gone . . . and he eliminated all the days up to Monday and decided that he wouldn't be hanged . . . and the judge came and hung him on Tuesday (laugh).

The subject told the experimenter that the dream seemed to relate to logic problems he was given in class recently. The quality of the experience is vaguely reminiscent of the "Zeno paradox" problem in which, through verbal distortion of physical laws (not unlike visual illustrations or "impossible figures" which cannot be duplicated in concrete objects), a fast running rabbit never catches up to the sluggish tortoise. Thus we have an example of the dream as *recreation* both in the reproductive, mnesic sense, and in the active, playful sense. But to the pragmatic and skeptical individual, that dreaming may involve mental effort, even attempts at solution, does not constitute evidence of "real" progress (e.g., actual solutions to problems) measured against objective criteria external to the dream. This kind of evidence comes basically in two kinds: anecdotal evidence of dreamed solutions (none accompanied by objective evidence that the subject was actually asleep and dreaming), and empirical evidence of a connection between problem related dream content and some kind of adaptive change in behavior (evidence extremely difficult to come by).

Inferences about the problem solving capacity of dreaming come from anecdotal evidence of "solutions". I am talking about symbolic activity that goes beyond clever *representation* of a problem (assuming that the cleverness is in the dreamwork rather than in the interpreter's "thoughtwork") to a literal or symbolic solution of the problem (a solution which the individual upon awakening may not realize is a solution). Sometimes an inference that a dream provides a "solution" seems strained, requiring a kind of intuitive appreciation.

For example, one of my students recounted a dream narrated by his friend's girlfriend. Apparently, she was quite attached to the friend, but he was about to move in with some other people which would mean that she would be left behind. The night of the final departure, she dreamed that she got up in the middle of the night and went into the living room of the house where she and a boyfriend and three other college men were staying temporarily. In actuality, the living room was the center of the social life of the house, and included a coffee table on which was a collection of pipes and assorted tobaccos belonging to the men. In the dream, the girlfriend gathers up the pipes, cleans them, and puts them in a pan of water. When the men return to try to light up, they can't get them lit. If we are comfortable with a Freudian attitude toward fantasy, interpreting this dream event should provide little problem. For those who do not carry around with them comfortable *a priori* assumptions about dream content, the dream merely seems intuitively to offer a kind of solution. Perhaps the answer lies in cutting the men down, making them less masculine in the sense of less mature, independent, adventuresome. Perhaps such a solution carried with it an additional "benefit": a way of expressing resentment, of getting back. Or perhaps the dream is less a solution than a representation of the actual personally disturbing state of affairs; a young lady tries to do something special for the men she wants to stay with. She tries to make something special (the pipes which are the center of attention in the central room of the house) even better (clean the pipes), but in doing so she makes things worse. She is incompetent in spite of her efforts, and thus there is no solution.

This kind of dream fragment illustrates the difficulty with anecdotal "evidence". We know little or nothing about the person, have an inadequate sample of dream content, know next to nothing of the presleep situation, and are without external criteria by which we could judge whether the dreamed events actually do constitute an adaptive sort of solution. (Perhaps she is most insightful into the psychology of her male friends. Perhaps if she actually carried out the pipe cleaning task and it failed, as in the dream, but the men realized how much she cared and were taken by her devotion, and *agreed to keep her*, we might be more impressed with the inference that this dream represents a kind of social psychological "solution".)

Another issue is the best rate problem. If only one out of a hundred dreams can be considered, against external criteria, to be a reasonably good solution to a problem, does this constitute a better than average hit rate? Better than waking thoughts? How representative of the population of *solution* dreams to total dreams (including dreams that attempted solutions, dreams that merely represent the problem, dreams that are irrelevant) are recalled dreams? How attentive are we to solution dreams vs. other dreams? Perhaps solution dreams are extremely rare but more likely to be recalled, remembered, and recounted, thus giving us a biased view of the usefulness or adaptiveness of dreaming, perhaps not. We just don't know.

Krippner and Hughes (1970) describe many examples of more obvious solution dreams. For example, Elias Howe, inventor of the sewing machine, took advantage of a dreamed solution to a problem. The obvious place for the hole in the needle was near the top rather than the tip. Perhaps out of a functional set characteristic of the relative inflexibility of waking thought under the stress of invention, Howe's progress was stymied. Then he had a dream in which savages demanded he invent a functional sewing machine within 24 hours. He could not do it so he was sentenced to death by spears with eye-shaped holes in the tips. Howe responded to the dreamed solution, made the appropriate needle, and had himself a workable sewing machine. If true, this would be an example of a better idea during dreaming than was available during wakefulness. Perhaps we have many such "better ideas", but fail to recognize them because of the dramatic, symbolic transformations that obscure their meaning. According to Dement, "perhaps only the most perceptive dreamers possess the ability to recognize a solution that is presented in disguised or symbolic fashion." "One can easily imagine Kekule shrugging as he awakened from the dream of the six circling snakes: 'What nonsense! I must forget about snakes and concentrate on chemistry'" (Dement, 1972, p. 101).

What problems are dreams most suited to?

This example of dreamwork brings up an issue that has not been given sufficient attention: if dreaming can be relevant to problems, if dreams can sometimes attain solutions to problems, then what kinds of problems are more likely to yield solutions during dreaming? Regardless of whether the content of the problem is personal, interpersonal, or intellectual, are there certain kinds of problems for which dreaming can compete with waking thought? There is no specific answer to this question, and I doubt that I can dream one up. I say this because it is my impression that the kind of problems that dreams are relatively more efficient in dealing with are those problems that are best solved in the language of imagery rather than in the language of words or mathematics, and the question I just posed is more amenable to verbal and mathematical language than to imagery.

In a book called *Conceptual Blockbusting,* Adams (1974) discusses the numerous ways that problem solving can be blocked by false and misleading assumptions or habits that constitute a narrow, stereotyped, safe, and uninspired approach to intellectual challenges. A major block to problem solving is the incorrect selection from a set of possible languages. For example, I borrow from Adams (1974, p. 4) who borrowed from Koestler who borrowed from Duncker who suggested the following problem:

> One morning, exactly at sunrise, a Buddhist monk began to climb a tall mountain. A narrow path, no more than a foot or two wide, spiraled around the mountain to a glittering temple at the summit. The monk ascended at varying rates of speed, stopping many times along the way to rest and eat dried fruit he carried with him. He reached the temple shortly before sunset. After several days of fasting and meditation, he began his journey back along the same path, starting at sunrise and again walking at varying speeds with many pauses along the way. His average speed descending was, of course, greater than his average climbing speed. Prove that there is *a spot* along the path that the monk will occupy on both trips at precisely the same time of day.

Now, as Adams points out, if you try to solve this problem with a verbal or mathematic mode of thought, you will have enormous difficulty. However, if you visualize the scene of a monk starting out at dawn at the bottom, and a monk starting out at the top of the mountain *simultaneously*, the solution is transparent. Clearly there are problems in literature, music, mathematics, and science whose solutions are most amenable to visual imagery. I would suggest that dreaming is better suited to deal with these kinds of problems. In addition, it is likely that factors such as motivation, intelligence, and temporal position of the dream will contribute to the probability that a dream will yield a solution. Thus, the hypothesis that dreaming is a problem solving process needs to be stated in a more specific way: dreaming *may* demonstrate problem solving capability, but under *certain conditions* (e.g., strong interest, relatively high intelligence, REM sleep, etc.), and for *certain kinds of problem solving* more than for others (e.g., imagery related problems). And of course, the likelihood that dream material will be used (aside from its unconscious influences) will depend on dream recall factors, a receptive attitude toward phenomenological "data", and the ability of the individual to recognize a solution or potential solution.

At this point we need to come to terms with the hypothetical capacity of dreaming to express what Piaget would call formal operations. If dreaming represents a shift toward right hemisphere and paleocortical processes, then it follows that dreaming will tend not to be about abstractions that normally are expressable in words. That is, the deep structure of (what Freud called dream thoughts) will tend to follow the rules of concrete operations, prelogical thought, sensorimotor (enactive) apprehension. The content of dreams will have more to do with intuitive, affective, and infantile motivation and knowledge. This view of dreaming would certainly be consistent with comparative and developmental, phylogenetic, and psychodynamic views of dreaming as a lower or more ancient, instinctive form of thinking. Note that this view does not detract from the psychobiological importance of the dreaming process, but it does impose a limitation upon what the dream can best accomplish. This view is consistent with the idea that cognitive structures suppressed during development continue to exist, in latent form, either separately or in combination. Representation in dreams of the earliest of these structures, derived from universal infant capacity and experience, may be thought of as the manifestation of the collective unconscious.

While Freud emphasized the effects of the ontogenetically primitive influences on the thought, affect, and behavior of adults, Piaget reminds us that influences proceed in the other direction.[1] In short, experiences organized early in life along the principles of sensorimotor, prelogical, and concrete operational information processing may be influenced by later experiences; open to the influence of daily life, they may be educated and modified. Thus, regressive thought during dreaming, that is, thought operating primarily according to earlier rules of information processing, may indeed be quite relevant to current concerns. Conceptualizing the dream as relevant only (or basically) to primitive concerns may be a theoretical artifact which reflects a data base provided by individuals for whom the early aspects of the ontogenetic continuum are more or less cut off from current functioning (e.g., suppressed, repressed, ignored, etc.). But in the healthy individual, all the ontogenetic levels of information processing can be relevant to all levels of experience. This notion of the interrelatedness of developmental experience is aptly expressed by Piaget: "Affective life, like intellectual life, is a continual adaptation, and the two are not only parallel but interdependent, since feelings express the interest and the value given to actions of which intelligence provides the structure. Since affective life is adaptation, it also implies the continual assimilation of present situations to earlier ones — assimilations which give rise to affective schemas or relatively stable modes of feeling or reacting — and continual accommodation of these schemas to the present situation" (Piaget, 1962, p. 205).

Consider a rather simple example of the way that dreaming might solve a problem. College women were asked to draw a person. This is clearly not a convergent thinking task because there is no one answer. (It is interesting to note that two of the subjects did treat the problem as a convergent task in the sense that they drew portraits of the person requesting the picture rather than making up something from their heads.) The range of competence,

---

[1] Freud derived his basic theoretical principles largely from neurotic patients. This accounts for the notion of thought processes ("complexes") split off (repressed) and having a prelogical life of their own more or less refractory to the modifying influence of later development. The continuing influence of such complexes would be to render behavior more "regressive" especially under stress or during sleep.

style, message in the drawings was remarkable. As with dreams, it is not clear to what extent any one represents situational states (e.g., mood) or traits (e.g., drawing ability, temperament). Also, like dreams, the drawings seemed to do two things at once; deal with an objective situation (requirement for producing a likeness of a person) but deal with it in a very subjective-expressive manner. Consider one of the drawings which is shown in Figure 10-1. The subject has followed directions to draw a person but note the underlying ("left-handed"!) message. Unlike some of the other productions which appear to express a more cerebral point, this drawing appears to express a more infantile motivation (aggression) within a perfectly acceptable social context. Thus, this play on words (like the dreamwork of latent thoughts) constitutes a creative if not intellectually sophisticated reaction to a mildly intrusive challenge. Even if the dreaming process rarely went beyond creative playfulness, like artistic productiveness it would be worthy of study as an important aspect of human information processing.

For Freud, all dreams could be understood as attempted solutions to problems. Thus, to understand the meaning of a dream meant the translation of dream symbolism in order to reveal the underlying problem. According to Freud (1955) there were two major kinds of

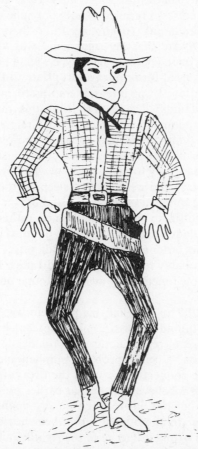

Figure 10-1 Draw-A-Person sketch made by a female undergraduate.

problem, a physiological need to maintain sleep in the face of other motives, and psychological needs or motives (usually of an infantile libidinal or aggressive nature). Like the "Draw" example in the Draw-A-Person Test, there are other examples from waking behavior which exemplify the assumed problem-solving representational processes of dreaming. Perhaps the best known example is the urinary symbolism in a cartoon published in a Hungarian paper and reproduced in Freud's *Interpretation of Dreams* (1955, p. 368). The cartoon, which portrays the "dream" of a French nurse, shows in successive frames an increasingly prodigious flow of urine made by the infant for whom she is responsible. The last frame shows the nurse awakening to the incessant cries of the infant. Presumably, the louder the infant cries, the greater the urine output fantasied in the dream. Two points are made. First, the dream directly translates the intensity of the real stimulus into the increasing size and spatial dimensions of the fantasy. Second, the need to maintain sleep contributes motivation to create a kind of instrumental solution; it is a kind of magical thinking which substitutes recognition (or re-cognition) for action.

I would like to suggest that while the need to maintain sleep may operate on dreaming, other somatic needs may override such a need, and in doing so, may influence the dreaming process in particularly novel and interesting ways. Consider the following example. One night I woke up just after three in the morning. I knew I was dreaming rather intensely but, aside from a few vague memories, I recalled vividly only one thing. I was dreaming something about the "right of mandamus" (pronounced like "handedness", i.e., man·da·mus). Simultaneously, I became aware that my right hand was without feeling, undoubtedly because I had been sleeping on it. (Perhaps had my *left* hand been "asleep", the dreamwork would have been of a nonverbal form more appropriate to the right hemisphere.) While shaking it to restore circulation, I was intensely impressed by the symbolic translation of right hand by "right of mandamus". That is, at the time, this translation seemed quite appropriate because, to me, "mandamus" was a word that referred to "hand". While this is technically incorrect, in my semiwake state it appeared profoundly true. (How often do we write something down while in some altered state of consciousness, something that appears to be of profound significance, only to review it somewhat embarrassingly in a more sober state!) I wrote down the phrase and went back to sleep. In the morning, I read the written phrase and could not see the connection between it and the recalled problem with my hand. What had seemed so insightful to me earlier seemed rather alien in the morning. The dictionary tells us that mandamus (pronounced man·da·mus) is a prerogative writ issued to enforce performance, a court order as in writ of mandamus. Of course, my "right" referred both to writ (order) and probably to right hand. And I must have learned the meaning of mandamus though it was now functionally available to me only in terms of its intuitive or better, its organismic sense.

A number of points can be made. First, my problem was an *acute* organismic one, to restore circulation. This required an organismic enforcement of performance, namely to awaken. Second, while a dream representing this organismic need was insufficient, it did constitute a kind of "solution" albeit of probably epiphenomenal significance. Third, why was I so impressed with the connection between the dream fragment and my bodily state while so unimpressed later? I believe that at that earlier point during the night my right hemisphere had relatively greater influence over my cognitive processes. What I am suggesting is that under certain conditions, verbal behavior that requires left hemisphere integrity is under relatively strong influence of the right hemisphere. What seems to make little sense from a critical, analytic perspective makes a good deal of sense from a subjective, intuitive perspective. And while the surface structure of the phrase may indeed be technically incorrect, the deep structure meaning may be quite valid. The process by which valid intuitive-organismic insights are successfully translated into recognizable surface structure is determined by a number of factors such as organismic state, verbal skills, prior experience, and recall. For example, I may have "chosen " mandamus because its dictionary meaning was available but not normally (during left hemisphere-dominated wakefulness) accessible, and because mandamus was associated with other related meanings: man(damus) (sound of the French word for hand), and *mand*(amus) (Skinner's term for "an utterance which procures a specific type of reinforcement from the hearer" (Keller and Schoenfeld, 1950, p. 384).[2] Perhaps Freud was profoundly correct to insist that while the surface structure of dreamwork is of great importance to our understanding of the whole of cognition, we should not dismiss potentially deeper truths about human nature often revealed through incomprehensible translation (Foulkes and Vogel, 1974).

Let us return to the issue of just how primitive is the dreaming process. If we assume that, especially during later REM periods, there is increased communication between left and right hemisphere (GILD hypothesis), or if we assume that right hemisphere dominance during dreaming determines more the mode of translation than the deep structure of dream thoughts, then it follows that dreaming may not always be a form of lower or more primitive thought. Dreaming may, under certain conditions (e.g., level of intelligence, motivation, time of night, etc.), involve the dramatization of formal operations. That is to say, there may be occasions when the latent content, the dream thoughts, may be mature rather than prelogical.

This view is consistent with the notion of "regression in the service of the ego", of dreaming as a different rather than necessarily a lower form of thought. It is also congruent with Piaget's view of the interconnectedness of mature and immature thought processes. To the degree that this view is correct, the big problem is how to translate from the concrete imagery of the recalled dream to the formal operations which are translated by the dreamwork. Verification of the hypothesis that formal operations can play a role in determining the dreams of intelligent adults will require more direct assessment of the activity of the left hemisphere during REM sleep (e.g., single cell recording, EEG recording). At present, we simply cannot evaluate in a scientifically satisfactory way the relative merits of these two opposing views of information processing during REM sleep.

Sometimes there is a question about whether dreams provide solutions. This is because a solution may be represented in any number of ways, many of which are quite frequent in dreams. For example, if the solution to a presleep unsolved problem is "unicorn" and the subject dreams of a unicorn (or a horse with a dunce cap on or some other unicorn-like object) is one reasonably confident that the dream contains the solution? Unicorns are extremely rare in dreams. However, suppose that the answer to an unsolved problem is "football". The appearance of a football (or any related imagery) would not constitute credible evidence of a solution; football imagery is frequent in dreams, especially of male college students.

Therefore, without a control for the base rate of solution-related symbolism, it is difficult to determine whether the individual dreamer has solved the problem or is pre-

[2] This was the first psychology textbook I ever read.

occupied with something quite different. Nevertheless, Dement (1972) provides a delightful anecdotal example of an apparent solution to the question: which word best represents the following sequence: H I J K L M N O? One student, whose incorrect waking solution was "alphabet", reported a number of dreams with water imagery (ocean, swimming, rain). Perhaps, this subject has an intuitive apprehension of the solution (H to O, or "water") which tends to be suppressed during wakefulness. Fromm (1951) talks about dreams revealing insights and sensitivities not obvious during wakefulness. He suggests that we pay more attention to these often-wasted resources.

One of my favorite solution dreams was one reported to me by my wife, Leslie. We and another couple were playing an alphabet game which included an especially difficult challenge to come up with the names of famous people whose initials (of first and last name) were A.A., E.E., O.O., etc. When these combinations appeared in the game, anyone thinking of a solution was virtually guaranteed a bundle of points. The EE combination was especially frustrating since, unlike UU, it seemed solvable but, unlike AA, no solution came to mind. (I must admit that at the time, the name Erik Erikson completely eluded both of us.) To appreciate the motivation behind the dream one must realize that Leslie is both competitive and verbally gifted (e.g., at anagrams), and loves to be challenged by anything resembling a puzzle. That night, preoccupied with the EE combination whose solution still eluded her, she dreamed that she was *changing* seats during a performance of a dance or acting troupe. Upon awakening she realized that the man sitting at the end of the row of seats was her 10th grade maths teacher, a person she had not thought of more than once in 11-12 years. Pondering the dream she suddenly recalled that his last name was *E*wing, but she didn't remember his first name. About a month later we discovered (by looking him up in a yearbook) that his first name was *E*arl! Though not exactly the kind of content discussed by clinically oriented theorists, this dream is suggestive of a process whereby current incentives are integrated with more remote (normally available but inaccessible) schemata to produce a solution to a problem (see Breger, 1967).

Perhaps in my attempt to reinforce through anecdote the value of dreaming, I have misrepresented the extent to which dreaming makes an intellectual contribution to adaptation. It is more likely that rather than problem solution, dreams more frequently provide alternative views, new perspectives, judgements reflecting intuitive rather than rational intelligence. Barzun best articulates this sentiment when commenting on Pascal's distinction between two categories of functioning: the geometric or scientific vs. the "subtle" mind. "Pascal goes on to describe the instantaneous synthesis by which the trained mind of the second category (*esprit de finesse*) grasps a situation and judges it. I have purposely avoided saying: 'grasps a problem and solves it', because it is precisely our self-immolation to science which misleads us into making a problem out of every situation. Our poets, painters, and novelists themselves talk of 'solving problems' in their respective arts. This is nonsense. They encounter difficulties, they are perplexed, but they face no problems in the sense of stated requirements which can completely be satisfied." And Barzun goes on to raise a serious and sobering challenge to the scientific researcher. Quoting Pascal: "When the scientists want to deal geometrically with these matters of finesse, beginning with definitions and going on to principles, they make themselves ridiculous, for such is not the way to reason in those cases — not because the mind does not proceed by reasons, but because it does this tacitly, naturally, artlessly. The full expression of it is beyond all men and the awareness of it belongs to few" (Barzun, 1959, p. 246).

2. EMPIRICAL EVIDENCE

At this point we move from anecdotes about uncontrolled events to more precise information obtained under controlled conditions. The question to be asked is whether the nature of the content of the dreaming process reflects presleep problems in an active and *adaptive* manner. The question is *not* whether dreaming is better than thinking, or whether individuals need dreaming. Comparisons between the effect on behavior of intervals filled with dreaming vs. wakeful thoughts would be useful to answer the former question; assessment of the effect of REM deprivation might be useful to determine the latter question. What is asked here is, given that dreaming does occur, in what sense or under what conditions can it be said to promote adaptive change (e.g., better mood, more incisive appreciation, deeper insight, intellectual apprehension, etc.)? Such a question requires that one assess the degree of adaptive behavior associated with different kinds of dream content. Ideally, after controlling for presleep baseline performance, attentional and motivational variables, quality of sleep (e.g., REM characteristics), quality of dream recall, and stage of sleep upon awakening, any such association can be (at least tentatively) taken as evidence of an adaptive *psychological* change. There are any number of hypotheses that lend themselves to testing the general notion of dream adaptation. A rather simple and straightforward hypothesis is that, given a presleep stress of nontraumatic proportions, it is better to dream about the situation than not to dream about it. If problems are "worked through" during dreaming, then individuals who dream about a stress should feel better in the morning for having dreamed about it than individuals who do not dream about it. We are assuming that the prediction holds for reasonably healthy individuals (since there is no reason to suppose that adaptive behavior during dreaming is marked while absent during wakefulness). I know of only three studies designed to test this idea in an empirical manner.

Correlational evidence

The first was reported by Kramer and Roth (1973). Their research was guided by the general idea that sleep and dreaming have a mood regulatory function. Consequently, they looked at correlations between *changes* in mood scale scores from evening to morning and (a) dream content and (b) REM and other sleep parameters. The strongest relationships between mood and dream content appeared to involve mood dimensions (e.g., happy) and number of dream characters. The strongest relationship between mood and sleep physiology appeared to involve information processing and energic aspects of mood (e.g., clear thinking, sleepy) and parameters such as sleep time. They concluded that "the unhappy, friendly, and aggressive subscales appear to be more related to the psychology [dream content aspect] of sleep while the clear thinking, sleepy and dizzy subscales may bear more a relationship to the physiology of sleep" (p. 570).

In planning the experiment to be discussed next (Cohen and Cox, 1975), I was not aware of this important preliminary report by Kramer and Roth (1973). Nevertheless, that earlier study must be considered the intellectual forerunner of the latter study which, in its broad outline, is essentially confirmatory.

Recall the manipulations used in the Cohen and Cox (1975) study. Subjects were randomly assigned either to a positive (friendly, sociable, highly informative situation during which the subject passes an IQ test) or a stress condition (isolation, little information, perfunctory treatment, and failing the IQ test). For purposes of this discussion we will ignore the positive condition (which was apparently not a "problem" for most subjects). Dream content from the 21 subjects exposed to the stress condition came from both REM and NREM awakenings (though most of the material is REM content). Of these subjects, 10 had dreams that showed evidence of literal or symbolic incorporation of experiment-related elements (laboratory, experiment, experimenter, etc.), and 11 did not show such evidence.

The left panel of Figure 10-2 shows the comparability of presleep affect scores (both are on the dysphoric side of the zero or "neutral" point) between the two subgroups. Note the marked and statistically significant ($p < .01$) difference in postsleep mood between the two groups. The nonincorporators are still, on the average, affectively dysphoric while the incorporators rate their mood as clearly on the euphoric side of zero. Actually, all but one incorporator showed a positive change from presleep baseline ratings, compared to only four of the 11 nonincorporators. The difference between subgroups in the apparent effect of dream content on adaptive change could not be attributed to a number of potentially competing variables: quality of affect reported for the dreams during the night, REM density, REM latency, number of awakenings, stage of sleep upon final awakening, success at filling out the dream diary sheet.

Only one variable, amount of dream material (number of dream units × number of dreams recalled) elicited by experimental awakenings, was also associated with adaptive change in mood ($r_{pb} = .51$), the relationship being almost as strong as that between incorporation and change ($r_{pb} = .59$). In the original paper we argued that the adaptive effect was really due to the content rather than success at dream recall. The rationale was as follows: "Perhaps good recallers feel that they are performing adequately, and therefore rate their postsleep affect more positively. If that is true, then why is there no relationship between success on the dream diary task and affect change, or between valence of affect reported in the dreams and affect changes? Perhaps amount and type of dream material are

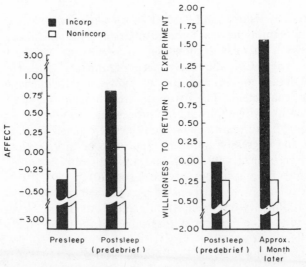

Figure 10-2 Changes in affect and attitude toward experimental participation for incorporator and nonincorporator subjects.

correlated with each other and with affect change because they are both products of the same underlying process: adaptation. There is evidence that amount of dream material is determined by the salience (subjective impact) of the experienced dream which in turn is determined by the 'psychological work' exerted by subjects who confront the presleep 'problem'. Thus, one could argue that evidence of incorporation *should* be correlated with amount of dream recall, and that controlling for amount of dream recall could lead one to reject a true hypothesis (Type II error)" (Cohen and Cox, 1975, p. 104). We then went on to do just that: control for amount of dream recall. We selected five incorporators who could be matched in terms of amount of dream recall to the five nonincorporators who produced *the most* dream material. Despite the virtual equivalence of dream material and the very small samples, the relationship between incorporation and adaptive change in affect, seen in the larger sample, was even stronger ($r_{pb} = .62$), though (due to attenuated N) just missing the .05 level of significance ($p < .07$).

These results do suggest that, given a class of problems, some types of dream content are better than others. This is not particularly surprising in that, given certain kinds of problems, certain kinds of waking thought are more effective in getting the individual closer to a solution. The obvious thing is to spend some time thinking about the problem rather than about something else.

The notion of incubation is venerable. Perhaps paying more attention to dream content, psychologists will learn more about incubation, that is, the way the mind works during altered states of attending and thinking. Can we define more specifically what it is about incorporator dreams that promoted adaptation? The quality of the data (including our unfortunate decision to go for NREM as well as REM awakenings) placed definite limits on the analyses that could be made. We did find one interesting association between affect change and the presence of cognitive effort (preoccupation with a problem, effort to figure out an ambiguity, etc.). This quality was associated with the greatest pre- to postsleep change. This preliminary finding suggests a possible avenue of approach to a problem which has hardly been given the empirical attention it deserves in the light of all the theoretical speculation about what dreams are supposed to accomplish.

There is one further set of findings regarding the apparent impact of attending to the presleep problem. Note that after awakening but *prior to debriefing*, incorporators felt better in the experimental situation. However, in terms of ratings of their willingness to return to the laboratory the following semester as unpaid subjects in a different experiment, there was no difference between the incorporator and nonincorporator subgroups. That is, despite feeling better, the incorporators seemed to have about the same *attitude* regarding the situation as did the nonincorporators. The right panel of Figure 10-2 shows that the two subgroups *prior to debriefing* are statistically comparable in mean ratings regarding the question about returning to the lab, they indicated "not sure" (roughly the midpoint of the scale). After these and other ratings about the experiment were obtained the subjects were debriefed regarding the artificial nature of the stress manipulations.

Approximately one month later, we were able to contact a large subsample of the original subjects in order to get follow-up information on the impact of the experiment. The objective of the follow-up was not to test hypotheses but merely to get information regarding the effect of a stress manipulation such as the one used in the experiment. However, serendipitously, we obtained results confirming the earlier findings. During the telephone interview, which had not been anticipated by the subject, he was asked the same question regarding willingness to return to a laboratory as an unpaid subject. Of the eight nonincorporators whom we were able to contact, only two indicated a greater willingness to return compared to their earlier (predebriefing) ratings, and two were less willing. There was no overall change in mean willingness from initial to second testing. However, of the seven incorporators whom we were able to contact, *all seven* indicated a greater willingness to return than originally indicated. The difference in change between the two subgroups was significant ($p < .01$) and fairly strong ($r_{pb} = .61$), and even *stronger* when smaller subgroups matched for amount of recall were selected ($r_{pb} = .77$). Suppressing my enthusiasm, I wrote in sober journalese: "These clearly tentative findings suggest that, for certain dimensions (e.g., attitude toward research) perhaps more than others (e.g., affect), the dreaming process provides a necessary but insufficient predisposition which, interacting with certain situational events (e.g., post-sleep debriefing), promotes a long-term change beyond the confines of the experiment" (Cohen and Cox, 1975, p. 107). Another possibility is that the mood induced by incorporative dreaming, not the dreaming *per se*, interacted with the debriefing to produce a lasting change of attitude. That is, individuals who felt better in the morning may have been more receptive to the debriefing. Thus, dreaming may have had a more indirect role in attitude change.

Experimental evidence

In the next issue of the same journal which published the Cohen and Cox study, another study appeared with what seems like diametrically opposite results. DeKoninck and Koulack (1975) reported that individuals demonstrating *less* adaptation to a postsleep stress film that had been shown the previous night were those subjects with more dream incorporation of film elements. This experimentally sophisticated study is of sufficient importance to require some detailed discussion. The investigators started out with the hypothesis that, if dreaming *per se* (rather than REM sleep) is an adaptive process, then adaptation to presleep stress should be associated with anxious, stress-related material. Twenty-four paid, male undergraduate volunteer subjects were randomly assigned to one of four experimental groups (four subjects each) and one control group (eight subjects). The first night was used to adapt the subjects to the laboratory. The second night yielded baseline data including REM dream content from each REM period. On the third night, subjects saw a stressful film prior to sleep and after sleep the next morning. REM content was collected throughout this night as well. Control group subjects were shown the film initially during the morning, and later, after an interval of normal wakefulness, during the evening.

Two groups got part of the film sound track during sleep (just above auditory threshold) on night 2 (prior to seeing the film). Two groups got the sound track during sleep on night 3, after viewing the film. The four experimental (sleep) groups were arranged so that comparisons could be made of sound vs. no sound prior to film, sound vs. no sound after film, and film vs. no film. But note that these are not really independent comparisons of independent effects since some subjects got sound during two nights of sleep, some only during one.

The film was a graphic portrayal of some grisly shop accidents, one resulting in the death of a worker who is impaled by a board hurled at him by a circular saw. The stressfulness of the presleep film experience was documented by increases in dysphoric adjective check-list ratings. Two sleep measures were reported to be affected by the film (compared to nonfilm night measures); there was a significant increase in sleep onset latency (defined in terms of stage 1 onset) and a corresponding decrease in REM onset latency. No other sleep characteristic data were reported, e.g., number of arousals from REM or NREM sleep, total sleep time, etc.

Next, the investigators reported that film plus sound (night 3) induced significantly more film incorporation on night 3 than did film without sound. The additive effect of film plus sound is suggested by the apparent absence of a sound alone effect on either incorporation or anxiety for night 2 (prefilm) dream data. Next, the investigators reported an unexpected statistically nonsignificant negative point-biserial correlation of —.57 between incorporation (vs. nonincorporation) of film elements and adaptation (reduced anxiety) during the second (morning) showing of the stress film. In addition, there was a positive correlation (roughly of .30) between dream anxiety and film-related anxiety.

These findings, especially those regarding the negative correlation between dream incorporation and film adaptation, constitute a serious threat to the dreaming-adaptation hypothesis. However, for a number of reasons, both methodological and theoretical, I believe that a case can be made that the findings provide an insufficient test of the hypothesis.

First the methodological point: DeKoninck and Koulack have not provided sufficient information regarding the differential effect of film plus sound vs. film alone on the quality of sleep. Yet it is known that external stimuli may affect the quality of sleep, and adequacy of performance (e.g., LeVere et al., 1975; Strauch, Schneider-Duker, Zayer, Heine, Heine, Lang and Müller, 1975).[3] Since the negative correlation found between incorporation and adaptation must be based largely on the film-sound condition (since film alone on night 3 had no effect in increasing incorporation over prefilm conditions on night 2), there is a definite possibility that the subjects in the film plus sound group were inadvertently awakened more frequently, or were more vigilant with respect to the "external" situation than to the "internal" situation (a distinction I raised in Chapter 8 and which I will discuss shortly). Either way, more fitful, awakening-interrupted sleep may account for *both* higher levels of film related themes and dream anxiety, both of which tended to correlate with "failure to adapt". Failure to adapt, that is, relatively high anxiety ratings, could simply be the effect of fatigue and/or irritability, or suppressed irritability and fatigue, or any number of other factors either that are independent of the dreaming process or are associated with the disruption of the normal dreaming process. To accept these findings as evidence against the hypothesis is to agree that manipulations which distract and annoy the waking person during problem solving, to the point where the very idea of the problem causes anxiety or resentment, constitutes evidence that thinking about problems is not adaptive.

The second problem with this otherwise methodologically sophisticated study is more theoretical in nature and has to do with the notion of external vs. internal threat and attention. Others have found such a distinction useful.[4] I have already commented on the artificial nature of many of the stress conditions used to test hypotheses about adaptation. I believe that we must distinguish between threats that relate to physical discomfort, even threats to survival (i.e., *external* threat) and threats to personality, self-esteem (i.e., *internal* threat). Perhaps largely inadvertently, sleep researchers are beginning to provide sleep data which tend to make such a distinction meaningful. We know that some animals do not have

---

[3] In fact, there is evidence that some "negative" conditions (e.g., heat) may produce performance deficits even in the absence of change in total sleep time (Herbert, 1975).

[4] For example, there is evidence that alcohol consumption is related to internal or ego threat rather than to external threat, e.g., threat of shock (see Higgins and Marlatt, 1975).

secure sleeping arrangements, e.g., ungulates. Their sleep tends to be more fitful, full of awakenings, and short relative to what would be predicted on the basis of correlations between sleep time and other biological variables (e.g., brain size, metabolism, etc.). In many ways, the sleep of individuals who anticipate danger (or external demand) can be described as "ungulate sleep". We may even speculate that the dreams of such an individual will, because of a continued vigilance, be more apt to contain evidence of incorporation of the external situation. And for individuals whose sleep is disrupted and who are constantly "re-minded" about the external threat (i.e., "minded" away from internal concerns normally processed during normal sleep), such a state of affairs will be associated with both incorporation and "failure to adapt". What I am again suggesting is that we distinguish between a need for REM sleep, which normally processes information about internal problems, and a need for *more* sleep, which is associated with "low ego strength" or with sleep-disrupting conditions.

What is the evidence from sleep data that there is a difference between external and internal threat? If I may use the Cohen and Cox (1975) stress condition as a reasonable model of internal threat, and the DeKoninck and Koulack (1975) mutilation film as an example of external threat, there are many differences which may provide replicable empirical bases for the distinction. First, while Cohen and Cox found a great deal of evidence of stress-related incorporation DeKoninck and Koulack did not; the film *per se* was not sufficient (without the sound) to impress the dreaming subject. Second, Cohen and Cox found rather modest effects of stress on sleep latency (not on stage 2) while DeKoninck and Koulack found a sizable effect for the film: thus the paucity of film-related elements in the dreams is all the more striking. One has to wonder what the subjects, shown the film, would have dreamed about had they not been "bullied" by the soundtrack into dreaming about the film! Third, while Cohen and Cox found that dream affect was more clearly related to *pre*sleep mood and not to postsleep mood, the opposite finding was reported by DeKoninck and Koulack. Another interesting fact is that the film-plus-sound group in the DeKoninck and Koulack study showed a nonsignificant *increase* in incorporations during the night compared to an *opposite* trend for the film only group. This suggests that the film-plus-sound group did not have a normal night's sleep since a normal night's sleep is associated with a tendency to dream less and less about the immediate situation and more about temporally more remote kinds of things. Thus, the "normal" process of dreaming was probably altered during the experiment. (It should be noted that the authors were aware of this and other problems, and adopted the customary due caution in discussing the implications of their results.)

In short, while the evidence for the adaptive hypothesis is certainly rather tentative, strong evidence for the null hypothesis seems equally tentative. Perhaps it will not seem overly self-serving to suggest that one of the most challenging and interesting, though largely unrecognized, problems in cognitive psychology today is the establishment of an empirical basis for the hypothesis that dreaming is not only a form of expression, but that it can be instrumentally adaptive.

There is any number of ways to approach, from the perspective of dream content, the hypothesis that the REM dreaming process makes a contribution to subsequent (waking) behavior. I mention two studies, one exploratory and one in progress. Both illustrate some of the problems that beset the researcher who stubbornly adheres to the hypothesis that dreaming can be adaptive.

The first study was an attempt to concretize in the laboratory the idea that dreaming is a process by which two sets of information, not obviously related, are *integrated* through dreaming to produce a novel and more useful "emergent" resultant. The idea that dreaming involves the integration of recent experiences into already established informational structures is a hardy one. It has been developed in theory by those with a major interest in the information processing, mind-as-computer view (e.g., Dewan, 1969), those with primarily a clinical orientation (e.g., Breger, 1967), and those who have adopted both views (e.g., Greenberg and Pearlman, 1974; Shapiro, 1967).

The question posed by the study I now describe was basically this: if an individual is given a problem, is the probability of coming to a solution increased by (a) an additional task that is ostensibly unrelated but is in fact an actual clue, and (b) dream pre-occupation with the task, the clue, or even better, both task and clue? The problem presented to the subject was the Duncker (1968) "X-ray problem". A 3×5 card with the diagram shown in Figure 10-3 was presented to the subject while he was asked the following question: "Given a human being with an inoperable stomach tumor, and rays that destroy organic tissue at sufficient intensity, by what procedure can one free him of the tumor by these rays and at the same time avoid destroying the healthy tissue which surrounds it?"

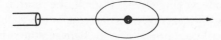

Figure 10-3 X-ray problem stimulus used in the study.

After working on the problem for 10 minutes, a subject who had not arrived at a solution was assigned to either one of two conditions. In the "ball and dowel" or clue condition, he was asked to assemble as fast as possible a tinker toy-like unit. The materials included a wooden ball painted black about 1.5 inches in diameter, and six dowel sticks each about 12 inches long which could be inserted into holes equally spaced along the "equator" of the ball. The subject was asked to assemble the ball and dowel unit as fast as possible. He was given four trials and was timed on each. Ostensibly, this was merely another task, but in fact, the completed array provided a physical analogue of the solution to the X-ray problem (i.e., a convergence onto the "tumor" [ball] of individual "rays" [dowels] none of which is sufficiently intense to damage surrounding tissue). Prior to sleep, no subject spontaneously caught on to the clue.

In the "block stacking" or nonclue condition, the subject was asked to build a tower of nine (1 cubic inch) WAIS blocks. He was to do this twice while facing the table on which the blocks were spread, and twice behind his back. Again, each trial was timed. Of course, there was no relationship between the configuration erected by the subject and the X-ray problem.

A total of 44 male subjects was introduced to the X-ray problem in the evening prior to sleep, and 25 in the morning prior to normal daily activity. Of the evening subjects, 11 (or 25%) solved the problem prior to the second task. Of the morning subjects, 6 (or 24%) solved the problem. These subjects in both groups were dismissed with ambivalent thanks. The remaining subjects in each group were then given the second task, and depending on the group, either spent the night in the sleep lab (evening or sleep group) or spent the day in their usual activities (morning or wake group). Subjects were asked to keep the X-ray problem in mind, and were aware that they would get a second chance to solve the problem when they returned.

TABLE 10-1.   X-ray Problem Results

Tally of *S*s who did not solve problem initially	Groups tested after			
	Sleep		Wake	
	Ball and dowel	Block stack	Ball and dowel	Block stack
Total run	18	15	11	8
Solutions	0	3	1	0
Percentage	0	20	9	0

Table 10-1 shows the number of subjects who had not initially solved the problem but who did solve the problem on the second trial (roughly 8-9 hours later). First, note how few subjects did attain the solution on the second try. Second, note that of the three subjects in the sleep condition who did solve the problem, all three were in the block stacking subgroup. So much for clever hypotheses about dream integration of problem and incidental but related information! Third, the difference between the sleep and wake groups was slight, but comforting to those who suspect that at least some problems are best handled during sleep (or at least facilitated by intervening sleep). Fourth, the results, such as they are, were not related to ratings made by subjects of their interest in the X-ray problem. There was no difference between the solvers and nonsolvers, or between the subjects of the ball and dowel vs. the block stacking conditions. The ratings of all subjects, on the average, indicated something between "somewhat" interested and "quite" interested in the X-ray problem.

Finally, perhaps a word ought to be said about the nature of the REM dream content of subjects who did solve the X-ray problem in the morning. The following comments will be brief because of the small magnitude of the results, because the quality of the dream material was not particularly high, and because there was no ostensible evidence of the kind of integration of information that we hoped would be forthcoming.

It is interesting, however, to speculate about the nature of the incubation process, as revealed by dreams, in conjunction with an unsolved task. For example, one of the subjects reported (after the third REM period was interrupted to retrieve material) an experience about a pit for a fire. He indicated interest in this project and said that it seemed as though he were learning something, something related to "survival". The construction of the pits included a consideration of "ventilation". Later in the report, the subject described how the soil was prepared by the action of the worms: ". . . that turn the soil . . . a *concentration in one place* would really make the soil loose . . . as opposed to the hard packed area around it. . . ." Throughout the report, the subject gave evidence of intellectual effort during the dream.

Another subject who solved the problem in the morning reported (after the second REM period was interrupted) an apparently conflictful interaction with the experimenter. "I told you (the experimenter) that I had a real dumb answer to the . . . problem. . . . Have you ever seen that movie 'Fantastic Voyage' where they shrink the man down and *shoot him into* the blood system? I told you to shrink the man down and shoot him into the blood system. . . ." The next REM report included a description of two little kids fighting over a golf ball after having chased it down the street. The dream also included an episode where the family car, surrounded by other cars in a parking lot, was hit, but not damaged, by another moving car. If one thinks of these events, as well as those in the dream of the previous subject, as objects and vectors, a small stretch of the imagination suggests a subjective preoccupation with the characteristics of the X-ray problem. More than this I really cannot (nor would like to) add.

One should be clear about the formidable difficulties in the testing of the hypothesis that dreaming can be an adaptive process. The hypothesis requires that we know something about the kinds of problems that are most likely to be dealt with actively (rather than merely reflectively) during REM dreaming. Having such information would maximize the likelihood of obtaining confirmatory results given the validity of the hypothesis. Assuming that such problems will be characterized by at least some complexity and personal relevance, it is clear that most tasks or problems used in the laboratory (at least in the typical REM deprivation studies published to date) do not meet the minimal requirements of personal relevance and complexity. Thus, if a problem does not fascinate the subject, appeal to conscious or unconscious needs, concerns, and talents, and if the problem tends to require information processing alien to the dreaming mode, then it will be all too easy to obtain evidence for the null hypothesis. We cannot simply balance failures with successes giving equal weight to each set of findings on the assumption that sufficient attention has been paid in each study to the kinds of requirements suggested above. A formidable problem is the selection of a problem that meets these requirements. It should not be so easy that few subjects remain to sleep on it, or so hard that no amount of waking or sleep and dreaming will provide opportunities for successful "incubation". Ideally, one would hope to find a problem which is highly motivating and sufficiently complex that a good percentage of subjects will go to sleep thinking about it and wake up either with a solution or a better idea. Under such conditions, an association between dream content incorporation of task-relevant themes and improved performance on the task during postsleep performance would provide the strongest kind of evidence that dreaming may, under certain conditions, play an active, adaptive role in problem solving. Perhaps we are dealing with a rare event which, because of its salience, is more readily recalled. Such a bias would naturally lead people to overestimate the frequency and importance of dream solutions to problems. We simply do not know.

We have sought a relationship between dream incorporation and postsleep behavior that would support the adaptive hypothesis of dreaming. But we have not yet tried to gain some control over incorporation by influencing the dreaming process *on-line*. Direct experimental manipulation of dreaming is fraught with methodological problems. Because of its potential power, the logic of such a technique deserves some elaboration. Let us assume that under many conditions, dreaming about a "problem" conveys some advantage to the dreamer with respect to the postsleep solution. The solution of a convergent problem is the correct answer. If the convergent problem is in the form of a series of steps, e.g., a series of mathematical equations, a solution may be in the form of more rapid movement through the series. The solution to a divergent problem is a better idea. Therefore, the experimenter must select or develop tasks on which performance can be assessed for progress if not answers.

Next, it is desirable to have a task that is graded with respect to intrinsic interest. If we want to compare the postsleep performance of a group that dreams about the task with that of a group which does not dream about the task, then a task of moderate interest must be chosen. If the task is uninteresting (irrelevant), neither group will be motivated to dream about it, i.e., it will not be a current concern. If the task is extremely interesting or important to the subjects, then task incorporation will be highly probable for both groups thereby precluding the relevant comparison. In other words, when stimulus control over the dreaming process is desired, then maximal differentiation between the experimental and control groups will require the use of tasks that are of medium interest.

Stimulus control presents a formidable problem to the investigator. The stimulus must be relevant to the task (in order to remind the subject to dream about the problem), but not so intrusive that it disrupts the sleep process. In addition, the status of the stimulus must be determined. If the stimulus introduced during REM sleep is part of the presleep task or problem, the subject may dream the stimulus rather than dream *about* the stimulus. In other words, the stimulus will tend to reduce the degrees of freedom regarding what to dream about. At present, it seems desirable to use a stimulus that has been conditioned as a discriminative stimulus (S^D) that elicits thinking about the problem. This can be accomplished during the presleep situation by using a series of trials that are initiated by the cue but which allow complete freedom to the subject once the cue is removed. Ideally, the cue should be inherently uninteresting and nonintrusive, thereby maximizing the difference between it (the nonfocal) and the task (focal). In short, to maximize stimulus control over dreaming *about* a problem, the problem should be of modest difficulty, modest interest, and conditioned to an otherwise meaningless or impersonal cue.

Figure 10-4 shows a hypothetical set of conditions which might affect the probability of dreaming about the task. The abscissa represents the motivation to think about the task. This motivation is a combined function of task difficulty and subject interest, both of which can be influenced by the experimenter (e.g., selecting subjects who are likely to show interest, stopping the subject at a crucial point, paying subjects for solutions, etc.). A threshold assumption is offered merely as a didactic device in order to clarify the point I am making with respect to the interaction of interest and cue manipulation. It is assumed that at some point (the S^D threshold) along the interest dimension the subject will be far more likely to dream about the task *if the task-related cue (S^D) is presented*. At some point further along the dimension, the probability of dreaming about the task is suddenly increased even by an irrelevant stimulus (S^Δ). The irrelevant stimulus may be physically the same as the cue, but is conditioned in the presleep situation to elicit some task-irrelevant behavior. However, by

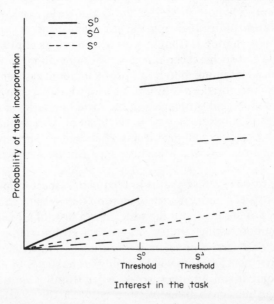

Figure 10-4 Hypothetical effect of task interest on the probability of task incorporation in dreams.

virtue of the high level of interest in the task (vs. lower interest in the irrelevant behavior), and the association of the two to the experimental situation in general, the task-irrelevant stimulus will elicit dreaming about the task. Finally, the figure shows a gradual increase (unaffected by thresholds) in the probality of dreaming about the task in the absence of any stimulation (s_0). This probability is determined by subject and situational factors existing in the presleep situation which continue to influence cognition during REM dreaming.

The figure demonstrates that differentiation between the experimental (cue) and control (noncue stimulus) groups is maximized at some point between the two thresholds along the dimension of task interest. Even if the threshold assumption is untenable, it remains to determine the critical points at which maximization of differentiation in task-relevant dreaming is accomplished. This is as formidable a problem as that of determining the mechanics of stimulation that will maximize detection and minimize the risk of distorting, disrupting, or terminating sleep. These are interrelated problems. It is possible that an intrusive stimulus may induce dreaming that is more relevant to the intrusion than to the task.

In order to determine the validity of the cue and the success in maintaining the integrity of sleep, it is necessary to assess the content of dreams. Once it can be established that the cue stimulus is maximizing the probability of task-relevant dreaming compared to the task-irrelevant stimulus, the two stimuli can be used in the absence of awakenings. If there is a difference in performance on the postsleep task between the cue and noncue stimulation groups, it can be assumed that task-relevant dreaming played a role. In this way, it can no longer be argued that group differences are determined by what the subject remembered about his dream (during the interviews) and how he felt about those experiences.

The attempt to gain experimental control over dream content by use of conditioned discriminative stimuli presented during sleep is derived from traditional psychological methodology. Nevertheless, it is clear from our preliminary experiences that alternative approaches may be more effective, given the ephemeral nature of the dependent variable. One such alternative which we intend to explore is the use of periodic REM deprivation to enhance the probability of task-relevant dreaming. Fiss (1969) reported that the continual interruption of REM periods eventuated in two reactions. First, REM periods were attenuated as though the subject were attempting to avoid interruption. Second, cognitive activity was intensified. For the present discussion, the intensification of cognition is most pertinent. Fiss reported that TAT stories obtained upon awakening from interrupted REM periods became more affectively charged and more focused on the current problems of the individual. This effect was not apparent in stories associated with awakenings made at the estimated ends of the REM period. In carrying out some recent experimental work we have noticed that REM deprivation appears to sharpen subjects' REM dream preoccupation with both laboratory themes and cognitive tasks presented after REM awakenings or presleep. While not analogous to the Fiss method of REM interruption, the following REM deprivation technique might be useful for purposes of exploring the adaptive hypothesis of dreaming.[5]

The experimental paradigm is outlined in Figure 10-5. The central idea is that an increase in REM pressure produced by awakenings accompanied by experimentally controlled cognitive activity will increase REM dream preoccupation with that specific activity. The process is facilitated by the fact that, as REM pressure builds up, the duration between task activity and REM period is diminished. The top right-hand section of Figure 10-5

[5] The idea was suggested to me by Les Bell.

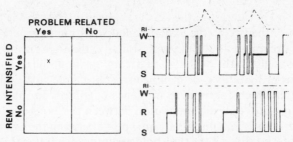

Figure 10-5 REM intensification method for increasing problem-relevant dream focus. The right side of the figure shows a segment of a hypothetical night including time in NREM sleep (S), REM (R), and wakefulness induced experimentally (W). The top section shows the increase and attenuation of REM sleep intensification (RI) induced experimentally. The lower section shows the control condition whose subjects are awakened at the end, rather than at the onset, of REM periods, as well as during NREM sleep. Note the relative absence of an increase in REM intensification. The left side of the figure shows the 2 (degree of REM intensification) × 2 (relevance vs. irrelevance of awakening activity to morning problem) design. In principle, the design should permit the assessment of the effect of enhanced dream focus on elements of a postsleep problem with control for number of REM periods, REM%, number of awakenings, total sleep time, distribution of REM periods, amount of experience during awakenings with the elements of the problem, sleep stage from which subjects finally awaken, etc.

represents this increase in temporal proximity between waking activity and onset of REM periods.

The novel aspect of the design is that after some criterion of pressure is fulfilled by the subject, he is allowed to remain in REM sleep for 15 minutes. This permits both an extended dreaming of the activity and a reduction of REM pressure. After 15 minutes, the REM period is then interrupted by an awakening during which the cognitive activity of the subject is again controlled by the experimenter. What follows is a repetition of the REM deprivation-relief procedure throughout the remainder of the night. By controlling the relevance to a postsleep problem of the cognitive activity occurring during the awakenings, the design permits an evaluation of the comparative effects of REM intensification *per se* vs. intensification plus relevant cognitive activity. A REM intensification-task irrelevant group provides a control for the distribution of REM periods, number of awakenings, etc. In addition, two control groups are utilized to evaluate the effects of task-relevant cognitive activity *per se* in the context of an equal number of REM periods, and equal percentage of REM sleep, total sleep time, number of awakenings, etc.

The experimental program would occur in two sequential steps. The first would constitute a test of the prediction that REM intensification is in fact associated with an increase and a sustained high level of REM dream preoccupation with specific aspects of cognitive activity occurring during the awakenings (as opposed to the laboratory situation in general). The prediction requires that the REM dream reports be evaluated for task relevance. The REM dreams of the control group, given an equal number of awakenings, would also be evaluated to provide a baseline level of preoccupation. The right side of Figure 10-5 provides a schematic representation of the sleep dynamics expected under experimental (deprivation-relief) and control conditions (nondeprivation).

Once it can be established that enhanced task-relevant dream focus occurs under experimental conditions, the 2 × 2 design shown on the left side of Figure 10-5 would be used. Dream reports would not be retrieved so that the effect of reporting can be eliminated. Thus, this experiment would test the hypothesis that the effect of REM dream preoccupation with problem-relevant elements will facilitate postsleep performance on that problem.

The proposed design is not entirely satisfactory. For example, one could question the generalizability of a hypothetical advantage of dreaming about problem-related elements during *recovery* rather than normal REM. The design does permit an evaluation of recovery REM effects *per se*, but the ecological validity of the findings will be somewhat ambiguous. Nevertheless, I believe that positive findings would constitute a significant empirical basis for the hypothesis that problem-relevant dreaming confers an advantage with respect to problem solving during wakefulness. In addition, the design eliminates problems associated with introducing exogenous cues (e.g., assuring that the cue is perceived without disrupting sleep) while retaining the advantage of experimental control over dream content.

At the end of Chapter 1, I quoted from Rechtschaffen on the mystery of sleep. Here I bow out with a quote from Jouvet: "Dreaming itself, particularly the question of its evolutionary origin and what function it serves, is still one of the great mysteries of biology. With the discovery of its objective accompaniments and the intriguing phenomenon of paradoxical sleep, however, it seems that we have set foot on a new continent that holds promise of exciting explorations" (1967, p. 72).

REFERENCES

ABRAMS, R., TAYLOR, M.A. and GAZTANAGA, P., Manic-depressive illness and paranoid schizophrenia, *Archives of General Psychiatry* 31, 640-642 (1974).

ADAMS, J.L., *Conceptual Blockbusting: A Guide to Better Ideas*, San Francisco: Freeman, 1974.

ADELSON, J., Creativity and the dream, *Merrill-Palmer Quarterly* 6, 91-97 (1959).

ADLER, A., *The Practice and Theory of Individual Psychology*, New York: Harcourt, 1927.

ADRIEN, J., Lesions of the locus coeruleus complex, and of the raphe nuclei in the newborn kitten, in M.H. Chase, W.C. Stern & P.L. Walter (Eds.), *Sleep Research, Vol. 4*, Brain Information Service/Brain Research Institute: Los Angeles, 1975. p. 69 (Abstract).

ADRIEN, J., BOURGOIN, S. and HAMON, M., Lesion of the anterior raphe nuclei in the newborn rat: Neurophysiology — biochemistry, in M.H. Chase, W.C. Stern & P.L. Walter (Eds.), *Sleep Research, Vol. 4*, Brain Information Service/Brain Research Institute: Los Angeles, 1975. p. 70.

AGNEW Jr., H.W. and WEBB, W.B., The displacement of stages 4 and REM sleep within a full night of sleep, *Psychophysiology* 5, 142-148 (1968).

AGNEW, J.W., WEBB, W.B. and WILLIAMS, R.L., the first night effect: An EEG study of sleep, *Psychophysiology* 2, 263-266 (1966).

AKISKAL, H.S. and McKINNEY Jr., W.T., Overview of recent research in depression, *Archives of General Psychiatry* 32, 285-305 (1975).

ALBERT, M.L., SILVERBERG, R., RECHES, A. and BERMAN, M., Cerebral dominance for consciousness, *Archives of Neurology* 33, 453-454 (1976).

ALLEN, S.R., OSWALD, I., LEWIS, S. and TAGNEY, J., The effects of distorted visual input on sleep, *Psychophysiology* 9, 498-504 (1972).

ALLISON, T. and CICCHETTI, D.V., Sleep in mammals: Ecological and constitutional correlates, *Science* 194, 732-734 (1976).

ALLISON, T., VAN TWYVER, J. and GOFF, W.R., Electrophysiological studies of the echidna, *Tachyglossus aculeatus*, I. Waking and sleep, *Archives of Italian Biology* 110, 145-184 (1972).

ALLPORT, G.W., *Personality: A Psychological Interpretation*, Holt: New York, 1937.

AMATRUDA III, T.T., BLACK, D.A., McKENNA, T.M., McCARLEY, R.W. and HOBSON, J.A., Sleep cycle control and cholinergic mechanisms: Differential effects of carbochol injections at pontine brain stem sites, *Brain Research* 98, 501-515 (1975).

ANDERS, T.F., Maturation of sleep patterns in the newborn infant, in E.D. Weitzman (Ed.), *Advances in Sleep Research, Vol. 3*, Spectrum Publications: New York, 1975.

ANDERS, T.F. and ROFFWARG, H.P., The relationship between internal and neonatal sleep, *Neuropädiatrie* 4, 64-75 (1973).

ANTROBUS, J.S., ANTROBUS, J.S. and SINGER, J.L., Eye movements accompanying daydreaming, visual imagery, and thought suppression, *Journal of Abnormal and Social Psychology* 69, 244-252 (1964).

ANTROBUS, J., DEMENT, W. and FISHER, C., Patterns of dreaming and dream recall: An EEG study, *Journal of Abnormal and Social Psychology* 69, 341-344 (1964).

ARBUTHNOTT, G., FUXE, K. and UNGERSTEDT, U., Central catecholamine turnover and self stimulation behavior, *Brain Research* 27, 406-413 (1971).

ARKIN, A.M., TOTH, M.F., BAKER, J. and HASTEY, J.M., The degree of concordance between the content of sleep talking and mentation recalled in wakefulness, *Journal of Nervous and Mental Disease* 151, 375-393 (1970).

AUERBACH, S.M., KENDALL, P.C., CUTTLER, H.F. and LEVITT, N.R., Anxiety, locus of control, type of preparatory information, and adjustment to dental surgery, *Journal of Consulting and Clinical Psychology* 44, 809-818 (1976).

AUSTIN, M.D., Dream recall and the bias of intellectual ability, *Nature* 231, 59-60 (1971).

AYALA, F.J. and DOBZHANSKY, T. (Eds.), *Studies in the Philosophy of Biology: Reduction and Related Problems*, University of California Press: Berkeley, 1974.

BAEKELAND, F., Exercise deprivation: Sleep and psychological reactions, *Archives of General Psychiatry* 22, 365-369 (1970).

BAEKELAND, F., KOULACK, D. and LASKY, R., Effects of a stressful presleep experience on electro-encephalograph — recorded sleep, *Psychophysiology* 4, 436-443 (1968).

BAKAN, D., *The Duality of Human Existence*, Rand McNally: Chicago, 1966.

BAKAN, P., The eyes have it, *Psychology Today* 96, 64-67 (1971).

BAKAN, P., The right brain is the dreamer, *Psychology Today* 9, 66-68 (1976).

BAKAN, P. and PUTNAM, W., Right-left discrimination and brain lateralization, *Archives of Neurology* 30, 334-335 (1974).

BAKKER, R.T., Dinosaur renaissance, *Scientific American* 232, 58-78 (1975).

BALDESSARINI, R.J., An overview of the basis for amine hypotheses in affective illness, in J. Mendels (Ed.), *The Psychobiology of Depression*, Spectrum Publications: New York, 1975.

BARBER, B., Factors underlying individual differences in rate of dream reporting (Doctoral dissertation, Yeshiva University, 1969), *Dissertation Abstracts International* 30, 1351 (1969).

BARBER, T.X., Imagery and "hallucinations": Effects of LSD contrasted with the effects of "hypnotic" suggestions, in S.J. Segal (Ed.), *Imagery: Current Cognitive Approaches*, Academic Press: New York, 1971.

BARBER, T.X., WALKER, P.C. and HAHN Jr., K.W., Effects of hypnotic induction and suggestions on nocturnal dreaming and thinking, *Journal of Abnormal Psychology* 82, 414-427 (1973).

BARDWICK, J., *Psychology of Women: A Study of Biosocial Conflicts*, Harper & Row: New York, 1971.

BARRETT, T.R. and EKSTRAND, B.R., Effect of sleep on memory: III. Controlling for time-of-day effects, *Journal of Experimental Psychology* 96, 321-327 (1972).

BARTLETT, F.C., *Remembering*, Cambridge University Press: Cambridge, England, 1932.

BARZUN, J., *The House of Intellect*, Harper & Brothers: New York, 1959.

BEAUMASTER, E.J.B., Individual differences in rapid eye movement (REM) sleep, Unpublished MA thesis, Queen's University, 1968.

BEAUMONT, J.G. and DIMOND, S.J., Brain disconnection and schizophrenia, *British Journal of Psychiatry* 123, 661-662 (1973).

BECKER, M. and HERTER, G., Effects of meditation upon SREM, in M. Chase, W. Stern & P. Walter (Eds.), *Sleep Research, Vol. 2*, Brain Information Service/Brain Research Institute: Los Angeles, 1973. p. 90.

BELL, A.I. and STROEBEL, C.F., The scrotal sac and testes during sleep: Physiological correlates and mental content, in W.P. Koella & P. Levin (Eds.), *Sleep: Physiology, Biochemistry, Psychology, Pharmacology, Clinical Implications*, S. Karger: Basel, Switzerland, 1973.

BELL, A.I., STROEBEL, C.F. and PRIOR, D.D., Interdisciplinary study. Scrotal sac and testes psychophysio-logical and psychological observations, *Psychoanalytic Quarterly* 40, 415-434 (1971).

BELL, R.Q., A reinterpretation of the direction of effects in studies of socialization, *Psychological Review* 75, 81-95 (1968).

BEM, D.J. and ALLEN, A., On predicting some of the people some of the time: The search for cross situational consistencies in behavior, *Psychological Review* 81, 506-520 (1974).

BEM, S.L. and LENNEY, E., Sex typing and the avoidance of cross-sex behavior, *Journal of Personality and Social Psychology* 33, 48-54 (1976).

BENOIT, O. and ADRIEN, J., PGO activity as a criterion of paradoxical sleep: A critical review, in G. Lairy & P. Salzarulo (Eds.), *The Experimental Study of Human Sleep: Methodological Problems*, Elsevier: Amsterdam, 1975.

BERGER, R.J., Experimental modification of dream content by meaningful verbal stimuli, *British Journal of Psychiatry* 109, 722-740 (1963).

BERGER, R.J. and MEIER, G.W., The effects of selective deprivation of states of sleep in the developing monkey, *Psychophysiology* 2, 354-371 (1966).

BERGER, R.J. and OSWALD, I., Eye movements during active and passive dreams, *Science* 137, 601 (1962).

BERGER, R.J. and SCOTT, T.D., Increased accuracy of binocular depth perception following REM sleep periods, *Psychophysiology* 8, 763-768 (1971).

BERTINI, M., REM sleep as a psychophysiological 'agency' of memory organization, in W.P. Koella & P. Levin (Eds.), *Sleep: Physiology, Biochemistry, Psychology, Pharmacology, Clinical Implications*, S. Karger: Basel, Switzerland, 1973.

BERTINI, M., Sleep-awake differentiation in a developmental context, in P. Levin & W.P. Koella (Eds.), *Sleep 1974: Instinct, Neurophysiology, Endocrinology, Episodes, Dreams, Epilepsy and Intracranial Pathology*, S. Karger: Basel, Switzerland, 1975.

BEUTLER, L.E., KARACAN, I., ANCH, A.M., SALIS, P.J., SCOTT, F.B. and WILLIAMS, R.L., MMPI and MIT discriminators of biogenic and psychogenic impotence, *Journal of Consulting and Clinical Psychology* 43, 899-903 (1975).

BLOCH, V. and FISHBEIN, W., Sleep and psychological functions: Memory, in G. Lairy & P. Salzarulo (Eds.), *The Experimental Study of Human Sleep: Methodological Problems*, Elsevier: Amsterdam, 1975.

BLOCK, J., Conceptions of sex role: Some cross-cultural and longitudinal perspectives, *American Psychologist* 28, 512-526 (1973).

BLODGETT, J.C., The effect of introduction of reward upon the maze performance of rats, *University of California Publications on Psychology* 4, 113-134 (1929).

BOKERT, E., The effects of thirst and related auditory stimulation on dream reports, Paper presented to the Association for the Psychophysiological Study of Sleep, Washington, D.C., 1965.

BONIME, W., *The Clinical Use of Dreams*, Basic Books: New York, 1962.

BOUHUYS, A.L. and VAN DEN HOOFDAKKER, R.H., Effects of lesions in the raphe system on sleep in the rat, in P. Levin & W.P. Koella (Eds.), *Sleep 1974: Instinct, Neurophysiology, Endocrinology, Episodes, Dreams, Epilepsy and Intracranial Pathology*, S. Karger: Basel, Switzerland, 1975.

BOWE-ANDERS, C., HERMAN, J.H. and ROFFWARG, H.P., Effects of goggle-altered color perception on sleep, *Perceptual and Motor Skills* 38, 191-198 (1974).

BOWERS, K.S., Situationism in psychology: An analysis and a critique, *Psychological Review* 80, 307-336 (1973).

BOYLE, E., APARICIO, A.M., KAYE, J. and ACKER, M., Auditory and visual memory losses in aging populations, *Journal of the American Geriatrics Society* 23, 284-286 (1975).

BRAZIER, M.A.B., Absence of dreaming or failure to recall?, *Experimental Neurology* 4, 98-106 (1967).

BREGER, L., Function of dreams, *Journal of Abnormal Psychology Monograph* 72, 1-28 (1967).

BREGER, L., HUNTER, J. and LANE, R.W., The effect of stress on dreams, *Psychological Issues* 7, 1-210 (1971).

BREMER, F., A further study of the inhibitory processes induced by the activation of the preoptic hypnogenic structures, *Archives of Italian Biology* 113, 79-88 (1975).

BRENNEIS, B., Male and female modalities in manifest dream content, *Journal of Abnormal Psychology* 76, 434-442 (1970).

BREWER, W.F., There is no convincing evidence for operant or classical conditioning in adult humans, in W.B. Weimer & D.S. Palermo (Eds.), *Cognition and the Symbolic Processes*, Lawrence Erlbaum Associates: Hillsdale, New Jersey, 1974.

BROUGHTON, R., Biorhythmic variations in consciousness and psychological functions, *Canadian Psychological Review* 16, 217-239 (1975).

BROVERMAN, D.M., KLAIBER, E.L., KOBAYASHI, Y. and VOGEL, W., Roles of activation and inhibition in sex differences in cognitive abilities, *Psychological Review* 75, 23-50 (1968).

BROWN, J., *Mind, Brain, and Consciousness*, Academic Press: New York, 1977.

BUDZYNSKI, T.H., Biofeedback and the twilight states of consciousness, in G.E. Schwartz & D. Shapiro (Eds.), *Consciousness and Self Regulation: Advances in Research, Vol. 1*, Plenum: New York, 1976.

BUGELSKI, B.R., The definition of the image, in S.J. Segal (Ed.), *Imagery: Current Cognitive Approaches*, Academic Press: New York, 1971.

BUSS, A.H., *Psychopathology*, Wiley: New York, 1966a.

BUSS, A.H., The effect of harm on subsequent aggression, *Journal of Experimental Research in Personality* 1, 249-255 (1966(b)).

BUSS, A.H. and PLOMIN, R., *A Temperament Theory of Personality Development*, Wiley: New York, 1975.

BUTCHER, J.N. (Ed.), *MMPI: Research Developments and Clinical Applications*, McGraw-Hill: New York, 1969.

BYRNE, D., Repression-sensitization as a dimension of personality, in B.A. Maher (Ed.), *Progress in Experimental Personality Research*, Academic Press: New York, 1964.

BYRNE, D., STEINBERG, M.A. and SCHWARTZ, M.S., Relationship between repression-sensitization and physical illness, *Journal of Abnormal Psychology* 73, 154-155 (1968).

CARLSON, N.R., *Physiology and Behavior*, Allyn & Bacon: Boston, 1977.

CARLSON, R., Sex differences in ego functioning: Exploratory studies of agency and communion, *Journal of Consulting and Clinical Psychology* 37, 267-277 (1971(a)).

CARLSON, R., Where is the person in personality research? *Psychological Bulletin* 75, 203-219 (1971(b)).

CARRINGTON, P., Dreams and schizophrenia, *Archives of General Psychiatry* 26, 343-350 (1972).

CARSON, R.C., Appendix A: Interpretive manual to the MMPI, in J.N. Butcher (Ed.), *MMPI: Research Developments and Clinical Applications*, McGraw-Hill: New York, 1969.

CARTWRIGHT, R.D., Dreams, reality, and fantasy, in J. Fisher & L. Breger (Eds.), *The Meaning of Dreams: Recent Insights from the Laboratory* (California Research Symposium No. 3), Bureau of Research, California Dept. of Mental Hygiene: Sacramento, California, 1969.

CARTWRIGHT, R.D., Sleep fantasy in normal and schizophrenic persons, *Journal of Abnormal Psychology* 80, 275-279 (1972).

CARTWRIGHT, R.D., The influence of a conscious wish on dreams: A methodological study of dream meaning and function, *Journal of Abnormal Psychology* 83, 387-393 (1974).

CARTWRIGHT, R.D., Is REM 4 really dreamier than REM 1?, in M.H. Chase, W.C. Stern, & P.L. Walter (Eds.), *Sleep Research, Vol. 4*, Brain Information Service/Brain Research Institute: Los Angeles, 1975, p. 181.

CARTWRIGHT, R.D. and MONROE, L.J., The relation of dreaming and REM sleep: The effects of REM deprivation under two conditions, *Journal of Personality and Social Psychology* 10, 69-74 (1968).

CARTWRIGHT, R.D., BERNICK, N., BOROWITZ, G. and KLING, A., Effect of an erotic movie on sleep and dreams of young men, *Archives of General Psychiatry* 20, 262-271 (1969).

CARTWRIGHT, R.D., MONROE, L.J. and PALMER, C., Individual differences in response to REM deprivation, *Archives of General Psychiatry* 16, 297-303 (1967).

CHASE, M.H. (Ed.), *The Sleeping Brain*, Brain Information Service/Brain Research Institute: Los Angeles, 1972.

CHERNIK, D.A., Effect of REM sleep deprivation on learning and recall by humans, *Perceptual and Motor Skills* 34, 283-294 (1972).

CHUTE, D.L. and WRIGHT, D.C., Retrograde state dependent learning, *Science* 180, 878-880 (1973).

CLARIDGE, G.S., *Personality and Arousal*, Pergamon: Oxford, 1967.

CLAUSEN, J., SERSEN, E. and LIDSKY, A., Variability of sleep measures in normal subjects, *Psychophysiology* 11, 509-516 (1974).

CLEMES, S.R. and DEMENT, W.C., Effect of REM deprivation on psychological functioning, *Journal of Nervous and Mental Disease* 144, 485-491 (1967).

COHEN, D.B., Current research on the frequency of dream recall, *Psychological Bulletin* 73, 433-440 (1970).

COHEN, D.B., Dream recall and short term memory, *Perceptual and Motor Skills* 33, 867-871 (1971).

COHEN, D.B., Dream recall and total sleep time, *Perceptual and Motor Skills* 34, 456-458 (1972(a)).

COHEN, D.B., Presleep experience and home dream reporting: An exploratory study, *Journal of Consulting and Clinical Psychology* 38, 122-128 (1972(b)).

COHEN, D.B., A comparison of genetic and social contributions to dream recall frequency, *Journal of Abnormal Psychology* 82, 368-371 (1973(a)).

COHEN, D.B., Sex role orientation and dream recall, *Journal of Abnormal Psychology* 82, 246-252 (1973(b)).

COHEN, D.B., Effect of personality and presleep mood on dream recall, *Journal of Abnormal Psychology* 83, 151-156 (1974(a)).

COHEN, D.B., Presleep mood and dream recall, *Journal of Abnormal Psychology* 83, 45-51 (1974(b)).

COHEN, D.B., On the etiology of neurosis, *Journal of Abnormal Psychology* 83, 473-479 (1974(c)).

COHEN, D.B., Toward a theory of dream recall, *Psychological Bulletin* 81, 138-154 (1974(d)).

COHEN, D.B., Eye movements during REM sleep: The influence of personality and presleep conditions, *Journal of Personality and Social Psychology* 32, 1090-1093 (1975).

COHEN, D.B., Dreaming: Experimental investigation of representational and adaptive properties, in G.E. Schwartz & D. Shapiro (Eds.), *Consciousness and Self-Regulation: Advances in Research, Vol. 1*, Plenum: New York, 1976.

COHEN, D.B., Changes in REM dream content during the night: Implications for a hypothesis about changes in cerebral dominance across REM periods, *Perceptual and Motor Skills* 44, 1267-1277 (1977(a)).

COHEN, D.B., Neuroticism and dreaming sleep: A case for interactionism in personality research, *British Journal of Social and Clinical Psychology* 16, 153-163 (1977(b)).

COHEN, D.B., Remembering and forgetting dreaming, in J.F. Kihlstrom & F.J. Evans (Eds.), *Functional Disorders of Memory*, in press.

COHEN, D.B. and COX, C., Neuroticism in the sleep laboratory: Implications for representational and adaptive properties of dreaming, *Journal of Abnormal Psychology* 84, 91-108 (1975).

COHEN, D.B. and MACNEILAGE, P.F., A test of the salience hypothesis of dream recall, *Journal of Consulting and Clinical Psychology* 42, 699-703 (1974).

COHEN, D.B. and WOLFE, G., Dream recall and repression: Evidence for an alternative hypothesis, *Journal of Consulting and Clinical Psychology* 41, 349-355 (1973).

COHEN, D.B., McGRATH, M.J., BELL, L.W., HANLON, M.J. and SIMON, M., REM motivation induced by brief REM deprivation: The influence of cognition, gender, and personality, *Journal of Personality and Social Psychology* 36, 741-751 (1978).

COHEN, H., EDELMAN, A., BOWEN, R. and DEMENT, W.C., Sleep and self stimulation in the rat, in M.H. Chase, W.C. Stern & P. Walter (Eds.), *Sleep Research, Vol. 4*, Brain Information Service/Brain Research Institute: Los Angeles, 1972.

CORBALLIS, M.C. and BEALE, I.L., *The Psychology of Left and Right*, Lawrence Erlbaum Associates: New Jersey, 1976.

CORY, T.L., ORMISTON, D.W., SIMMEL, E. and DAINOFF, M., Predicting the frequency of dream recall, *Journal of Abnormal Psychology* 84, 261-266 (1975).

COURSEY, R.D., BUCHSBAUM, M. and FRANKEL, B.L., Personality measures and evoked responses in chronic insomniacs, *Journal of Abnormal Psychology* 84, 239-249 (1975).

CRAIK, F.I.M. and BLANKSTEIN, K.R., Psychophysiology and human memory, in P.H. Venables & M.J. Christie (Eds.), *Research in Psychophysiology*, Wiley: London, 1975.

DAVIDSON, R.J., SCHWARTZ, G.E., PUGASH, E. and BROMFIELD, E., Sex differences in pattern of EEG asymmetry, *Biological Psychology* 4, 119-138 (1976).

DAVIS, J.M., Critique of single amine theories: Evidence of a cholinergic influence in the major mental illnesses, in D.X. Freedman (Ed.), *Biology of the Major Psychoses: A Comparative Analysis (Research Publications: Association for Research in Neurons and Mental Disease, Vol. 54)*, Raven Press: New York, 1975.

DAVIS, J.M. and JANOWSKY, D., Clinical pharmacological strategies, in J. Mendels (Ed.), *The Psychobiology of Depression*, Spectrum Publications: New York, 1975.

DAWSON, T.J., "Primitive" mammals, in C.C. Whittow (Ed.), *Comparative Physiology of Thermoregulation, Vol. III*, Academic Press: New York, 1973.

DE ANDRES, I., NAVA, B.E., GUTIERREZ-RIVAS, E. and REINOSO-SUAREZ, F., Comparative study of sleep-wakefulness cycle between a dog's implanted head and its receptor, in M.H. Chase, W.C. Stern, & P.L. Walter (Eds.), *Sleep Research, Vol. 4*, Brain Information Service/Brain Research Institute: Los Angeles, 1975. p. 2.

DEKONINCK, J.M. and KOULACK, D., Dream content and adaptations to a stressful situation, *Journal of Abnormal Psychology* 84, 250-260 (1975).

DEKONINCK, J.M., KOULACK, D. and OCZKOWSKI, G., Decrease in field dependence following rapid eye movement sleep, *Bulletin of the Psychonomic Society* 1, 257-258 (1973).

DE LA PEÑA, A., ZARCONE, V. and DEMENT, W.C., Correlation between measure of the rapid eye movements of wakefulness and sleep, *Psychophysiology* 10, 488-500 (1973).

DEMENT, W.C., The effect of dream deprivation, *Science* 131, 1705-1707 (1960).

DEMENT, W.C., *Some Must Watch while Some Must Sleep*, W.H. Freeman: San Francisco, 1972.

DEMENT, W., Report IV (b): Comments to Report IV, in G.C. Lairy & P. Salzarulo (Eds.), *The Experimental Study of Human Sleep: Methodological Problems*, Elsevier: Amsterdam, 1975.

DEMENT, W. and KLEITMAN, N., The relation of eye movements during sleep to dream activity: An objective method for the study of dreaming, *Journal of Experimental Psychology* 53, 339-346 (1957).

DEMENT, W.C. and MITLER, M.M., An introduction to sleep, in O. Petre-Quadens & J.D. Schlag (Eds.), *Basic Sleep Mechanisms*, Academic Press: New York, 1974.

DEMENT, W. and WOLPERT, E., The relation of eye movements, body motility, and external stimuli to dream content, *Journal of Experimental Psychology* 55, 543-553 (1958).

DEMENT, W.C., COHEN, H., FERGUSON, J. and ZARCONE, V., A sleep researcher's odyssey: The function and clinical significance of REM sleep, in L. Madow & L.H. Snow (Eds.), *The Psychodynamic Implications of the Physiological Studies on Dreams*, Charles Thomas: Springfield, Illinois, 1970.

DEMENT, W., HENRY, P., COHEN, H. and FERGUSON, J., Studies on the effect of REM deprivation in humans and animals, in S.S. Kety & E.V. Evarts (Eds.), *Sleep and Altered States of Consciousness*, Williams & Wilkins: Baltimore, 1967.

DEMENT, W., KAHN, E. and ROFFWARG, H.P., The influence of the laboratory situation on the dreams of the experimental subject, *Journal of Nervous and Mental Disease* 140, 119-131 (1965).

DESJARDINS, J., HEALEY, T. and BROUGHTON, R., Early evening exercise and sleep, in M.H. Chase, W.C. Stern & P. Walter (Eds.), *Sleep Research, Vol. 3*, Brain Information Service/Brain Research Institute: Los Angeles, 1974.

DEWAN, E.M., The programming (P) hypothesis for REMs, *Physical Science Research Papers*, No. 388, Air Force Cambridge Research Laboratories, Project 5628, 1969.

DIMOND, S.J., FARRINGTON, L. and JOHNSON, P., Differing emotional response from right and left hemispheres, *Nature* 261, 690-692 (1976).

DOMINO, G., Compensatory aspects of dreams: An empirical test of Jung's theory, *Journal of Personality and Social Psychology* 34, 658-662 (1976(a)).

DOMINO, G., Primary process thinking in dream reports as related to creative achievement, *Journal of Consulting and Clinical Psychology* 44, 929-932 (1976(b)).

DONNELLY, E.F., MURPHY, D.L. and SCOTT, W.H., Perception and cognition in patients with bipolar and unipolar depressive disorders, *Archives of General Psychiatry* 32, 1128-1131 (1975).

DRUCKER-COLIN, R.R., SPANIS, C.W., COTMAN, C.W. and McGAUGH, J.L., Proteins and REM sleep, in P. Levin & W.P. Koella (Eds.), *Sleep 1974: Instinct, Neurophysiology, Endocrinology, Episodes, Dreams, Epilepsy and Intracranial Pathology*, S. Karger: Basel, Switzerland, 1975.

DULANY, D.E., On the support of cognitive theory in opposition to behavior theory: A methodological problem, in W.B. Weimer & D.S. Palermo (Eds.), *Cognition and the Symbolic Processes*, Lawrence Erlbaum Associates: New Jersey, 1974.

DUNCKER, K., On problem solving, excerpted in P.C. Wason & P.N. Johnson-Laird (Eds.), *Thinking and Reasoning*, Penguin: Baltimore, 1968.

ECCLES, J.C., *The Understanding of the Brain*, McGraw-Hill: New York, 1973.

EMPSON, J.A.C. and CLARKE, P.R.F., Rapid eye movements and remembering, *Nature* 227, 287-288 (1970).

ENGEL, R.R., Report IV (A): Comments to report IV, in G.C. Lairy & P. Salzarulo (Eds.), *The Experimental Study of Human Sleep: Methodological Problems*, Elsevier: Amsterdam, 1975.

EPHRON, H.S. and CARRINGTON, P., Rapid eye movement sleep and cortical homeostasis, *Psychological Review* 75, 500-526 (1966).

EPSTEIN, A.W. and COLLIE, W.R., Is there a genetic factor in certain dream types?, *Biological Psychiatry* 11, 359-362 (1976).

ERIKSON, E.H., *Childhood and Society*, Norton: New York, 1952.

EVANS, F.J., COOK, M.R., COHEN, H.D., ORNE, E.C. and ORNE, M.T., Appetitive and replacement naps: EEG and behavior, *Science* 197, 687-689 (1977).

EVANS, F.J., GUSTAFSON, L.A., O'CONNELL, D.N., ORNE, M.T. and SHOR, R.E., Verbally induced behavioral responses during sleep, *Journal of Nervous and Mental Diseases* 150, 171-187 (1970).

EYSENCK, H.J., *The Biological Basis of Personality*, Charles Thomas: Springfield, Illinois, 1967.

EYSENCK, H.J., *The Structure of Human Personality*, Methuen: London, 1970.

EYSENCK, H.J., The learning theory model of neurosis — a new approach, *Behavior Research and Therapy* 14, 251-267 (1976).

EYSENCK, H.J. and RACHMAN, S., *The Causes and Cures of Neurosis*, Robert Knapp: San Diego, 1965.

FARLEY, F. and FARLEY, S.V., Extraversion and stimulus-seeking motivation, *Journal of Consulting Psychology* 31, 215-216 (1967).

FEINBERG, I., Effects of age on human sleep patterns, in A. Kales (Ed.), *Sleep: Physiology and Pathology: A Symposium*, Lippincott: Philadelphia, 1969.

FEINBERG, I., Some observations on the reliability of REM variables, *Psychophysiology* 11, 68-72 (1974).

FEINBERG, I. and EVARTS, E.V., Changing concepts of the function of sleep: Discovery of intense brain activity during sleep calls for revision of hypotheses as to its function, *Biological Psychiatry* 1, 331-348 (1969).

FEINBERG, I., KORESKO, R.L., HELLER, N. and STEINBERG, H.R., Sleep EEG and eye-movement patterns in young and aged normals and in patients with chronic brain syndromes, in W.B. Webb (Ed.), *Sleep: An Active Process: Research and Commentary*, Scott Foresman: Glenview, Illinois, 1973.

FENIGSTEIN, A., SCHEIER, M.F. and BUSS, A.H., Public and private self-consciousness: Assessment and theory, *Journal of Consulting and Clinical Psychology* 43, 522-527 (1975).

FERNSTROM, J.D. and WURTMAN, R.J., Nutrition and the brain, *Scientific American* 230, 84-91 (1974).

FIRTH, H. and OSWALD, I., Eye movements and visually active dreams, *Psychophysiology* 12, 602-606 (1975).

FISHBEIN, W. and ANTROBUS, J.S., Review of Grieser, C., Greenberg, R. and Harrison, R.H., The adaptive function of sleep: The differential effects of sleep and dreaming on recall, *Journal of Abnormal Psychology* 80, 280-286 (1972); in M.H. Chase, W.C. Stern & P.L. Walter (Eds.), *Sleep Research, Vol. 3*, Brain Information Service/Brain Research Institute: Los Angeles, 1974. p. 315.

FISHBEIN, W. and GUTWEIN, B.M., Paradoxical sleep and memory storage processes, *Behavioral Biology* 19, 425-464 (1977).

FISHBEIN, W. and KASTANIOTIS, C., Augmentation of REM sleep after learning, in M.H. Chase, W.C. Stern & P.L. Walter (Eds.), *Sleep Research, Vol. 2*, Brain Information Service/Brain Research Institute: Los Angeles, 1973, p. 94.

FISHBEIN, W., SCHAUMBURG, H. and WEITZMAN, E.D., Rapid eye movements during sleep in dark-reared kittens, *Journal of Nervous and Mental Disease* 143, 281-283 (1966).

FISHER, C., Dream and perception, *Journal of the American Psychoanalytic Association* 2, 389-445 (1954).

FISHER, C., Dreams, images, and perception: A study of unconscious and preconscious relationships, *Journal of the American Psychoanalytic Association* 4, 5-48 (1956).

FISHER, C., A study of the preliminary stages of the construction of dreams and images, *Journal of the American Psychoanalytic Association* 5, 5-60 (1957).

FISHER, C., Introduction to Poetzl's, Aller's, and Teller's works in translation, *Psychological Issues* 2, 1-40 (1960(a)).

FISHER, C., Subliminal and supraliminal influences on dreams, *American Journal of Psychiatry* 116, 1009-1017 (1960(b)).

FISHER, C., Psychoanalytic implications of recent research on sleep and dreaming, *Journal of the American Psychoanalytic Association* 13, 197-303 (1965).

FISHER, C., Dreaming and sexuality, in R.M. Lowenstein, L.M. Newman, M. Schur & A.J. Solnit (Eds.), *Psychoanalysis: A General Psychology*, International Universities Press: New York, 1966.

FISHER, J., The twisted pear and the prediction of behavior, *Journal of Consulting Psychology* 23, 400-405 (1959).

FISS, H., The need to complete one's dreams, in J. Fisher & L. Breger (Eds.), *The Meaning of Dreams: Recent Insights from the Laboratory, Research Symposium No. 3*, Bureau of Research, California Department of Mental Hygiene: Sacramento, 1969.

FISS, H., KLEIN, G.S. and SHOLLAR, E., "Dream intensification" as a function of prolonged REM period interruption, *Psychoanalysis and Contemporary Science* 3, 399-424 (1974).

FOULKES, D., *The Psychology of Sleep*, Scribner: New York, 1966.

FOULKES, D., Dreams of the male child: Four case studies, *Journal of Child Psychology and Psychiatry* 8, 81-87 (1967).

FOULKES, D., Personality and dreams, *International Psychiatry Clinics*, 7, 147-153 (1970).

FOULKES, D. and FLEISHER, S., Mental activity in relaxed wakefulness, *Journal of Abnormal Psychology* 84, 66-75 (1975).

FOULKES, D. and GRIFFIN, M.L., An experimental study of "creative dreaming", paper presented to the annual meeting of the Association for the Psychophysiological Study of Sleep, Cincinnati, June, 1976.

FOULKES, D. and POPE, R., Primary visual experience and secondary cognitive elaboration in state REM: A modest confirmation and extension, *Perceptual and Motor Skills* 37, 107-118 (1973).

FOULKES, D. and RECHTSCHAFFEN, A., Presleep determinants of dream content: Effects of two films, *Perceptual and Motor Skills* 19, 983-1005 (1964).

FOULKES, D. and VOGEL, G., Mental activity at sleep onset, *Journal of Abnormal and Social Psychology* 70, 231-243 (1965).

FOULKES, D. and VOGEL, G.W., The current status of laboratory dream research, *Psychiatric Annals* 4, 19-23, 27 (1974).

FOULKES, D., SPEAR, P.S. and SYMONDS, J.D., Individual differences in mental activity at sleep onset, *Journal of Abnormal Psychology*, 71, 280-286 (1966).

FRANKS, J.J., Toward understanding understanding, in W.B. Weimer & D.S. Palermo (Eds.), *Cognition and the Symbolic Processes*, Lawrence Erlbaum Associates: Hillsdale, New Jersey, 1974.

FREEDMAN, D.G., *Human Infancy: An Evolutionary Perspective*, Lawrence Erlbaum Associates: Hillsdale, New Jersey, 1974.

FREUD, S., *On Dreams*, Norton: New York, 1952.

FREUD, S., *The Interpretation of Dreams*, Basic Books: New York, 1955.

FROMM, E., *The Forgotten Language*, Grove Press: New York, 1951.

GAINOTTI, G., Emotional behavior and hemispheric side of lesion, *Cortex* 8, 41-55 (1972).

GALIN, D., Implications for psychiatry of left and right cerebral specialization, *Archives of General Psychiatry* 31, 572-583 (1974).

GALIN, D. and ORNSTEIN, R., Lateral specialization of cognitive mode: An EEG study, *Psychophysiology* 9, 412-418 (1972).

GALLUP, G.G., Self recognition in primates: A comparative approach to the bidirectional properties of consciousness, *American Psychologist* 32, 329-338 (1977).

GARDINER, R., GROSSMAN, W.I., ROFFWARG, H.P. and WEINER, H., The relationship of small limb movement during REM sleep for dreamed limb action, *Psychosomatic Medicine* 37, 147-159 (1975).

GARFIELD, S.L., *Clinical Psychology: The Study of Personality and Behavior*, Aldine: Chicago, 1974.

GASTAUT, H. and BROUGHTON, R., A clinical and polygraphic study of episodic phenomenon during sleep, *Recent Advances in Biological Psychiatry* 7, 197-221 (1965).

GAZZANIGA, M.S., One brain—two minds?, *American Scientist* 60, 311-317 (1972).

GESCHWIND, N., The apraxias: Neural mechanisms of disorders of learned movement, *American Scientist* 63, 188-195 (1975).

GIBBS, E.L. and WEIR, H., Amphetamine induced sleep in children with extreme spindles, *Clinical Electroencephalography* 4, 127 (1973).

GILLIN, J.C. and WYATT, R.J., Schizophrenia: Perchance a dream, *International Review of Neurobiology* 17, 297-342 (1975).

GILLIN, J.C., BUCHSBAUM, M.S., JACOBS, L.S., FRAM, D.H., WILLIAMS, R.B., VAUGHAN, T.B., MELLON, E., SNYDER, F. and WYATT, R.J., Partial REM sleep deprivation, schizophrenia and field articulation, *Archives of General Psychiatry* 30, 653-662 (1974).

GLICKSTEIN, M. and GIBSON, A.R., Visual cells in the pons of the brain, *Scientific American* 235, 90-98 (1976).

GLOBUS, G.G., Rapid eye movement cycle in real time, *Archives of General Psychiatry* 15, 654-659 (1966).

GLOTZBACH, S.E. and HELLER, H.C., Central nervous regulation of body temperature during sleep, *Science* 194, 537-539 (1976).

GOLDSTEIN, L., STOLTZFUS, N.W. and GARDOCKI, J.F., Changes in interhemispheric amplitude relationships in the EEG during sleep, *Physiology and Behavior* 8, 811-815 (1972).

GOLIN, S., HERRON, E., LAKOTA, R. and REINECK, L., Factor analytic study of the manifest anxiety, extraversion, and repression-sensitization scales, *Journal of Consulting Psychology* 31, 564-569 (1967).

GOODENOUGH, D.R., Some recent studies of dream recall, in H.A. Witkin & H.B. Lewis (Eds.), *Experimental Studies of Dreaming*, Random House: New York, 1967.

GOODENOUGH, D.R., LEWIS, H.B., SHAPIRO, A., JARET, L. and SLESER, F., Dream reporting following abrupt and gradual awakenings from different types of sleep, *Journal of Personality and Social Psychology* 2, 170-179 (1965).

GOODENOUGH, D.R., WITKIN, H.A., LEWIS, H.B., KOULACK, D. and COHEN, H., Repression, interference, and field dependence as factors in dream forgetting, *Journal of Abnormal Psychology* 83, 32-44 (1974).

GOTTLIEB, G., Conception of prenatal development: Behavioral embryology, *Psychological Review* 83, 215-234 (1976).

GREENBERG, R. and PEARLMAN, C.A., Cutting the REM nerve: An approach to the adaptive role of REM sleep, *Perspectives in Biology and Medicine* 17, 513-521 (1974).

GREENBERG, R., PEARLMAN, C., BROOKS, R., MAYER, R. and HARTMANN, E., Dreaming and Korsakoff's psychosis, *Archives of General Psychiatry* 18, 203-209 (1968).

GREENBERG, R., PEARLMAN, C., FINGAR, R., KANTROWITZ, J. and KAWLICHE, S., The effects of dream deprivation: Implications for a theory of the psychological function of dreaming, *British Journal of Medical Psychology* 43, 1-11 (1970).

GREENBERG, R., PILLARD, R. and PEARLMAN, C., The effect of dream deprivation on adaptation to stress, *Psychosomatic Medicine* 34, 257-262 (1972).

GRIESER, C., GREENBERG, R. and HARRISON, R.H., The adaptive function of sleep: The differential effects of sleep and dreaming on recall, *Journal of Abnormal Psychology* 80, 280-286 (1972).

GUILLEMINAULT, C., PERAITA, R., SOUQUET, M. and DEMENT, W.C., Apneas during sleep in infants: Possible relationship with sudden infant death syndrome, *Science* 190, 677-679 (1975).

GUR, R.E. and GUR, R.C., Defense mechanisms, psychomatic symptomatology, and conjugate lateral eye movements, *Journal of Consulting and Clinical Psychology* 43, 416-420 (1975).

GUR, R.C., SACKEIM, H.A. and GUR, R.E., Classroom seating and psychopathology: Some initial data, *Journal of Abnormal Psychology* 85, 122-124 (1976).

GUTMAN, D., Women and the conception of ego strength, *Merrill-Palmer Quarterly* 11, 17-26 (1965).

HALL, C.S., *The Meaning of Dreams*, McGraw-Hill: New York, 1966.

HALL, C.S., Caveat lector (Review of E. Hartmann, *The Biology of Dreaming*, Charles Thomas: Sprinfield, Illinois, 1967), *The Psychoanalytic Review* 54, 99-105 (1967).

HALL, C.S., Normative dream-content studies, in M. Kramer (Ed.), *Dream Psychology and the New Biology of Dreaming*, Charles Thomas: Springfield, Illinois, 1969.

HALL, C.S. and NORDBY, V.J., *The Individual and his Dreams*, Signet: New York, 1972.

HALL, C.S. and VAN DE CASTLE, R.L., *The Content Analysis of Dreams*, Appleton-Century-Crofts: New York, 1966.

HALPER, C., PIVIK, T. and DEMENT, W., An attempt to reduce the REM rebound following REM deprivation by the use of induced waking mentation, Paper presented at the meeting of the Association for the Psychophysiological Study of Sleep, Boston, March, 1969.

HAMPDEN-TURNER, C. and WHITTEN, P., Morals left and right, *Psychology Today* 74, 39-43 (1971).

HARDYCK, C. and PETRINOVICH, L.F., Left-handedness, *Psychological Bulletin* 84, 385-404 (1977).

HARPER, L.V., The scope of offspring effects: From caregiver to culture, *Psychological Bulletin* 82, 784-801 (1975).

HARTLEY, R., Sex-role pressures and socialization of the male child, *Psychological Reports* 5, 457-468 (1959).

HARTMANN, E., *The Functions of Sleep*, Yale University Press: New Haven, 1973.

HARTMANN, E. and STERN, W.E., Desynchronized sleep deprivation: Learning deficit and its reversal by increased catecholamines, *Physiology and Behavior* 8, 585-587 (1972).

HAURI, P., Effects of evening activity on early night sleep, *Psychophysiology* 4, 267 (1968).

HAURI, P., Evening activity, sleep mentation, and subjective sleep quality, *Journal of Abnormal Psychology* 76, 270-275 (1970).

HAURI, P., Categorization of sleep mental activity for psychophysiological studies, in G.C. Lairy & P. Salzarulo (Eds.), *The Experimental Study of Human Sleep: Methodological Problems*, Elsevier: Amsterdam, 1975.

HAURI, P., Dreams in patients remitted from reactive depression, *Journal of Abnormal Psychology* 85, 1-10 (1976).

HAURI, P. and VAN DE CASTLE, R.L., Psychophysiological parallels in dreams, *Psychosomatic Medicine* 35, 297-308 (1973(a)).

HAURI, P. and VAN DE CASTLE, R.L., Psychophysiological parallels in dreams, in M. Jovanović (Ed.), *The Nature of Sleep*, Gustav Fischer: Stuttgart, Germany, 1973(b).

HAWKINS, D.R., A Freudian view, in M. Kramer (Ed.), *Dream Psychology and the New Biology of Dreaming*, Charles Thomas: Springfield, Illinois, 1969.

HELD, R. and HEIN, A., Movement-produced stimulation in the development of visual guided behavior, *Journal of Comparative and Physiological Psychology* 56, 872-876 (1963).

HELLER, H.C., COLLIVER, G.W. and ANAND, P., CNS regulation of body temperature in euthermic hibernators, *American Journal of Physiology* 227, 576-589 (1974).

HERBERT, M., Performance after heat-disturbed sleep, in M.H. Chase, W.C. Stern & P.L. Walter (Eds.), *Sleep Research, Vol. 4*, Brain Information Service/Brain Research Institute: Los Angeles, 1975. p. 172.

HERNANDEZ-PEON, R., Neurophysiology, phylogeny, and functional significance of dreaming, *Experimental Neurology* 4, 106-125 (1967).

HERSCH, R.G., ANTROBUS, J.S., ARKIN, A.M. and SINGER, J.L., Dreaming as a function of sympathetic arousal, *Psychophysiology* 7, 329-330 (1970).

HERSEN, M., Personality characteristics of nightmare sufferers, *Journal of Nervous and Mental Disease* 153, 27-31 (1971).

HIATT, J.F. and KRIPKE, D.F., Ultradian rhythms in waking gastric activity, *Psychosomatic Medicine* 37, 320-325 (1975).

HIGGINS, R.L. and MARLATT, G.A., Fear of interpersonal evaluation as a determinant of alcohol consumption in male social drinkers, *Journal of Abnormal Psychology* 84, 644-651 (1975).

HISCOCK, M., Eye-movement asymmetry and hemispheric function: An examination of individual differences, *Journal of Psychology* 97, 49-52 (1977).

REFERENCES

HISCOCK, M. and COHEN, D.B., Visual imagery and dream recall, *Journal of Research in Personality* 7, 179-188 (1973).

HOBSON, J.A., The cellular basis of sleep cycle control, in E. Weitzman (Ed.), *Advances in Sleep Research, Vol. I*, Spectrum Publications: New York, 1974.

HOBSON, J.A., The sleep-dream cycle: A neurobiological rhythm, in H.L. Joachim (Ed.), *Pathobiology Annual*, Appleton-Century-Crofts, New York, 1975.

HOBSON, J.A., The reciprocal interaction model of sleep cycle control: Implications for PGO wave generation and dream amnesia, in R.R. Drucker-Colin & J. McGaugh (Eds.), *Sleep and Memory*, Academic Press: New York, 1977.

HOBSON, J.A., McCARLEY, R.W. and WYZINSKI, P.W., Sleep cycle oscillation: reciprocal discharge by two brain stem neuronal groups, *Science* 189, 55-58 (1975).

HOLT, R.R., On the nature and generality of mentality imagery, in P.W. Sheehan (Ed.), *The Function and Nature of Imagery*, Academic Press: New York, 1972.

HOPPE, K.D., Split brains and psychoanalysis, *The Psychoanalytic Quarterly* 46, 220-244 (1977).

HORN, J.M., TURNER, R.G. and DAVIS, L.S., Personality differences between both intended and actual social sciences and engineering majors, *British Journal of Educational Psychology* 45, 293-298 (1975).

HORNE, J.A. and PORTER, J.M., Time of day effects with standardized exercise upon subsequent sleep, *Electroencephalography and Clinical Neurophysiology* 40, 178-184 (1976).

HOSHINO, K. and POMPEIANO, O., Selective discharge of pontine neurons during postural atonia produced by an anticholinesterase in the decerebrate cat, *Archives of Italian Biology* 114, 244-277 (1976).

HUME, K.I. and MILLS, J.N., A split sleep investigation of the relative effects of time of day and duration of prior wakefulness on the sleep process, in M.H. Chase, W.C. Stern & P.L. Walter (Eds.), *Sleep Research, Vol. 4*, Brain Information Service/Brain Research Institute: Los Angeles, 1975. p. 266.

HYDEN, H., The question of a molecular basis for the memory traces, in K. Pribram & D. Broadbent (Eds.), *The Biology of Memory*, Academic Press: New York, 1970.

JACOBS, L., FELDMAN, M. and BENDER, M.B., Eye movements during sleep. I. The pattern in the normal human, *Archives of Neurology* 25, 151-159 (1971).

JASPER, H.H., Thalamic reticular system, in D.E. Sheir (Ed.), *Electrical Stimulation of the Brain: An Interdisciplinary Survey of Neurobehavioral Integrative Systems*, Hogg Foundation for Mental Health: Austin, Texas, 1961.

JENSEN, A.R., How much can we boost IQ and scholastic achievement?, *Harvard Educational Review, Reprint Series No. 2*, President and fellows of Harvard College, 1969.

JENSEN, A.R., *Genetics and Education*, Harper & Row: New York, 1972.

JERISON, H.J., *Evolution of the Brain and Intelligence*, Academic Press: New York, 1973.

JERISON, H.J., Paleoneurology and the evolution of mind, *Scientific American* 234, 90-91, 94-101 (1976).

JOHN, E.R., A model of consciousness, in G.E. Schwartz & D. Shapiro (Eds.), *Consciousness and Self-Regulation: Advances in Research, Vol. 1*, Plenum: New York, 1976.

JOHNS, M.W., MASTERSON, J.P., PADDLE-LEDINEK, J.E., WINIKOFF, M. and MALINEK, M., Delta-wave sleep and thyroid function in healthy young men, in M.H. Chase, W.C. Stern & P.L. Walter (Eds.), *Sleep Research, Vol. 4*, Brain Information Service/Brain Research Institute: Los Angeles, 1975. p. 277.

JOHNSON, H. and ERIKSEN, C.W., Preconscious perception: A re-examination of the Poetzl phenomenon, *Journal of Abnormal and Social Psychology* 62, 497-503 (1961).

JOHNSON, L.C., Are stages of sleep related to waking behavior?, *American Scientist* 61, 326-338 (1973(a)).

JOHNSON, L.C., The effect of total, partial, and stage sleep deprivation on EEG patterns and performance, in N. Burch & H.L. Altschuler (Eds.), *Behavior and Brain Electrical Activity*, Plenum: New York, 1973(b).

JONES, B.M. and PARSONS, O.A., Alcohol and consciousness: Getting high, coming down, *Psychology Today* 8, 53-58 (1975).

JOUVET, M., The states of sleep, *Scientific American* 216, 62-72 (1967).

JOUVET, M., Commentary, in W.B. Webb (Ed.), *Sleep: An Active Process*, Scott, Foresman: Glenview, Illinois, 1973.

JOUVET, M., The role of monoaminergic neurons in the regulation and function of sleep, in O. Petre-Quadens & J.D. Schlag (Eds.), *Basic Sleep Mechanisms*, Academic Press: New York, 1974.

JOUVET, M., Cholinergic mechanisms and sleep, in P.G. Waser (Ed.), *Cholinergic Mechanisms*, Raven Press: New York, 1975.

JOVANOVIĆ, U.J., The sleep-waking cycle in healthy test subjects, *Waking and Sleeping* 1, 7-26 (1976).

JUNG, C.G., *Modern Man in Search of a Soul*, Harcourt, Brace & World: New York, 1933.

JUNG, C.G., Approaching the unconscious, in C.G. Jung & M-L. von Franz (Eds.), *Man and his Symbols*, Aldus Books: London, England, 1964.

JUS, A., JUS, K., VILLENEUVE, A., PIRES, A., LACHANCE, R., FORTIER, J. and VILLENEUVE, R., Studies on dream recall in chronic schizophrenic patients after prefrontal labotomy, *Biological Psychiatry* 6, 275-293 (1973).

KAHN, E. and FISHER, C., The sleep characteristics of the aged male, *Journal of Nervous and Mental Disease* 148, 477-494 (1969).

KAHN, E., DEMENT, W., FISHER, C. and BARMACK, J.E., Incidence of color in immediately recalled dreams, *Science* 137, 1054-1055 (1962).

KALES, A., WILSON, T., KALES, J.D., JACOBSON, A., PAULSON, M.J., KOLLAR, E. and WALTER, R.D., Measurements of all night sleep in normal elderly persons: Effects of aging, *Journal of the American Geriatrics Society* 15, 405-414 (1967).

KANNER, A.D., Femininity and masculinity: Their relationships to creativity in male architects and their independence from each other, *Journal of Consulting and Clinical Psychology* 44, 802-805 (1976).

KARACAN, I., GOODENOUGH, D.R., SHAPIRO, A. and STARKER, S., Erection cycle during sleep in relation to dream anxiety, *Archives of General Psychiatry* 15, 183-189 (1966).

KARACAN, I., WOLFF, S.M., WILLIAMS, H.L., HURSCH, C.J. and WEBB, W.B., The effects of fever on sleep and dreams, *Psychosomatics* 9, 331-339 (1968).

KELLER, F.S. and SCHOENFELD, W.N., *Principles of Psychology: A Systematic Text in the Science of Behavior*, Appleton-Century-Crofts: New York, 1950.

KESSLER, S., Genetic factors in narcolepsy, in C. Guilleminault, W.C. Dement, & P. Passouant (Eds.), *Narcolepsy*, Spectrum Publications: New York, 1976.

KINSBOURNE, M., Eye and head turning indicates cerebral lateralization, *Science* 176, 539-541 (1972).

KLEITMAN, N., *Sleep and Wakefulness*, University of Chicago Press: Chicago, 1963.

KLEITMAN, N., The basic rest-activity cycle and physiological correlates of dreaming, *Experimental Neurology Supplement* 4, 2-4 (1967).

KLEITMAN, N., The basic rest-activity cycle in relation to sleep and wakefulness, in A. Kales (Ed.), *Sleep: Physiology and Pathology*, Lippincott: Philadelphia, 1969.

KLINGER, E., *Structure and Functions of Fantasy*, Wiley-Interscience: New York, 1971.

KLINGER, E., Consequences of commitment to and disengagement from incentives, *Psychological Review* 82, 1-25 (1975).

KLINGER, E., GREGOIRE, K.C. and BARTA, S.G., Physiological correlates of mental activity: Eye movements, alpha, and heart rate during imaginary, suppression, concentration, search, and choice, *Psychophysiology* 10, 471-477 (1973).

KOPPEL, B.S., ZARCONE, V., DE LA PEÑA, A. and DEMENT, W.C., Changes in selective attention as measured by the visual averaged evoked potential following REM deprivation in man, *Electroencephalography and Clinical Neurophysiology* 32, 322-325 (1972).

KOSSLYN, S.M. and POMERANTZ, J.R., Imagery, propositions, and the form of internal representation, *Cognitive Psychology* 9, 52-76 (1977).

KOULACK, D., Effects of somatosensory stimulation on dream content, *Archives of General Psychiatry* 20, 718-725 (1969).

KOULACK, D., Rapid eye movements and visual imagery during sleep, *Psychological Bulletin* 78, 155-158 (1972).

KOULACK, D., Effects of a hypnogogic type situation and a dull task on subsequent REM-rebound: A preliminary report, in M.H. Chase, W.C. Stern & P.L. Walter (Eds.), *Sleep Research, Vol. 2*, Brain Information Service/Brain Research Institute: Los Angeles, 1973, p. 167.

KRAMER, M. and ROTH, T., A comparison of dream content in laboratory dream reports of schizophrenic and depressive patient groups, *Comprehensive Psychiatry* 14, 325-329 (1973).

KRAMER, M. and ROTH, T., Dreams and dementia: A laboratory exploration of dream recall and dream content in chronic brain syndrome patients, *International Journal of Aging and Human Development* 6, 169-178 (1975).

KRAMER, M., BALDRIDGE, B.J., WHITMAN, R.M., ORNSTEIN, P.H. and SMITH, P.C., An exploration of the manifest dream in schizophrenic and depressed patients, *Diseases of the Nervous System* 30, 126-130 (1969).

KRAMER, M., ROTH, T. and CZAYA, J., Dream development within a REM period, in P. Levin & W.P. Koella (Eds.), *Sleep 1974: Instinct, Neurophysiology, Endocrinology, Episodes, Dreams, Epilepsy and Intracranial Pathology*, S.Karger: Basel, Switzerland, 1975.

KRAMER, M., WHITMAN, R.M., BALDRIDGE, B.J. and ORNSTEIN, P.H., The pharmacology of sleep: A review, in G.J. Martin & B. Kisch (Eds.), *Enzymes and Mental Health*, Lippincott: Philadelphia, 1966.

KRAMER, M., WHITMAN, R.M., BALDRIDGE, B.J. and ORNSTEIN, P.H., Dream content in male schizophrenic patients, *Disease of the Nervous System* 31, 51-58 (1970).

KRIPPNER, S. and HUGHES, W., Dreams and human potential, *Journal of Humanistic Psychology* 10, 1-20 (1970).

KRUGLANSKI, A.W., Much ado about the "volunteer artifacts", *Journal of Personality and Social Psychology* 28, 348-354 (1973).

KUPFER, D.J., REM latency: A psychobiological marker for primary depression, *Biological Psychiatry* 11, 159-174 (1976).

KUPFER, D.J., PICKAR, D., HIMMELHOCH, J.M. and DETRE, T.P., Are there two types of unipolar depression?, *Archives of General Psychiatry* 32, 866-871 (1975).

LAGERKVIST, P., *The Dwarf*, Hill & Wang: New York, 1945.

LAIRY, G.C., Dream and delusion symptoms, in P. Levin & W.P. Koella (Eds.), *Sleep 1974: Instinct, Neurophysiology, Endocrinology, Episodes, Dreams, Epilepsy and Intracranial Pathology*, S. Karger: Basel, Switzerland, 1975.

LAMSTEIN, S., ROFFWARG, H. and HERMAN, J., Middle ear muscle activity (MEMA): A low threshold phasic phenomenon, paper presented at the second International Sleep Research Congress, Edinburgh, Scotland, July, 1975.

LAVIE, P. and GIORA, Z., Spiral aftereffect durations following awakening from REM and nonREM sleep, *Perception and Psychophysics* 1, 19-20 (1973).

LAVIE, P. and KRIPKE, D.F., Ultradian rhythms: The 90-minute clock inside us, *Psychology Today* 8, 54-56 (1975).

LAVIE, P., LEVY, C.M. and COOLIDGE, F.L., Ultradian rhythms in the perception of the spiral aftereffect, *Physiological Psychology* 3, 144-146 (1975).

LAZARUS, R.S. and ALFERT, E., The short-circuiting of threat by experimentally altering cognitive appraisal, *Journal of Abnormal and Social Psychology* 69, 195-205 (1964).

LECAS, J-C., Changes in paradoxical sleep accompanying instrumental learning in the cat, *Neuroscience Letters* 3, 349-355 (1976).

LECONTE, P. and HENNEVIN, E., Caractéristiques temporelles de l'augmentation de sommeil paradoxal consecutif à l'apprentissage chez le rat, *Physiology and Behavior* 11, 677-686 (1973).

LECONTE, P., HENNEVIN, E. and BLOCH, V., Duration of paradoxical sleep necessary for the acquisition of conditional avoidance in the rat, *Physiology and Behavior* 13, 675-681 (1974).

LEHMANN, D. and KOUKKOU, M., Learning and EEG during sleep in humans, in W.P. Koella & P. Levin (Eds.), *Sleep 1974: Physiology, Biochemistry, Psychology, Pharmacology, Clinical Implications*, S. Karger: Basel, Switzerland, 1973.

LENARD, H.G. and SCHULTE, F.J., Polygraphic sleep study in craniopagus twins, *Journal of Neurology, Neurosurgery and Psychiatry* 35, 756-762 (1972).

LENNEBERG, E.H., *Biological Foundations of Language*, Wiley: New York, 1967.

LERNER, B., Dream function reconsidered, *Journal of Abnormal Psychology* 72, 85-100 (1967).

LEVERE, T.E., MORLOCK, G.W. and HART, F.D., Waking performance decrements following minimal sleep disruption: The effects of habitation during sleep, *Physiological Psychology* 3, 147-154 (1975).

LEVIS, D.J., Learned helplessness: A reply and an alternative S-R interpretation, *Journal of Experimental Psychology: General* 105, 47-65 (1976).

LEVY, J., Lateral specialization of the human brain: Behavioral manifestations and possible evolutionary basis, in J.A. Kiger (Ed.), *Proceedings of the 32nd Annual Biology Colloquium on the Biology of Behaviors*, Oregon State University Press: Corvallis, 1972.

LEWIN, I. and GLAUBMAN, H., The effect of REM deprivation: Is it detrimental, beneficial or neutral?, *Psychophysiology* 12, 349-353 (1975).

LEWIS, H.B., GOODENOUGH, D.R., SHAPIRO, A. and SLESER, I., Individual differences in dream recall, *Journal of Abnormal Psychology* 71, 52-59 (1966).

LEWIS, S.A., The neurochemical approach to sleep: From the outside, looking in, in G.C. Lairy & P. Salzarulo (Eds.), *The Experimental Study of Human Sleep: Methodological Problems*, Elsevier: Amsterdam, 1975.

LEYGONIE, F., HOUZEL, D., GUILHAUME, A. and BENOIT, O., Intrasleep organization in neurotic children, in P. Levin & W.P. Koella (Eds.), *Sleep 1974: Instinct, Neurophysiology, Endocrinology, Episodes, Dreams, Epilepsy and Intracranial Pathology*, S. Karger: Basel, Switzerland, 1975.

LINDEN, E.R., BERN, D. and FISHBEIN, W., Retrograde amnesia: Prolonging the fixation phase of memory consolidation by paradoxical sleep deprivation, *Physiology and Behavior* 14, 409-412 (1975).

LIPSITT, L.P., Learning capacities of the human infant, in J.F. Rosenblith, W. Allinsmith, & J.P. Williams (Eds.), *The Cause of Behaviors: Readings in Child Development and Educational Psychology* (3rd ed.), Allyn & Bacon: Boston, 1972.

LUGARESI, E., COCCAGNA, G., FARNETI, P., MANTOVANI, M. and CIRIGNOTTA, F., Snoring, *Electroencephalography and Clinical Neurophysiology* 39, 59-64 (1975).

LUND, R., Personality factors and desynchronization of circadian rhythms, *Psychosomatic Medicine* 36, 224-228 (1974).

MAAS, J.W., Biogenic amines and depression, *Archives of General Psychiatry* 32, 1357-1361 (1975).

MACCOBY, E.E. and JACKLIN, C.N., *The Psychology of Sex Differences*, Stanford University Press: Stanford, 1974.

MAGNI, F., MORUZZI, G., ROSSI, G.F. and ZANCHETTI, P., EEG arousal following inactivation of the lower brain stem by selective injection of barbiturate into the vertebral circulation, *Archives of Italian Biology* 97, 33-46 (1959).

MANDLER, G., *Mind and Emotion*, Wiley: New York, 1975.

MARKS, D.F., Individual differences in the vividness of visual imagery and their effect on function, in P.W. Sheehan (Ed.), *The Function and Nature of Imagery*, Academic Press: New York, 1972.

McCABE, M.S. and STROMGREN, E., Reactive psychosis, *Archives of General Psychiatry* 32, 447-454 (1975).

McCANNE, T.R. and SANDMAN, C.A., Human operant heart rate conditioning: The importance of individual differences, *Psychological Bulletin* 83, 587-601 (1976).

McCARLEY, R.W. and HOBSON, J.A., Neuronal excitability modulation over the sleep cycle: A structural and mathematical model, *Science* 189, 58-60 (1975).

McGINTY, D.J., HARPER, R.M. and FAIRBANKS, M.K., Neuronal unit activity and the control of sleep states, in E.D. Weitzman (Ed.), *Advances in Sleep Research, Vol. 1*, Spectrum Publications: New York, 1974.

McGRATH, M.J. and COHEN, D.B., REM sleep facilitation of adaptive waking behavior: A review of the literature, *Psychological Bulletin* 85, 24-57 (1978).

McNEIL, T., Prebirth and postbirth influence on the relationship between creativity and recorded mental illness, *Journal of Personality* 39, 391-406 (1971).

MEDDIS, R., The function of sleep, *Animal Behavior* 23, 676-691 (1975).

MENDELSON, J.H., SIGER, L. and SOLOMON, P., Psychiatric observations on congenital and acquired deafness: Symbolic and perceptual processes in dreams, *American Journal of Psychiatry* 116, 883-888 (1960).

MENDELSON, W.B., REICHMAN, J. and OTHMER, E., Serotonin inhibition and sleep, *Biological Psychiatry* 10, 459-464 (1975).

MILNER, P.M., *Physiological Psychology*, Holt, Rinehart, & Winston: New York, 1970.

MISCHEL, W., *Personality and Assessment*, Wiley: New York, 1968.

MOISEEVA, N.I., The characteristics of EEG activity and the subjective estimation of time during dreams of different structure, in M.H. Chase, W.C. Stern and P.L. Walter (Eds.), *Sleep Research, Vol. 4*, Brain Information Service/Brain Research Institute: Los Angeles, 1975. p. 161.

MOLINARI, S. and FOULKES, D., Tonic and phasic events during sleep: Psychological correlates and implications, *Perceptual and Motor Skills, Monograph Supplement No. 1* 29, 343-368 (1969).

MONEY, J. and TUCKER, P., *Sexual Signatures: On being a Man or a Woman*, Little, Brown: Boston, 1975.

MONROE, L.J., Psychological and physiological differences between good and poor sleepers, *Journal of Abnormal Psychology* 72, 255-264 (1967).

MORRISON, A.R. and BOWKER, R.M., PGO spikes: A sign of startle reflex activation, in M.H. Chase, W.C. Stern & P.L. Walter (Eds.), *Sleep Research, Vol. 4*, Brain Information Service/Brain Research Institute: Los Angeles, 1975. p. 36.

MORUZZI, G., Neural mechanisms of the sleep-waking cycle, in O. Petre-Quadens & J.D. Schlag (Eds.), *Basic Sleep Mechanisms*, Academic Press: New York, 1974.

MOSCOWITZ, E. and BERGER, R.J., Rapid eye movements and dream imagery: are they related? *Nature* 224, 613-614 (1969).

MOSES, J.M., HORD, D.J., LUBIN, A., JOHNSON, L.C. and NAITOH, P., Dynamics of nap sleep during a 40 hour period, *Electroencephalography and Clinical Neurophysiology* 39, 627-633 (1975(a)).

MOSES, J.M., JOHNSON, L.C., NAITOH, P. and LUBIN, A., Sleep stage deprivation and total sleep loss: Effects on sleep behavior, *Psychophysiology* 12, 141-146 (1975(b)).

MURPHY, G., *Personality: A Biosocial Approach to Origins and Structure*, Harper & Brothers: New York, 1947.

MYSLOBODSKY, M. and WEINER, M., Pharmacological implications of hemispheric asymmetry, *Life Sciences* 19, 1467-1478 (1976).

MYSLOBODSKY, M.S., BEN-MAYOR, V., YEDID-LEVY, B. and MINZ, M., Interhemispheric asymmetry of electrical activity of the brain in sleep and "cerebral dominance", *Bulletin of the Psychonomic Society* 7, 465-467 (1976).

NAKAZAWA, Y., KOTORII, M., KOTORII, T., TACHIBANA, H. and NAKANO, T., Individual differences in compensatory rebound of REM sleep, with particular reference to their relationship to personality and behavioral characteristics, *Journal of Nervous and Mental Disease* 161, 18-25 (1975(a)).

NAKAZAWA, Y., KOTORII, M., ARIKAWA, K., HORIKAWA, S. and HASUZAWA, H., Personality characteristics and sleep variables, *Folia Psychiatrica et Neurologica Japonica* 29, 101-109 (1975(b)).

NAKAZAWA, Y., TACHIBANA, H., KOTORII, M. and OGATA, M., Effects of L-Dopa on natural night sleep and on rebound of REM sleep, *Folia Psychiatrica et Neurologica Japonica* 27, 223-230 (1973).

NAQUET, R., From cat to man, from physiology to psychophysiology, the "as if" thinking, in G.C. Lairy & P. Salzarulo (Eds.), *The Experimental Study of Human Sleep: Methodological Problems*, Elsevier: Amsterdam, 1975.

NEISSER, U., Cultural and cognitive discontinuity, in Anthropological Society of Washington, *Anthropology and Human Behavior*, Gaus: Washington, D.C., 1962.

NEISSER, U., *Cognitive Psychology*, Appleton-Century-Crofts: New York, 1967.

NEWTON, P.M., Recalled dream content and the maintenance of body image, *Journal of Abnormal Psychology* 76, 134-139 (1970).

NISBETT, R.E. and WILSON, T.D., Telling more than we can know: Verbal reports on mental processes, *Psychological Review* 84, 231-259 (1977).

NOTON, D. and STARK, L., Eye movements and visual perception, *Scientific American* 224, 35-43 (1971).

OKUMA, T., SUNAMI, Y., FUKUMA, E., TAKEO, S. and MOTOIKE, M., Dream content study on chronic schizophrenics and normals by REMP-awakening technique, *Folia Psychiatrica et Neurologica Japonica* 24, 151-162 (1970).

ORNITZ, E.M., FORSYTHE, A.B. and DE LA PEÑA, A., Effect of vestibular and auditory stimulation on the REMs of REM sleep in autistic children, *Archives of General Psychiatry* 29, 786-791 (1973).

ORNITZ, E.M., RITVO, E.R., BROWN, M.B., LAFRANCHI, S., PARMELEE, T. and WALTER, R.D., The EEG and rapid eye movements during REM sleep in normal and autistic children, *Electroencephalography and Clinical Neurophysiology* 26, 167-175 (1969).

OSWALD, I., Is sleep related to synthetic purpose?, in W.P. Koella & P. Levin (Eds.), *Sleep: Physiology, Biochemistry, Psychology, Pharmacology, Clinical Implications*, S. Karger: Basel, Switzerland, 1973.

OSWALD, I., Pharmacology of sleep, in O. Petre-Quadens & J.D. Schlag (Eds.), *Basic Sleep Mechanism*, Academic Press: New York, 1974.

OSWALD, I., TAYLOR, A.M. and TREISMAN, M., Discriminative responses to stimulation during human sleep, *Brain* 83, 440-453 (1960).

OVERTON, D.A., State-dependent retention of learned responses produced by drugs: Its relevance to sleep and learning and recall, in W.P. Koella & P. Levin (Eds.), *Sleep: Physiology, Biochemistry, Psychology, Pharmacology, Clinical Implications*, S. Karger: Basel, Switzerland, 1973.

PAIVIO, A., *Imagery and Verbal Processes*, Holt, Rinehart & Winston: New York, 1971.

PAIVIO, A., YUILLE, J.C. and MADIGAN, S., Concreteness, imagery, and meaningfulness values for 925 nouns, *Journal of Experimental Psychology* 76 (1968).

PAPPENHEIMER, J.R., The sleep factor, *Scientific American* 235, 24-29 (1976).

PAPPENHEIMER, J.R., KOSKI, G., FENCL, V., KARNOVSKY, M.L. and KRUEGER, J., Extraction of sleep-promoting factor S from cerebrospinal fluid and from brains of sleep deprived animals, *Journal of Neurophysiology* 38, 1299-1311 (1975).

PARMEGGIANI, P.L., FRANZINI, C. and LENZI, P., Preoptic heating and respiratory frequency during sleep, in M.H. Chase, W.C. Stern & P.L. Walter (Eds.), *Sleep Research, Vol. 4*, Brain Information Service/Brain Research Institute: Los Angeles, 1975, p. 65.

PARMEGGIANI, P.L., FRANZINI, C. and LENZI, P., Respiratory frequency as a function of preoptic temperature during sleep, *Brain Research* 111, 253-260 (1976).

PAUL, K. and DITTRICHOVA, J., Sleep patterns following learning in infants, in P. Levin & W.P. Koella (Eds.), *Sleep 1974: Instinct, Neurophysiology, Endocrinology, Episodes, Dreams, Epilepsy and Intracranial Pathology*, S. Karger: Basel, Switzerland, 1975.

PEARLMAN, C.A. and BECKER, M., Brief posttrial REM sleep deprivation impairs discrimination learning in rats, *Physiological Psychology* 1, 373-376 (1973).

PEARLMAN, C.A. and GREENBERG, R., Posttrial REM sleep: A critical period for consolidation of shuttlebox avoidance, *Animal Learning and Behavior* 1, 49-51 (1973).

PETRE-QUADENS, O., Sleep in the human newborn, in O. Petre-Quadens & J.D. Schlag (Eds.), *Basic Sleep Mechanisms*, Academic Press: New York, 1974.

PETRE-QUADENS, O. and SCHLAG, J.D., *Basic Sleep Mechanisms*, Academic Press: New York, 1974.

PHILLIPS, F., CHEN, C.N., CRISP, A.H., KOVAL, J., McGUINNESS, B., KALUCY, R.S., KALUCY, E.C. and LACEY, J.H., Isocaloric diet changes and electroencephalographic sleep, *Lancet* 2, 723-725 (1975).

PIAGET, J., *Play, Dreams and Imitation*, Norton: New York, 1962.

PIVIK, T. and FOULKES, D., "Dream deprivation": Effects on dream content, *Science* 153, 1282-1284 (1966).

PIVIK, T. and FOULKES, D., NREM mentation: Relation to personality orientation time, and time of night, *Journal of Consulting and Clinical Psychology* 144-151 (1968).

POMPEIANO, O. and MORRISON, A.R., Vestibular influences during sleep: Abolition of the rapid eye movements during desynchronized sleep after vestibular lesions, *Archives of Italian Biology* 103, 569-575 (1965).

POMPEIANO, O. and VALENTINUZZI, M., A mathematical model for the mechanism of rapid eye movements induced by an anticholinesterase in the decerebrate cat, *Archives of Italian Biology* 114, 103-154 (1976).

POTTER, W. and HERON, W., Sleep during perceptual deprivation, *Brain Research* 40, 534-539 (1972).

PREVOST, G., DEKONINCK, J. and PROULX, G., Stage REM rapid eye movements following visual inversion: Further investigation and replication, Paper presented to the Second International Sleep Research Congress, Edinburgh, Scotland, July 1975.

PRINZ, P.N., OBRIST, W.D. and WANG, H.S., Sleep patterns in healthy elderly subjects: Individual differences as related to other neurobiological variables, in M.H. Chase, W.C. Stern & P.L. Walter (Eds.), *Sleep Research, Vol. 4*, Brain Information Service/Brain Research Institute: Los Angeles, 1975, p. 132.

RECHTSCHAFFEN, A., Discussion of W. Dements's "Experimental dream studies", in J.H. Masserman (Ed.), *Science and Psychoanalysis*, Grune & Stratton: New York, 1964.

RECHTSCHAFFEN, A., Dream reports and dream experiences, *Experimental Neurology Supplement* 4, 4-15 (1967).

RECHTSCHAFFEN, A., The control of sleep, in W.A. Hunt (Ed.), *Human Behavior and its Control*, Schenkman Press: Cambridge, Massachusetts, 1971.

RECHTSCHAFFEN, A., The psychophysiology of mental activity during sleep, in J. McGuigan & R.A. Schoonover (Eds.), *The Psychophysiology of Thinking*, Academic Press: New York, 1973.

RECHTSCHAFFEN, A. & KALES, A. (Eds.), *A Manual of Standardized Terminology, Techniques and Scoring System for Sleep Stages of Human Subjects*, HEW Neurological Information Network: Bethesda, 1968.

RECHTSCHAFFEN, A. and MONROE, L.J., Laboratory studies of insomnia, in A. Kales (Ed.), *Sleep: Physiology and Pathology*, Lippincott: Philadelphia, 1969.

RECHTSCHAFFEN, A. and VERDONE, P., Amount of dreaming: Effect of incentive, adaptation to laboratory, and individual differences, *Perceptual and Motor Skills* 19, 947-958 (1964).

RECHTSCHAFFEN, A., HAURI, P. and ZEITLIN, M., Auditory awakening thresholds in REM and NREM sleep stages, *Perceptual and Motor Skills* 22, 927-942 (1966).

RECHTSCHAFFEN, A., WATSON, R., WINCOR, M.Z., MOLINARI, S. and BARTA, S.G., The relationship of phasic and tonic periorbital EMG activity to NREM mentation, *Sleep Research* 1, 114 (1972).

REITAN, R.M., Methodological problems in clinical neuropsychology, in R. Reitan & L.A. Davison (Eds.), *Clinical Neuropsychology: Current States and Applications*, Winston, Washington, D.C., 1974.

REITAN, R.M. and DAVISON, L.A. (Eds.), *Clinical Neuropsychology: Current Status and Applications*, Winston, Washington, D.C., 1974.

RISBERG, J., HALSEY, J.H., WILLS, E.L. and WILSON, E.M., Hemispheric specialization in normal man studied by bilateral measurements of the regional cerebral blood flow, *Brain* 98, 511-524 (1975).

ROBERTS, W.W. and ROBINSON, T.C.L., Relaxation and sleep induced by warming the preoptic region and anterior hypothalamus in cats, *Experimental Neurology* 25, 282-294 (1969).

ROFFWARG, H.P., DEMENT, W.C., MUZIO, J.N. and FISHER, C., Dream imagery: Relationship to rapid eye movements of sleep, *Archives of General Psychiatry* 7, 235-238 (1962).

ROFFWARG, H.P., MUZIO, J. and DEMENT, W.C., The ontogenetic development of the human sleep dream cycle, *Science* 152, 604-618 (1966).

ROSENBAUM, D.A., The theory of cognitive residues: A new view of fantasy, *Psychological Review* 79, 471-486 (1972).

ROSSI, E.L., The dream-protein hypothesis, *American Journal of Psychiatry* 130, 1094-1097 (1973).

ROUTTENBERG, A., Neural mechanisms of sleep: Changing view of reticular formation function, *Psychological Review* 73, 481-499 (1966).

SACHS, J., UNGAR, J., WASER, P.G. and BORBÉLY, A.A., Factors in cerebrospinal fluid affecting motor activity in the rat, *Neuroscience Letters* 2, 83-86 (1976).

SALAMY, J., Instrumental responding to internal cues associated with REM sleep, *Psychonomic Science* 18, 342-343 (1970).

SALAMY, J., Effects of REM deprivation and awakening on instrumental performance during stage 2 and REM sleep, *Biological Psychiatry* 3, 321-330 (1971).

SARNAT, H.B. and NETSKY, M.G., *Evolution of the Nervous System*, Oxford University Press: New York, 1974.

SATINOFF, E., McEWEN Jr., G.N. and WILLIAMS, B.A., Behavioral fever in newborn rabbits, *Science* 193, 1139-1140 (1976).

SAUERLAND, E.K. and HARPER, R.M., The human tongue during sleep: Electromyographic activity of the genioglossus muscle, *Experimental Neurology* 51, 160-170 (1976).

SCHACTER, D.L., The hypnogogic state: A critical review of the literature, *Psychological Bulletin* 83, 452-481 (1976).

SCHECHTER, N., SCHMEIDLER, G.R. and STAAL, M., Dream reports and creative tendencies in students of the arts, sciences, and engineering, *Journal of Consulting Psychology* 29, 415-421 (1965).

SCHOENBERGER, G.A. and MONNIER, M., Isolation, partial characterization and activity of humoral "delta-sleep" transmitting factor, in H.M. van Praag & H. Meinardi (Eds.), *Brain and Sleep*, de Erven Bohn: Amsterdam, 1974.

SCHONBAR, R.A., Some manifest characteristics of recallers and nonrecallers of dreams, *Journal of Consulting Psychology* 23, 414-418 (1959).

SCHONBAR, R.A., Differential dream recall frequency as a component of life style, *Journal of Consulting Psychology* 29, 468-474 (1965).

SCHUBERT, F. and JOVANOVIĆ, U.J., Sleep behavior-especially falling asleep and awakenings during the night in adults in relation to personality variables, in U. Jovanović (Ed.), *The Nature of Sleep*, Gustav Fischer: Stuttgart, W. Germany, 1973.

SCHWARTZ, G.E., DAVIDSON, R.J. and MAER, F., Right hemisphere lateralization for emotion in the human brain: Interactions with cognition, *Science* 190, 286-288 (1975).

SCHWARTZ, M.S., KRUPP, N.E. and BYRNE, D., Repression-sensitization and medical diagnosis, *Journal of Abnormal Psychology* 78, 286-291 (1971).

SEARLEMAN, A., A review of right hemisphere linguistic capabilities, *Psychological Bulletin* 84, 503-528 (1977).

SELIGMAN, M.E.P., On the generality of the laws of learning, *Psychological Review* 77, 406-418 (1970).

SELIGMAN, M.E.P., *Helplessness: On Depression, Development and Death*, W.H. Freeman: San Francisco, 1975.

SEYFRIED, B.A. and HENDRICK, C., When do opposites attract? When they are opposite in sex and sex role attitudes, *Journal of Personality and Social Psychology* 25, 15-20 (1973).

SHAPIRO, A., Dreaming and the physiology of sleep: A critical review of some empirical data and a proposal for a theoretical model of sleep and dreaming, *Experimental Neurology Supplement* 4, 56-81 (1967).

SHAPIRO, A., GOODENOUGH, D.R., LEWIS, H.B. and SLESER, I., Gradual arousal from sleep: A determinant of thinking reports, *Psychosomatic Medicine* 27, 342-349 (1965).

SHAPIRO, C.M., GRIESEL, R.D., BARTEL, P.R. and JOOSTE, P.L., Sleep patterns after graded exercise, *Journal of Applied Physiology* 39, 187-190 (1975).

SILVERSTONE, T. and TURNER, P., *Drug Treatment in Psychiatry*, Routledge & Kegan Paul: London,1974.

SINGER, J.L., *The Inner World of Daydreaming*, Harper & Row: New York, 1975.

SINGER, J.L. and SCHONBAR, R., Correlates of daydreaming: A dimension of self awareness, *Journal of Consulting Psychology* 25, 1-6 (1961).

SITARAM, N., MENDELSON, W.B., DAWSON, S., WYATT, R.J. and GILLIN, J.C., Time dependent effects of physostigmine on normal human sleep and arousal, Paper presented at the annual meeting of the Association for the Psychophysiological Study of Sleep, Cincinnati, June, 1976.

SITARAM, N., WYATT, R.J., DAWSON, S. and GILLIN, J.C., REM sleep induction by physostigmine infusion during sleep, *Science* 191, 1281-1283 (1976).

SLATER, E. and COWIE, V., *The Genetics of Mental Disorders*, Oxford University Press: London, 1971.

SNYDER, F., Toward an evolutionary theory of dreaming, *American Journal of Psychiatry* 123, 121-136 (1966).

SNYDER, F., The phenomenology of dreaming, in L. Madow & L.H. Snow (Eds.), *The Psychodynamic Implications of the Physiological Studies on Dreams*, Charles Thomas: Springfield, Illinois, 1970.

SNYDER, F., Psychophysiology of human sleep, *Clinical Neurosurgery* 18, 503-536 (1971).

SNYDER, F., HOBSON, J.A., MORRISON, D.F. and GOLDFRANK, F., Changes in respiration, heart rate, and systolic blood pressure in human sleep, *Journal of Applied Physiology* 19, 417-422 (1964).

SPENCE, J.T., HELMREICH, R. and STAPP, J., Ratings of self and peers on sex role attributes and their relation to self esteem and conception of masculinity and femininity, *Journal of Personality and Social Psychology* 32, 29-39 (1975).

SPERRY, R.W., Hemisphere deconnection and unity in conscious awareness, *American Psychologist* 23, 723-733 (1968).

SPITZER, R.L. and FLEISS, J.L., A re-analysis of the reliability of psychiatric diagnosis, *British Journal of Psychiatry* 125, 341-347 (1974).

SROUFE, L.A. and WATERS, E., The ontogenesis of smiling and laughter: A perspective on the organization of development in infancy, *Psychological Review* 83, 173-189 (1976).

STARKER, S., Daydreaming stages and nocturnal dreaming, *Journal of Abnormal Psychology* 83, 52-55 (1974).

STEGIE, R., BAUST, W. and ENGEL, R.R., Psychophysiological correlates in dreams, in P. Levin & W.P. Koella (Eds.), *Sleep 1974: Instinct, Neurophysiology, Endocrinology, Episodes, Dreams, Epilepsy, and Intracranial Pathology*, S. Karger: Basel, Switzerland, 1975.

STEINER, S.S. and ELLMAN, S.J., Relation between REM sleep and intracranial self-stimulation, *Science* 177, 1122-1124 (1972).

STERN, W.C. and MORGANE, P.J., Theoretical view of REM sleep function: Maintenance of catecholamine systems in the central nervous system, *Behavioral Biology* 11, 1-32 (1974).

STOYVA, J. and KAMIYA, J., Electrophysiological studies of dreaming as the prototype of a new strategy in the study of consciousness, *Psychological Review* 75, 192-205 (1968).

STRAUCH, I., SCHNEIDER-DUKER, M., ZAYER, H., HEINE, H.W., HEINE, I., LANG, R. and MÜLLER, N., The influence of meaningful auditory stimuli on sleep behavior, in M.H. Chase, W.C. Stern & P.L. Walter (Eds.), *Sleep Research, Vol. 4*, Brain Information Service/Brain Research Institute: Los Angeles, 1975, p. 178.

STUSS, D., HEALEY, T. and BROUGHTON, R., Personality and performance measures in natural extreme short sleepers, in M.H. Chase, W.C. Stern & P.L. Walter (Eds.), *Sleep Research, Vol. 4*, Brain Information Service/Brain Research Institute: Los Angeles, 1975, p. 204.

TANAKA, M., Characteristics of poor sleep with the normal human being, *Folia Psychiatrica et Neurologica Japonica* 29, 149-167 (1975).

TART, C.T., Toward the experimental control of dreaming: A literature review, *Psychological Bulletin* 64, 81-91 (1965).

TART, C.T. and DICK, L., Conscious control of dreaming: I. The posthypnotic dream, *Journal of Abnormal Psychology* 76, 304-315 (1970).

TAUB, J.M., Dream recall and content following extended sleep, *Perceptual and Motor Skills* 3, 987-990 (1970(a)).

TAUB, J.M., Dream recall and content following various durations of sleep, *Psychonomic Science* 18, 82 (1970(b)).

TAUB, J.M., TANGUAY, P.E. and CLARKSON, D., Effects of daytime naps on performance and mood in a college student population, *Journal of Abnormal Psychology* 85, 210-217 (1976).

TAUBER, E.S., Phylogeny of sleep, in E. Weitzman (Ed.), *Advances in Sleep Research, Vol. 1*, Spectrum Publications: New York, 1974.

TORDA, C., Contribution to serotonin theory of dreaming (LSD infusion), *New York State Journal of Medicine*, May 1, 1135-1138 (1968).

TORDA, C., Dreams of subjects with loss of memory for recent events, *Psychophysiology* 6, 358-365 (1969).

TROSSMAN, H., RECHTSCHAFFEN, A., OFFENCRANTZ, W. and WOLPERT, E., Studies in psychophysiology of dreams: IV. Relations among dreams in sequence, *Archives of General Psychiatry* 3, 602-607 (1960).

TRUPIN, E.W., Correlates of ego-level and agency-communion in stage REM dreams of 11-13 year old children, in M.H. Chase, W.C. Stern & L.P. Walter (Eds.), *Sleep Research, Vol. 4*, Brain Information Service/Brain Research Institute: Los Angeles, 1975, p. 167.

TUCKER, D.M., ROTH, R.S., ARNESON, B.A. and BUCKINGHAM, V., Right hemisphere activation during stress, *Neuropsychologia* 15, 697-700 (1977).

TURNER, R.G., Consistency, self-consciousness, and the predictive validity of typical and maximal personality measures, *Journal of Research in Personality* 12, 117-132 (1978).

UNDERWOOD, B.J., Individual differences as a crucible in theory construction, *American Psychologist* 30, 128-134 (1975).

VALATX, J.L. and CHOUVET, G., Genetics of sleep-waking cycle, in P. Levin & W.P. Koella (Eds.), *Sleep 1974: Instinct, Neurophysiology, Endocrinology, Episodes, Dreams, Epilepsy and Intracranial Pathology*, S. Karger: Basel, Switzerland, 1975.

VAN DE CASTLE, R.L., Problems in applying methodology of content analysis, in M. Kramer (Ed.), *Dream Psychology and the New Biology of Dreaming*, Charles Thomas: Springfield, Illinois, 1969.

VAN DE CASTLE, R.L., Temporal patterns of dreams, in E. Hartmann (Ed.), *Sleep and Dreaming* (International Psychiatry Clinics, Vol. 7), Little & Brown: Boston, 1970.

VAN DE CASTLE, R.L. and SMITH, T.F., Dream content and body build, in M.H. Chase, W.C. Stern & P.L. Walter (Eds.), *Sleep Research, Vol. 1*, Brain Information Service/Brain Research Institute: Los Angeles, 1972, p. 127.

VAUGHN, C., The development and use of an operant technique to provide evidence for visual imagery in the rhesus monkey under sensory deprivation, University of Pittsburg: Doctoral dissertation, 1964.

VERDONE, P., Temporal reference of manifest dream content, *Perceptual and Motor Skills* 20, 1253 (1965).

VOGEL, G.W., REM deprivation, III. Dreaming and psychosis, *Archives of General Psychiatry* 18, 312-329 (1968).

VOGEL, G.W., Dreaming and schizophrenia, *Psychiatric Annals* 4, 63-65, 68-73, 77 (1974).

VOGEL, G.W., A review of REM sleep deprivation, *Archives of General Psychiatry* 32, 749-761 (1975).

VOGEL, G.W., GIESLER, D.D. and BARROWCLOUGH, B., Exercise as a substitute for REM sleep, *Psychophysiology* 7, 300-301 (1970).

VOGEL, G.W., McABEE, R., BARKER, K. and THURMOND, A., Endogenous depression improvement and REM pressure, *Archives of General Psychiatry* 34, 96-97 (1977).

WABER, D.P., Sex differences in cognition: A function of maturation rate?, *Science* 192, 572-573 (1976).

WACHTEL, P.L., Psychodynamic, behavior therapy, and the implacable experimenter: An inquiry into the consistency of personality, *Journal of Abnormal Psychology* 82, 324-334 (1973).

WALKER, P.C. and JOHNSON, R.F.Q., The influence of presleep suggestions on dream content: Evidence and methodological problems, *Psychological Bulletin* 81, 362-370 (1974).

WALKER, J.M. and BERGER, R.J., The ontogenesis of slow wave sleep and homoiothermy in the opossum, Paper presented at the annual meeting of the Association for the Psychophysiological Study of Sleep, Jackson Hole, Wyoming, 1974.

WALKER, J.M., GLOTZBACH, S.F., BERGER, R.J. and HELLER, H.C., Sleep and hibernation I: Electrophysiological observation, in M.H. Chase, W.C. Stern & P.L. Walter (Eds.), *Sleep Research, Vol. 4*, Brain Information Service/Brain Research Institute: Los Angeles, 1975, p. 67.

WALKER, J.P. and WALKER, J.B., Self-produced locomotion restores visual capacity after striate lesions, *Science* 187, 265-266 (1975).

WALTER, W.G., *The Living Brain*, Norton: New York, 1953.

WATSON, R., Mental correlates of periorbital PIPs during REM sleep, in M.H. Chase, W.C. Stern, & P.L. Walter (Eds.), *Sleep Research, Vol. 1*, Brain Information Service/Brain Research Institute: Los Angeles, 1972, p. 116.

WATSON, R., LIEBMANN, K. and WATSON, S., Comparison of NREM-PIP frequency in schizophrenic and non-schizophrenic patients, Paper presented at the annual meeting of the Association for the Psychophysiological Study of Sleep, Cincinnati, June 1, 1976(a).

WATSON, R., LIEBMANN, K. and WATSON, S., Individual differences in frequency of NREM PIPs and Rorschach scores, Paper presented at the annual meeting of the Association for the Psychophysiological Study of Sleep, Cincinnati, June, 1976(b).

WAXENBERG, S.E., DICKES, R. and GOTTESFELD, H., The Poetzl phenomenon reexamined experimentally, *Journal of Nervous and Mental Diseases* 135, 387-398 (1962).

WEBB, W.B., *Sleep: An Active Process: Research and Commentary*, Scott, Foresman: Glenview, Illinois, 1973.

WEBB, W.B. and AGNEW Jr., H.W., The effects of a chronic limitation of sleep length, *Psychophysiology* 11, 265-274 (1974).

WEBB, W.B. and FRIEDMAN, J., Attempts to modify the sleep patterns of the rat, *Physiology and Behavior* 6, 459-460 (1971).

WEBB, W.B. and FRIEL, J., Sleep stage and personality characteristics of "natural" long and short sleepers, *Science* 171, 587-588 (1971).

WEBB, W.B. and KERSEY, J., Recall of dreams and the probability of stage 1-REM sleep, *Perceptual and Motor Skills* 24, 627-630 (1967).

WEIMER, W.B. and PALERMO, D.S. (Eds.), *Cognition and the Symbolic Processes*, Lawrence Erlbaum Associates: Hillsdale, New Jersey, 1974.

WEINER, S. and EHRLICHMAN, H., Ocular motility and cognitive processes, *Cognition* 4, 31-43 (1976).

WEISZ, R. and FOULKES, D., Home and laboratory dreams collected under uniform sampling conditions, *Psychophysiology* 6, 588-596 (1970).

WEITZMAN, E.D., POLLACK, C.P. and McGREGOR, P.A., The effects of progressive, partial sleep deprivation on sleep stage, in M.H. Chase, W.C. Stern & P.L. Walter (Eds.), *Sleep Research, Vol. 4*, Brain Information Service/Brain Research Institute: Los Angeles, 1975, p. 246.

WEST, L.J., *Hallucinations*, Grune & Stratton, New York, 1962.

WHITE, R.W., Motivation reconsidered: The concept of competence, *Psychological Review* 66, 297-333 (1959).

WHITMAN, R.M., PIERCE, C.M., MAAS, J.W. and BALDRIDGE, B.J., The dreams of the experimental subject, *Journal of Nervous and Mental Disease* 134, 431-439 (1962).

WIGGINS, J.S., Personality structure, *Annual Review of Psychology* 19, 293-350 (1968).

WIGGINS, J.S., *Personality and Prediction: Principles of Personality Assessment*, Addison Wesley: Reading, Massachusetts, 1973.

WILLERMAN, L., *The Psychology of Individual and Group Differences*, W.H. Freeman: San Francisco, 1979.

WILLIAMS, H.L., The problem of defining depth of sleep, in S.S. Kety, E.V. Evarts & H.L. Williams (Eds.), *Sleep and Altered States of Consciousness* (Research publication of the Association for Research in Nervous and Mental Disease, Vol. 45), Williams & Wilkins: Baltimore, 1967.

WILLIAMS, H.L., Information processing during sleep, in W.P. Koella & P. Levin (Eds.), *Sleep: Physiology, Biochemistry, Psychology, Pharmacology, Clinical Implications*, S. Karger: Basel, Switzerland, 1973.

WILLIAMS, R.L., KARACAN, I. and HURSCH, C.J., *EEG of Human Sleep: Clinical Application*, Wiley: New York, 1974.

WILLIAMS, R.L., KARACAN, I., SALIS, P.J., THORNBY, J.I. and ANCH, A.M., Ontogenetic aspects of stages 1-REM and 4-Sleep, in P. Levin & W.P. Koella (Eds.), *Sleep 1974: Instinct, Neurophysiology, Endocrinology, Episodes, Dreams, Epilepsy and Intracranial Pathology*, S. Karger: Basel, Switzerland, 1975.

WILSON, W.P. and ZUNG, W.W.K., Attention, discrimination, and arousal during sleep, *Archives of General Psychiatry* 15, 523-528 (1966).

WILSON, W.P., ZUNG, W.W.K. and LEE, J.C.M., Arousal from sleep of male homosexuals, *Biological Psychiatry* 6, 81-84 (1973).

WINGET, C. and FARRELL, R.A., A comparison of the dreams of homosexual and non-homosexual males, Paper presented at the annual meeting of the Association for the Psychophysiological Study of Sleep, Bruges, Belgium, June, 1971.

WINGET, C., KRAMER, M. and WHITMAN, R.M., Dreams and demography, *Canadian Psychiatric Association Journal* 17, 203-208 (1972).

WINTROBE, M.M., THORN, G.W., ADAMS, R.D., BENNETT Jr., I.L., BRAUMWALD, E., ISSELBACHER, K.J. and PETERSDORF, R.G. (Eds.), *Harrison's Principles of Internal Medicine*, McGraw-Hill: New York, 1970.

WITKIN, H.A., Presleep experience and dreams, in J. Fisher & L. Breger (Eds.), *The Meaning of Dreams: Recent Insights from the Laboratory* (California Mental Health Research Symposium, No. 3), Sacramento, California: Bureau of Research, California Department of Mental Hygiene, 1969.

WITKIN, H.A., DYK, R.B., FATERSON, H.F., GOODENOUGH, D.R. and KARP, S.A., *Psychological Differentiation: Studies of Development*, Wiley: New York, 1962.

WOLPERT, E.A., Psychophysiological parallelism in the dream, in L.E. Abt & B.F. Reiss (Eds.), *Progress in Clinical Psychology, Vol. 10*, Grune & Stratton, 1969.

WOOD, P.B., Dreaming and social isolation, unpublished doctoral dissertation, University of South Carolina, 1962.

WURTMAN, R.J. and FERNSTROM, J.D., Control of brain monoamine synthesis by diet and plasma amino acids, *American Journal of Clinical Nutrition*, June, 638-647 (1975).

WYATT, R.J., The serotonin-catecholamine-dream bicycle: A clinical study, *Biological Psychiatry* 5, 33-64 (1972).

WYATT, R.J. and GILLIN, J.C., Biochemistry and human sleep, in R.L. Williams & I. Karacan (Eds.), *Pharmacology of Sleep*, Wiley: New York, 1976.

ZEPELIN, H. and RECHTSCHAFFEN, A., Mammalian sleep, longevity and energy metabolism, *Brain Behavior and Evolution* 10, 425-470 (1974).

ZIEGLER, A.J., Dream emotions in relation to room temperature, in W.P. Koella & P. Levin (Eds.), *Sleep: Physiology, Biochemistry, Psychology, Pharmacology, Clinical Implications*, S. Karger: Basel, Switzerland, 1973.

ZIMMERMAN, J., STOYVA, J. and METCALF, D., Distorted visual feedback and augmented REM sleep, *Psychophysiology* 7, 298 (1970).

ZIMMERMAN, W.B., Sleep mentation and auditory awakening thresholds, *Psychophysiology* 6, 540-549 (1970).

ZUCKERMAN, M., KOLIN, E.A., PRICE, L. and ZOOB, I., Development of a sensation-seeking scale, *Journal of Consulting Psychology* 28, 447-482 (1964).

NAME INDEX

SUBJECT INDEX